Depression and Bip

D0870401

The best-selling *Stahl's Essential Psychopharmacology* – fully revised and updated throughout – continues its tradition of being the preeminent source of information in its field. This third edition of *Depression and Bipolar Disorders* draws from the revised chapters in *Stahl's Essential Psychopharmacology* to form a resource that is essential reading for all clinicians involved in the treatment of depression and bipolar disorder. Straightforward reading for both professionals treating these conditions and students learning the mechanisms of drug reactions, this eminently readable book can be read cover to cover by experts and novices alike.

Stephen M. Stahl is Adjunct Professor of Psychiatry at the University of California at San Diego. He has conducted numerous research projects awarded by the National Institute of Mental Health, the Veterans Administration, and the pharmaceutical industry. Author of more than 350 articles and chapters, Dr. Stahl is an internationally recognized clinician, researcher, and teacher in psychiatry with subspecialty expertise in psychopharmacology.

Depression and Bipolar Disorder

Stahl's Essential Psychopharmacology

Third Edition

Stephen M. Stahl

University of California at San Diego

With Illustrations by
Nancy Muntner

Editorial Assistant
Meghan M. Grady

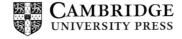

CAMBRIDGE
UNIVERSITY PRESS

CAMBRIDGE UNIVERSITY PRESS
Cambridge, New York, Melbourne, Madrid, Cape Town, Singapore, São Paulo, Delhi

Cambridge University Press
32 Avenue of the Americas, New York, NY 10013-2473, USA

www.cambridge.org
Information on this title: www.cambridge.org/9780521714129

© Stephen M. Stahl 2008

WM
171
S781d
2008

First published 2008

Printed in the United States of America

A catalog record for this publication is available from the British Library.

Library of Congress Cataloging in Publication Data

Stahl, S. M.
  Depression and bipolar disorder : Stahl's essential psychopharmacology,
3rd edition / Stephen M. Stahl ; with illustrations by Nancy Muntner ;
editorial assistant, Meghan M. Grady.
     p. ; cm.
  Includes bibliographical references and index.
  ISBN 978-0-521-88663-5 (hardback) – ISBN 978-0-521-71412-9 (paperback)
    1. Depression, Mental–Chemotherapy.   2. Manic-depressive illness–Chemotherapy.
3. Antidepressants.   I. Stahl, S. M. Stahl's essential psychopharmacology.   II. Title.
    [DNLM: 1. Mood Disorders–drug therapy.   2. Antidepressive Agents–therapeutic use.
WM 171 S781d 2008]
  RC537.S7358 2008
  616.85′27061–dc22
                                                                            2008004353

ISBN   978-0-521-88663-5   hardback
ISBN   978-0-521-71412-9   paperback

In memory of Daniel X. Freedman, mentor, colleague, and scientific father.

To Cindy, my wife, best friend, and tireless supporter.

To Jennifer and Victoria, my daughters, for their patience and understanding of the demands of authorship.

Contents

Preface to the Third Edition

This booklet is a set of the three chapters from the third edition of *Stahl's Essential Psychopharmacology* that deal exclusively with depression and bipolar disorders and their treatment with modern psychopharmacological agents. The knowledge base of psychopharmacology for depression and bipolar disorders has exploded since the publication of the second edition of *Essential Psychopharmacology*, and this third edition attempts to reflect these changes.

Some would argue that antidepressants have become the therapeutic market that is the largest and has the most prescribers anywhere in the world, and in fact, anywhere in medicine. Since all specialties prescribe these medications, with psychiatrists in fact a minority of prescribers, there is intense interest in this area of therapeutics. This therapeutic area of psychopharmacology occupies the largest single section of the full textbook, and since many readers may be interested in this area alone, we offer the three chapters on depression, bipolar disorders, antidepressants, and mood stabilizers as a stand-alone spinoff of the third edition of *Stahl's Essential Psychopharmacology*.

Psychopharmacology has not only experienced incredible growth since publication of the second edition of this textbook; it has also experienced a major paradigm shift from a limited focus on neurotransmitters and receptors to an emphasis as well on brain circuits, neuroimaging, genetics, and signal transduction cascades. The third edition of *Stahl's Essential Psychopharmacology* attempts to reflect this transformation in the field, and elements of this paradigm shift are incorporated into each of these chapters in this booklet. Many new antidepressants and mood stabilizers have been introduced in recent years, and many more are now in clinical testing, and these are covered in this new edition. These three chapters on mood disorders and their treatments have been extensively reorganized, rewritten, and illustrated with roughly twice the number of figures in every chapter. However, what has not changed is the didactic style of the first and second editions, which continues in this third edition.

The text is purposely written at a conceptual level rather than a pragmatic level and includes ideas that are simplifications and rules, while sacrificing precision and discussion of exceptions to rules. Thus, this is not a text intended for the sophisticated subspecialist in psychopharmacology. Also, it is not extensively referenced to original papers, but rather to textbooks and reviews and a few selected original papers, with only a limited reading list for each chapter. For those of you interested in specific prescribing information about the most common one hundred or so psychotropic drugs, this information is available in the companion textbook, *Essential Psychopharmacology Prescriber's Guide*. A spinoff of this book just on antidepressants is also available, called *Essential Psychopharmacology Prescriber's Guide of Antidepressants*. Mood stabilizers are available in a second spinoff, called *Essential Psychopharmacology of Antipsychotics and Mood Stabilizers*.

Now, you also have the option of going to Essential Psychopharmacology Online at www.essentialpsych.org. We are proud to announce the launch of this new website, which is due to premiere in the fall of 2008. Access to this website will allow you to search within the entire Essential Psychopharmacology series that includes not only this third edition of *Stahl's Essential Psychopharmacology*, but also *Essential Psychopharmacology Prescriber's Guide*. This site will be updated regularly and should therefore provide an up-to-date source for what you need to know about the essentials of psychopharmacology between publication of subsequent editions of these books.

Much of the new content in this text is based on updated lectures, courses, slides, and articles by the author. Many of the new illustrations are now available as animations on the Neuroscience Education Institute's website, as are the lectures, slides and articles, continuing medical education (CME) credits, tests, certifications, and much more. I invite you to explore this interactive reference by visiting the Neuroscience Education Institute's website at www.neiglobal.com. If you are interested in comprehensive materials, you can choose to have access to both websites.

In general, this text attempts to present the fundamentals of psychopharmacology in simplified and readily readable form. Thus, this material should prepare the reader to consult more sophisticated textbooks as well as the professional literature. The organization of the information here also applies principles of programmed learning for the reader, namely repetition and interaction, which has been shown to enhance retention.

Therefore, it is suggested that novices first approach this text by going through it from beginning to end, reviewing only the color graphics and the legends for these graphics. Virtually everything covered in the text is also covered in the graphics and icons. Once having gone through all the color graphics in these chapters, it is recommended that the reader then go back to the beginning of the book and read the entire text, reviewing the graphics at the same time. After the text has been read, the entire book can be rapidly reviewed again merely by referring to the various color graphics in the book. Finally, as a member of the Neuroscience Education Institute, you can utilize the content available online at www.neiglobal.com to obtain continuing medical education credits for this activity or as a helpful interactive reference. Many of the graphics are animated and available on this site. Also, you can search topics in the field covered in the Essential Psychopharmacology book series on Essential Psychopharmacology Online.

This mechanism of using the materials will create a certain amount of programmed learning by incorporating the elements of repetition, as well as interaction with visual learning through graphics. Hopefully, the visual concepts learned via graphics will reinforce abstract concepts learned from the written text, especially for those of you who are primarily "visual learners" (i.e., those who retain information better from visualizing concepts than from reading about them).

For those of you who are already familiar with psychopharmacology, this book should provide easy reading from beginning to end. Going back and forth between the text and the graphics should provide interaction. Following review of the complete text, it should be simple to review the entire book by going through the graphics once again. In addition, the Neuroscience Education Institute's website further expands the Essential Psychopharmacology learning experience and Essential Psychopharmacology Online allows quick searches of topics in this field.

For those of you interested in the specific updates made in the third edition, the mood disorder chapter expands the descriptions of unipolar and bipolar disorders and discusses the entire bipolar spectrum. Included are sections on matching the symptoms of the disorder under discussion to various hypothetically malfunctioning brain circuits. The antidepressant chapter includes extensive coverage not only of new drugs and several agents in late-stage testing, but also expanded coverage of "old" (and often neglected) drugs that remain valuable therapeutics but are off-patent and not promoted commercially. In this chapter are new sections on antidepressants and women; on trimonoamine modulators and brain stimulation therapies that may augment antidepressants; and a discussion of "symptom-based" antidepressant selection algorithms for combining antidepressants to treat residual symptoms and attain remission in major depressive disorder. The chapter on mood stabilizers explains not only the mechanism of action of agents used to treat bipolar disorder, but also the use of drugs in combinations to treat this disorder.

This is an incredibly exciting time for the fields of neuroscience and mental health, creating fascinating opportunities for clinicians to utilize current therapeutics and to antic-ipate future medications that are likely to transform the field of psychopharmacology. Best wishes for your first step on your journey into this fascinating field of psychopharmacology.

Stephen M. Stahl, MD, PhD

CME Information

Release/Expiration Dates

Original release date: March 2008
CME credit expiration date: original expiration February 2011 (if this date has passed, please contact NEI for updated information)

Target Audience

This activity was designed for health care professionals, including psychiatrists, neurologists, primary care physicians, pharmacists, psychologists, nurses, and others, who treat patients with psychiatric conditions.

Statement of Need

The content of this educational activity was determined by rigorous assessment, including activity feedback, expert faculty assessment, literature review, and new medical knowledge, which revealed the following unmet needs:

- Psychiatric illnesses such as mood disorders have a neurobiological basis and are primarily treated by pharmacological agents; understanding each of these, as well as the relationship between them, is essential in order to select appropriate treatment for a patient

- The field of psychopharmacology has experienced incredible growth; it has also experienced a major paradigm shift from a limited focus on neurotransmitters and receptors to an emphasis as well on brain circuits, neuroimaging, genetics, and signal transduction cascades

Learning Objectives

Upon completion of this activity, you should be able to:

- Apply neurobiologic and mechanistic evidence when selecting treatment strategies in order to match treatment to the individual needs of the patient

- Utilize new scientific data to modify existing treatment strategies in order to improve patient outcomes in mood disorders

Accreditation and Credit Designation Statements

The Neuroscience Education Institute is accredited by the Accreditation Council for Continuing Medical Education to provide continuing medical education for physicians.

The Neuroscience Education Institute designates this educational activity for a maximum of 24.0 *AMA PRA Category 1 Credits*TM. Physicians should only claim credit commensurate with the extent of their participation in the activity.

Activity Instructions

This CME activity is in the form of a printed book and incorporates instructional design to enhance your retention of the information and pharmacological concepts that are being presented. You are advised to go through the figures in this activity from beginning to end, followed by the text, and then complete the posttests and evaluations. The estimated time for completion of this activity is 24 hours.

Instructions for CME Credit

To receive a certificate of CME credit or participation, please complete the posttest (you must score at least 70% to receive credit) and evaluation available online only at http://www.neiglobal.com/ep3. If a score of 70% or more is attained, you can immediately print your certificate. There is a fee for the posttest (certificate included) for non-NEI members.

NEI Disclosure Policy

It is the policy of the Neuroscience Education Institute to ensure balance, independence, objectivity, and scientific rigor in all its educational activities. The Neuroscience Education Institute takes responsibility for the content, quality, and scientific integrity of this CME activity.

All faculty participating in any NEI-sponsored educational activity and all individuals in a position to influence or control content development are required by NEI to disclose to the activity audience any financial relationships or apparent conflicts of interest that may have a direct bearing on the subject matter of the activity. Although potential conflicts of interest are identified and resolved prior to the activity, it remains for the audience to determine whether outside interests reflect a possible bias in either the exposition or the conclusions presented.

Neither the Neuroscience Education Institute nor Stephen M. Stahl, MD, PhD has received any funds or grants in support of this educational activity.

Individual Disclosure Statements

Authors/Developers
Stephen M. Stahl, MD, PhD
Adjunct Professor, Department of Psychiatry
University of California, San Diego School of Medicine, San Diego, CA

Dr. Stahl has been a consultant, board member, or on the speakers bureau for the following pharmaceutical companies within the last three years: Acadia, Alkermes, Amylin, Asahi Kasei, Astra Zeneca, Avera, Azur, Biovail, Boehringer Ingelheim, BristolMyers Squibb, Cephalon, CSC Pharmaceuticals, Cyberonics, Cypress Bioscience, Dainippon, Eli Lilly, Forest, GlaxoSmithKline, Janssen, Jazz Pharmaceuticals, Labopharm, Lundbeck, Neurocrine Biosciences, NeuroMolecular, Neuronetics, Novartis, Organon, Pamlab, Pfizer, Pierre Fabre, sanofi-aventis, Schering-Plough, Sepracor, Shire, SK Corporation, Solvay, Somaxon, Takeda, Tethys, Tetragenix, Vanda Pharmaceuticals, and Wyeth.

Meghan Grady
Director, Content Development
Neuroscience Education Institute, Carlsbad, CA

No other financial relationships to disclose.

Editorial and Design Staff
Nancy Muntner
Director, Medical Illustrations
Neuroscience Education Institute, Carlsbad, CA

No other financial relationships to disclose.

Disclosed financial relationships have been reviewed by the Neuroscience Education Institute CME Advisory Board to resolve any potential conflicts of interest. All faculty and planning committee members have attested that their financial relationships do not affect their ability to present well-balanced, evidence-based content for this activity.

Disclosure of Off-Label Use

This educational activity may include discussion of unlabeled and/or investigational uses of agents that are not approved by the FDA. Please consult the product prescribing information for full disclosure of labeled uses.

Disclaimer

Participants have an implied responsibility to use the newly acquired information from this activity to enhance patient outcomes and their own professional development. The information presented in this educational activity is not meant to serve as a guideline for patient management. Any procedures, medications, or other courses of diagnosis or treatment discussed or suggested in this educational activity should not be used by clinicians without evaluation of their patients' conditions and possible contraindications or dangers in use, review of any applicable manufacturer's product information, and comparison with recommendations of other authorities. Primary references and full prescribing information should be consulted.

Sponsorship Information

Sponsored by Neuroscience Education Institute

Support

This activity is supported solely by the sponsor, Neuroscience Education Institute.

Mood Disorders

This chapter discusses disorders characterized by abnormalities of mood: namely, depression, mania, or both. Included are descriptions of a wide variety of mood disorders that occur over a broad clinical spectrum. Also included is an analysis of how abnormalities in regulation of the trimonoaminergic neurotransmitter system – comprising the three monoamine neurotransmitters norepinephrine (NE; also called noradrenaline, or NA), dopamine (DA), and serotonin (also called 5-hydroxytryptamine, or 5HT) – are hypothesized to explain the biological basis of mood disorders. The approach taken here is to deconstruct each mood disorder into its component symptoms, followed by matching each symptom to hypothetically malfunctioning brain circuits, each regulated by one or more of the neurotransmitters within the trimonoaminergic neurotransmitter system. The genetic regulation and neuroimaging of these hypothetically malfunctioning brain circuits are also briefly mentioned. The discussion of symptoms and circuits in this chapter is intended to set the stage for understanding the pharmacological concepts underlying the mechanisms of action and use of antidepressants and mood-stabilizing drugs reviewed in the following two chapters (Chapters 2 and 3).

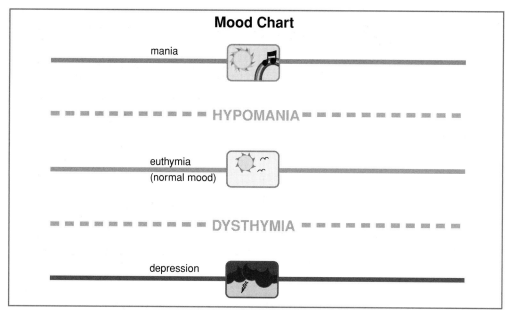

FIGURE 1-1 Mood chart. Disorders of mood can be mapped on a mood chart to track the course of illness, identify phase of illness, and aid in differential diagnosis. As shown in this chart, mood can range from mania at the top, to hypomania, to euthymia (normal mood) in the middle, and to dysthymia and depression at the bottom.

Clinical descriptions and criteria for the diagnosis of disorders of mood are mentioned only in passing. The reader should consult standard reference sources for this material. Here we discuss how the discovery of various neurotransmitters and brain circuits has influenced the understanding of symptoms in mood disorders. The goal of this chapter is to outline current ideas about the clinical and biological aspects of mood disorders in order to prepare the reader to understand the various treatments for these disorders discussed in later chapters.

Description of mood disorders

Disorders of mood are often called affective disorders, since affect is the external display of mood or emotion which is, however, felt internally. Depression and mania are often seen as opposite ends of an affective or mood spectrum. Classically, mania and depression are "poles" apart, thus generating the terms "unipolar" depression (i.e., as in patients who just experience the *down* or depressed pole) and "bipolar" [i.e., as in patients who at different times experience either the *up* (manic) pole or the *down* (depressed) pole]. In practice, however, depression and mania may occur simultaneously, in which case a "mixed" mood state exists. Mania may also occur in lesser degrees, known as "hypomania"; or a patient may switch so quickly between mania and depression that it is called "rapid cycling."

Mood disorders can be usefully visualized not only to distinguish different mood disorders from one another but also to summarize the course of illness for individual patients by showing them their disorders mapped onto a mood chart. Thus, mood ranges from hypomania to mania at the top, to euthymia (or normal mood) in the middle, to dysthymia and depression at the bottom (Figure 1-1). Mood abnormalities for the major diagnostic entities are summarized in Figure 1-2 and shown in more detail in Figures 1-3 through 1-29.

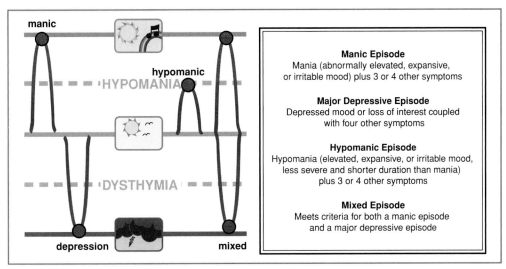

FIGURE 1-2 Mood episodes. Bipolar disorder is generally characterized by four types of illness episodes: manic, major depressive, hypomanic, and mixed. A patient may have any combination of these episodes over the course of illness; subsyndromal manic or depressive episodes also occur during the course of illness, in which case there are not enough symptoms or the symptoms are not severe enough to meet the diagnostic criteria for one of these episodes. Thus the presentation of mood disorders can vary widely.

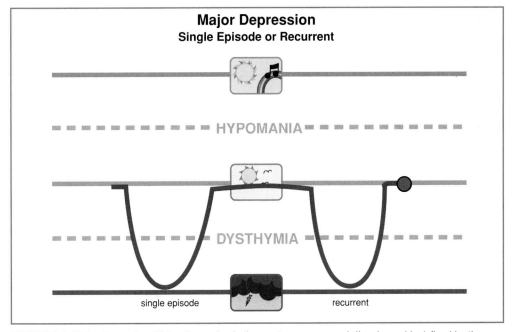

FIGURE 1-3 Major depression. Major depression is the most common mood disorder and is defined by the occurrence of at least a single major depressive episode, although most patients will experience recurrent episodes.

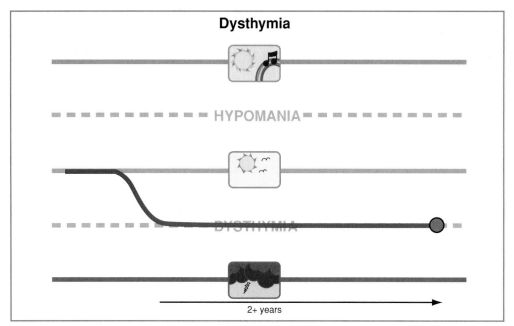

Dysthymia

2+ years

FIGURE 1-4 Dysthymia. Dysthymia is a less severe form of depression than major depression but long-lasting (over two years in duration) and is often unremitting.

The most common and readily recognized mood disorder is major depression (Figure 1-3) as a single episode or recurrent episodes. Dysthymia is a less severe but often longer-lasting form of depression (Figure 1-4). Patients with a major depressive episode who have poor inter-episode recovery, only to the level of dysthymia, which is then followed by another episode of major depression, are sometimes said to have "double depression," alternating between major depression and dysthymia but not remitting (Figure 1-5).

Bipolar I patients have full-blown manic episodes and/or mixed episodes of full mania plus simultaneous full depression, often followed by a full depressive episode (Figure 1-6). When mania recurs at least four times a year, it is called rapid cycling (Figure 1-17A). Bipolar I patients can also have rapid switches from mania to depression and back (Figure 1-17B). By definition, this occurs at least four times a year, but it can happen much more frequently than that.

Bipolar disorder is characterized by at least one hypomanic episode and one full depressive episode (Figure 1-8). Cyclothymic disorder is characterized by mood swings less severe than full mania and full depression but still waxing and waning above and below the boundaries of normal mood (Figure 1-9). There may be lesser degrees of variation from normal mood that are stable and persistent, including both depressive temperament (below normal mood but not a mood disorder) (Figure 1-10) and hyperthymic temperament (above normal mood but also not a mood disorder) (Figure 1-11). Temperaments are lifelong personality styles of responding to environmental stimuli; they can be heritable patterns present early in life and persisting thereafter and include such independent personality dimensions as novelty seeking, harm avoidance, and conscientiousness. Some patients may have mood-related temperaments that may render them vulnerable to mood disorders, especially bipolar spectrum disorders, later in life.

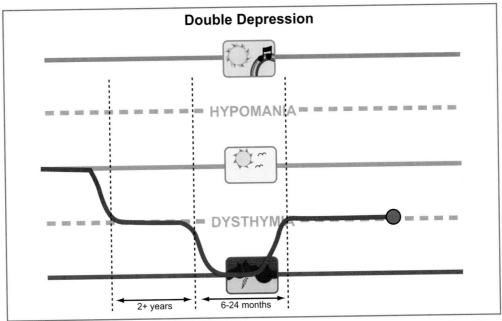

FIGURE 1-5 Double depression. Patients with unremitting dysthymia who also experience the superimposition of one or more major depressive episodes are described as having double depression. This is also a form of recurrent major depressive episodes with poor inter-episode recovery.

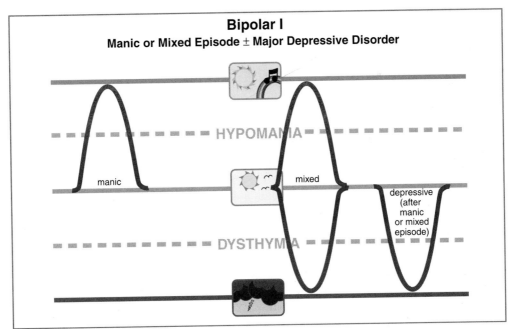

FIGURE 1-6 Bipolar I disorder. Bipolar I disorder is defined as the occurrence of at least one manic or mixed (full mania and full depression simultaneously) episode. Patients with bipolar I disorder typically experience major depressive episodes as well, although this is not necessary for the bipolar I diagnosis.

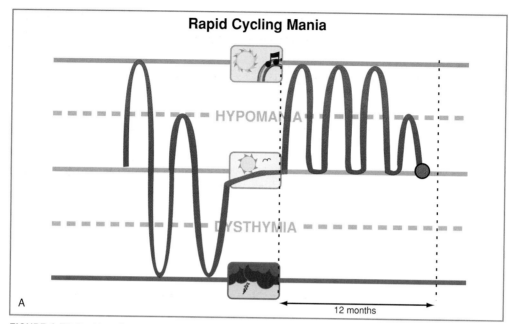

FIGURE 1-7A Rapid cycling mania. The course of bipolar disorder can be rapid cycling, which means that at least four episodes occur within a one-year period. This can manifest itself as four distinct manic episodes, as shown here. Many patients with this form of mood disorder experience switches much more frequently than four times a year.

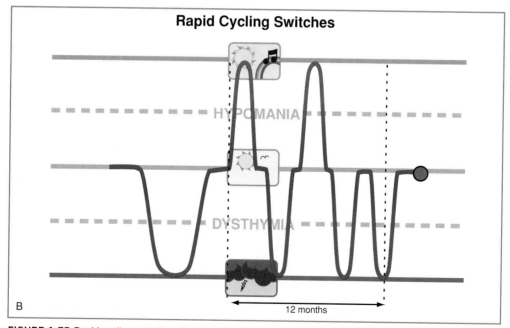

FIGURE 1-7B Rapid cycling switches. A rapid cycling course (at least four distinct mood episodes within one year) can also manifest as rapid switches between manic and depressive episodes.

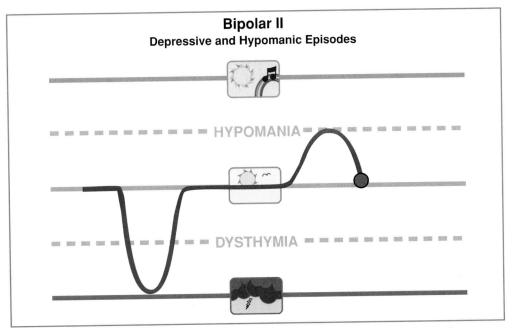

FIGURE 1-8 Bipolar disorder. Bipolar disorder is defined as an illness course consisting of one or more major depressive episodes and at least one hypomanic episode.

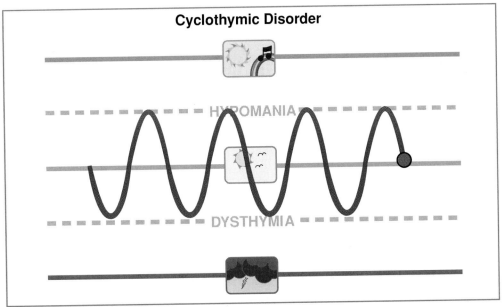

FIGURE 1-9 Cyclothymic disorder. Cyclothymic disorder is characterized by mood swings between hypomania and dysthymia but without any full manic or major depressive episodes.

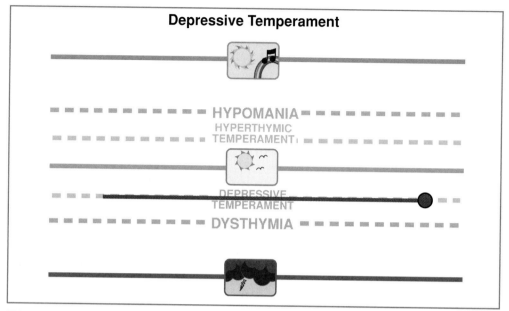

FIGURE 1-10 Depressive temperament. Not all mood variations are pathological. Individuals with depressive temperament may be consistently sad or apathetic but do not meet the criteria for dysthymia and do not necessarily experience any functional impairment. However, individuals with depressive temperament may be at greater risk for the development of a mood disorder later in life.

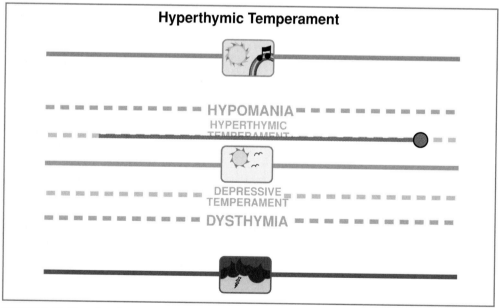

FIGURE 1-11 Hyperthymic temperament. Hyperthymic temperament, in which mood is above normal but not pathological, includes stable characteristics such as extroversion, optimism, exuberance, impulsiveness, overconfidence, grandiosity, and lack of inhibition. Individuals with hyperthymic temperament may be at greater risk for the development of a mood disorder later in life.

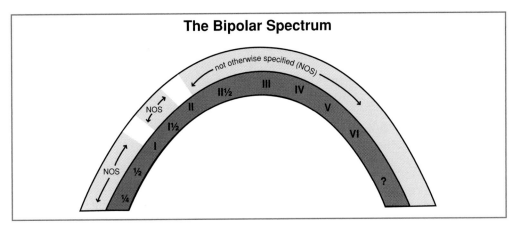

FIGURE 1-12 Bipolar spectrum. The only formal unique bipolar diagnoses identified in the *Diagnostic and Statistical Manual of Mental Disorders*, fourth edition (DSM-), are bipolar I, bipolar , and cyclothymic disorder, with all other presentations that include mood symptoms above the normal range lumped together in a single category called "not otherwise specified (NOS)." However, there is a huge variation in the presentation of patients within this bipolar NOS category. It may be more useful, instead, to think of these patients as belonging to a bipolar spectrum and to identify subcategories of presentations, as has been done by Akiskal and other experts and as illustrated in the next several figures.

The bipolar spectrum

From a strict diagnostic point of view, our discussion of mood disorders might now be complete. However, there is growing recognition that many or even most patients seen in clinical practice may have a mood disorder that is not well described by the categories outlined above. Formally, they would be called "not otherwise specified" or "NOS," but this creates a huge single category for many patients that belies the richness and complexity of their symptoms. Increasingly, such patients are seen as belonging in general to the "bipolar spectrum" (Figure 1-12) and, in particular, to one of several additional descriptive categories proposed by experts such as Akiskal (Figures 1-12 through 1-21).

Two forms of mood disorder often considered to be "not quite bipolar" may include bipolar ¼ and bipolar ½ (Figures 1-13 and 1-14). Bipolar ¼ (or 0.25) could designate an unstable form of unipolar depression that responds sometimes rapidly but in an unsustained manner to antidepressants. Such an uneven response is sometimes called antidepressant "poop out" (Figure 1-13). These patients have unstable mood but not a formal bipolar disorder, yet they can sometimes benefit from mood-stabilizing treatments added to robust antidepressant treatments. Bipolar ½ (or 0.5) may indicate a type of "schizobipolar" disorder, also sometimes called schizoaffective disorder, combining positive symptoms of psychosis with manic, hypomanic, and depressive episodes (Figure 1-14). The placement of these patients within the bipolar spectrum can provide a rationale for treating them with mood stabilizers and atypical antipsychotics as well as antidepressants.

Although patients with protracted or recurrent hypomania without depression are not formally diagnosed as having bipolar disorder, they are definitely part of the bipolar spectrum and may benefit from the mood stabilizers studied mostly in bipolar I disorder (Figure 1-15). Eventually such patients often develop a major depressive episode, and their diagnosis then changes to bipolar disorder. In the meantime, they can be treated for hypomania while being vigilantly watched for the onset of a major depressive episode.

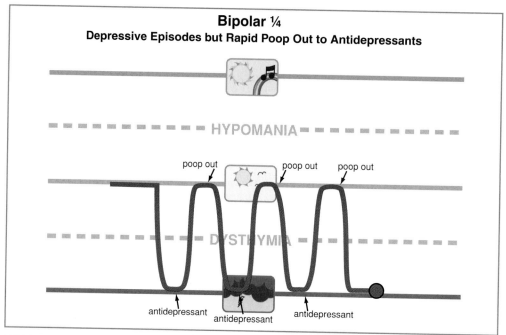

FIGURE 1-13 Bipolar ¹/₄. Some patients may present only with depressive symptoms yet exhibit rapid but unsustained response to antidepressant treatment (sometimes called rapid "poop out"). Although such patients may have no spontaneous mood symptoms above normal, they potentially could benefit from mood-stabilizing treatment. This presentation may be termed bipolar 0.25 (or bipolar 1/4).

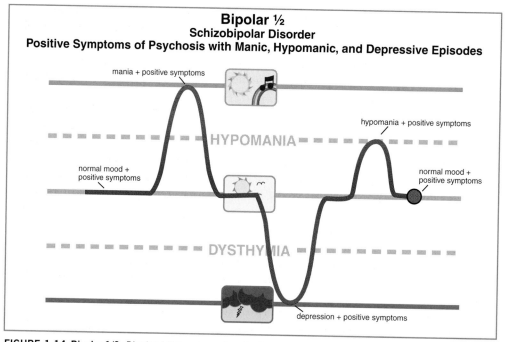

FIGURE 1-14 Bipolar 1/2. Bipolar 1/2 has been described as schizobipolar disorder, which combines positive symptoms of psychosis with manic, hypomanic, and depressive episodes.

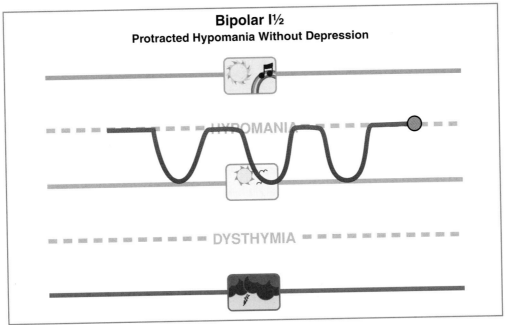

FIGURE 1-15 Bipolar I ½. A formal diagnosis of bipolar disorder requires the occurrence of not only hypomanic episodes but also depressive episodes. However, some patients may experience recurrent hypomania without having experienced a depressive episode – a presentation that may be termed bipolar ½. These patients may be at risk of eventually developing a depressive episode and are candidates for mood stabilizing treatment, although no treatment is formally approved for this condition.

Bipolar ½ is the designation for patients with cyclothymic temperament who develop major depressive episodes (Figure 1-16). Many patients with cyclothymic temperament are just considered "moody" and do not consult professionals until they experience a full depressive episode. It is important to recognize patients in this part of the bipolar spectrum because treatment of their major depressive episodes with antidepressant monotherapy may actually cause increased mood cycling or even induce a full manic episode, just as can happen in patients with bipolar I or depressive episodes.

In fact, patients who develop a manic or hypomanic episode on an antidepressant are sometimes called bipolar (Figure 1-17). According to formal diagnostic criteria, however, when an antidepressant causes mania or hypomania, the diagnosis is not bipolar disorder but rather "substance-induced mood disorder." Many experts disagree with this designation and feel that patients who have a hypomanic or manic response to an antidepressant do so because they have a bipolar spectrum disorder and can be more appropriately diagnosed as bipolar disorder (Figure 1-17) until they experience a spontaneous manic or hypomanic episode while taking no drugs, at which point their diagnosis would be bipolar I or , respectively. The bipolar designation is helpful in the meantime, reminding clinicians that such patients are not good candidates for antidepressant monotherapy.

A variant of bipolar disorder has been called bipolar ½ to designate a type of bipolar disorder associated with substance abuse (Figure 1-18). Although some of these patients can utilize substances of abuse to treat depressive episodes, others have previously experienced natural or drug-induced mania and take substances of abuse to induce mania. This combination of a bipolar disorder with substance abuse is a formula for chaos and can often be the story of a patient prior to seeking treatment from a mental health professional.

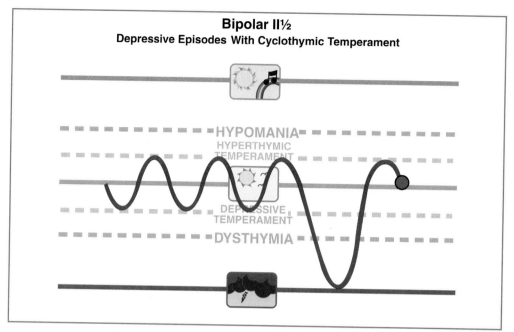

FIGURE 1-16 Bipolar $\frac{1}{2}$. Patients may present with a major depressive episode in the context of cyclothymic temperament, which is characterized by oscillations between hyperthymic or hypomanic states (above normal) and depressive or dysthymic states (below normal) upon which a major depressive episode intrudes (bipolar $\frac{1}{2}$). Individuals with cyclothymic temperament who are treated for the major depressive episodes may be at increased risk for antidepressant-induced mood cycling.

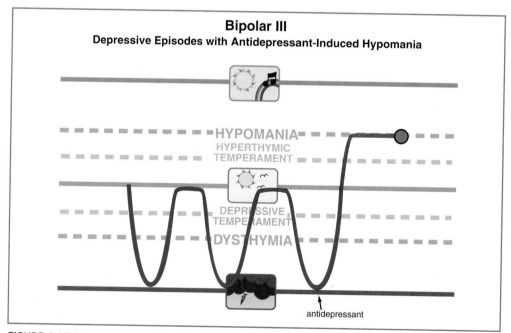

FIGURE 1-17 Bipolar . Although the *Diagnostic and Statistical Manual of Mental Disorders*, fourth edition (DSM-), defines antidepressant-induced (hypo)mania as a substance-induced mood disorder, some experts believe that individuals who experience substance-induced (hypo)mania are actually predisposed to these mood states and thus belong to the bipolar spectrum (bipolar).

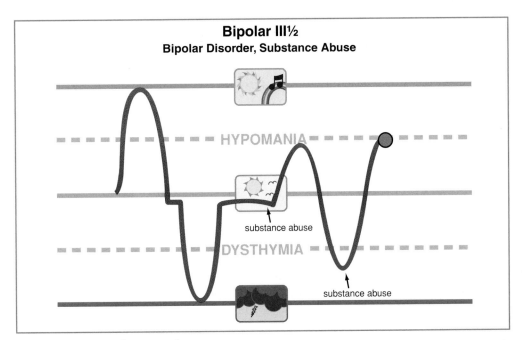

FIGURE 1-18 Bipolar $\frac{1}{2}$. Bipolar $\frac{1}{2}$ is bipolar disorder with substance abuse, in which the substance abuse is associated with efforts to achieve hypomania. Such patients should be evaluated closely to determine if (hypo)mania has ever occurred in the absence of substance abuse.

Bipolar disorder is the association of depressive episodes with a preexisting hyperthymic temperament (Figure 1-19). Patients with hyperthymia are often sunny, optimistic, high-output, successful individuals whose temperaments have been stable for years but who then suddenly collapse into a severe depression. In such cases, it may be useful to be vigilant to the need for more than antidepressant monotherapy if the patient is unresponsive to such treatment or develops rapid cycling, hypomanic, or mixed states in response to antidepressants. Despite not having a formal bipolar disorder, such patients may respond best to mood stabilizers.

Bipolar V disorder is depression with mixed hypomania (Figure 1-20). Formal diagnostic criteria for mixed states require full expression of both depression and mania simultaneously. In the real world, however, many depressed patients can have additional symptoms that qualify as only hypomania or even just a few or mild manic symptoms. Depression coexisting with full hypomania is represented in Figure 1-20 and requires mood stabilizer treatment, not antidepressant monotherapy.

Related states include mood states where full diagnostic criteria are not reached; these can range from full mixed states [both full mania diagnostic criteria (M) and full depression diagnostic criteria (D)] to depression with hypomania or only a few hypomanic symptoms (mD), as already discussed. In addition, other combinations of mania and depression range from full mania with only a few depressive symptoms (Md, sometimes also called "dysphoric" mania), to subsyndromal but unstable states characterized by some symptoms of both mania and depression but not diagnostic of either (md) (Table 1-1). All of these states differ from unipolar depression and belong in the bipolar spectrum; they may require treatment with the same agents used to treat bipolar I or disorder, with appropriate caution for antidepressant monotherapy. The fact that a patient is depressed does not mean that he or she should start

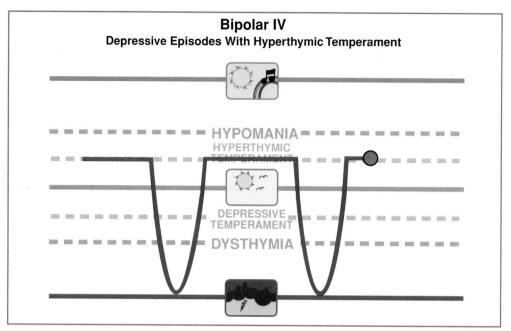

FIGURE 1-19 Bipolar . Bipolar is seen in individuals with long-standing and stable hyperthymic temperament into which a major depressive episode intrudes. Individuals with hyperthymic temperament who are treated for depressive episodes may be at increased risk for antidepressant-induced mood cycling and may instead respond better to mood stabilizers.

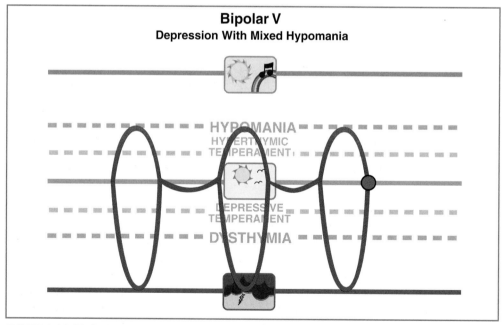

FIGURE 1-20 Bipolar V. Bipolar V is defined as major depressive episodes with hypomanic symptoms occurring during the major depressive episode but without the presence of discrete hypomanic episodes. Because the symptoms do not meet the full criteria for mania, these patients would not be considered to have a full mixed episode, but they nonetheless exhibit a mixed presentation and may require mood stabilizer treatment as opposed to antidepressant monotherapy.

TABLE 1-1 Mixed States of Mania and Depression

Description	Designation	Comment/Other Names
DSM- mixed	MD	Full diagnostic criteria for both mania and depression
Depression with hypomania	mD	Bipolar V
Depression with some manic symptoms	mD	Bipolar NOS
Mania with some depressive symptoms	Md	Dysphoric mania
Subsyndromal mania with subsyndromal depression	md	Prodrome or presymptomatic or state of incomplete remission

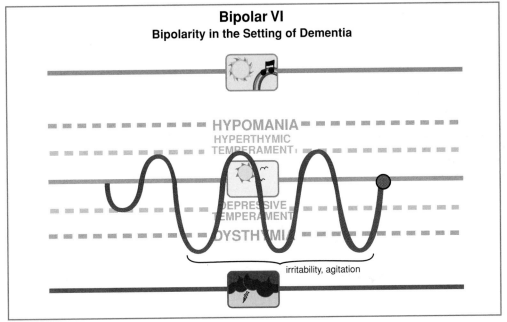

FIGURE 1-21 Bipolar . Another subcategory within the bipolar spectrum may be "bipolarity in the setting of dementia," termed bipolar . Mood instability here begins late in life, followed by impaired attention, irritability, reduced drive, and disrupted sleep. The presentation may initially appear to be attributable to dementia or be considered unipolar depression, but it is likely to be exacerbated by antidepressants and may respond to mood stabilizers.

treatment with an antidepressant. Patients with mixed states of depression and mania may be particularly vulnerable to the induction of activation, agitation, rapid cycling, dysphoria, hypomania, mania, or suicidality when treated with antidepressants, particularly without the concomitant use of a mood stabilizer or an atypical antipsychotic.

Finally, bipolar disorder (Figure 1-21) represents bipolarity in the setting of dementia, where it can be incorrectly attributed to the behavioral symptoms of dementia rather than recognized as a comorbid mood state and treated with mood stabilizers and even with atypical antipsychotics. Many more subtypes of mood disorders can be described within the bipolar spectrum. The important thing to take away from this discussion is that not all patients with depression have major depressive disorder requiring treatment with antidepressant monotherapy and that there are many states of mood disorder within the bipolar spectrum beyond just bipolar I and disorders.

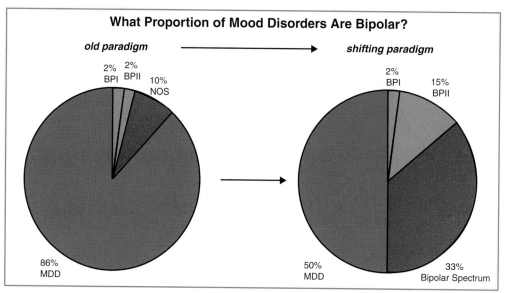

FIGURE 1-22 Prevalence of mood disorders. In recent years there has been a paradigm shift in terms of the recognition and diagnosis of patients with mood disorders. That is, many patients once considered to have major depressive disorder (old paradigm, left) are now recognized as having bipolar disorder or another form of bipolar illness within the bipolar spectrum (shifting paradigm, right).

Can unipolar depression be distinguished from bipolar depression?

One of the important developments in the field of mood disorder in recent years, in fact, is the recognition that many patients once considered to have major depressive disorder actually have a form of bipolar disorder, especially bipolar disorder or one of the conditions within the bipolar spectrum (Figure 1-22). Since symptomatic patients with bipolar disorder spend much more of their time in the depressed state than in the manic, hypomanic, or mixed state, this means that many depressed patients in the past were incorrectly diagnosed with unipolar major depression and treated with antidepressant monotherapy instead of being diagnosed as having a bipolar spectrum disorder and treated first with lithium, anticonvulsant mood stabilizers, and/or atypical antipsychotics prior to being given an antidepressant.

Up to half of patients once considered to have a unipolar depression are now considered to have a bipolar spectrum disorder (Figure 1-22), and although they would not necessarily be good candidates for antidepressant monotherapy, this is often the treatment that they receive when the bipolar nature of their condition is not recognized. Antidepressant treatment of unrecognized bipolar disorder may not only increase mood cycling, mixed states, and conversion to hypomania and mania, as mentioned above, but also contribute to the increase in suicidality of patients treated with antidepressants, with adults below twenty-five years of age being at greater risk for antidepressant-induced suicidality than older adults, adolescents more at risk than younger adults, and children more at risk than adolescents.

Thus it becomes important to recognize whether a depressed patient has a bipolar spectrum disorder or a unipolar major depressive disorder. How can this be done? In reality, these patients can have identical current symptoms (Figure 1-23), so obtaining the profile of current symptomatology is obviously not sufficient to distinguish unipolar from bipolar

TABLE 1-2 Is it unipolar or bipolar depression? Questions to ask

Who's your daddy?
■ What is your family history of:
  – Mood disorder
  – Psychiatric hospitalizations
  – Suicide
  – Anyone who took lithium, mood stabilizers, antipsychotics, antidepressants
  – Anyone who received ECT
These can be indications of a unipolar or bipolar spectrum disorder in relatives.

Where's your mama?
■ Additional history is needed about you from someone close to you, such as your mother or spouse. Patients may especially lack insight about their manic symptoms and underreport them.

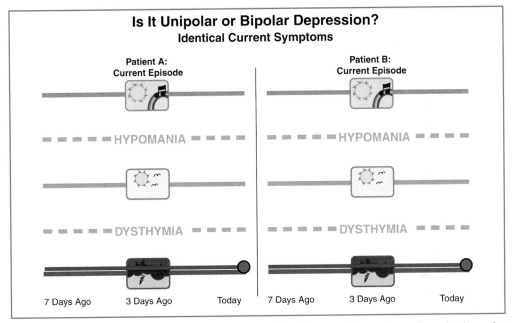

FIGURE 1-23 Unipolar versus bipolar depression presentation. The presenting symptoms of a major depressive episode in bipolar illness (Patient B) may be indistinguishable from those of a major depressive episode in unipolar depression (Patient A). Thus, the current presentation is not sufficient for making the differential diagnosis. The additional information needed includes family history, symptom and treatment-response history, and feedback from a friend or relative.

depression. The answer may be to ask the two questions shown in Table 1-2, namely, "Who's your daddy?" and "Where's your mama?"

What this means is "What is your family history?" since the existence of a first-degree relative with a bipolar spectrum disorder can strongly suggest that the patient also has a bipolar spectrum disorder rather than unipolar depression. This also means, "I need to get additional history from someone else close to you," since patients tend to underreport their manic symptoms, and the insight and observations of an outside informant such as a mother or spouse can give a past history quite different from the one the patient is reporting and thus help establish a bipolar spectrum diagnosis that patients themselves do not perceive or may deny.

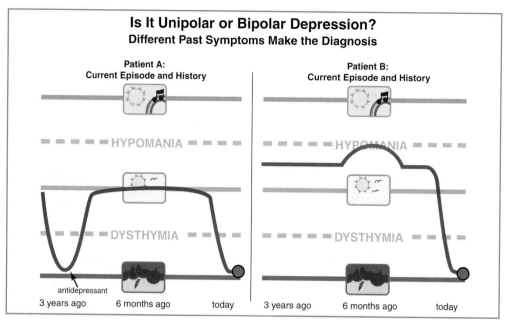

FIGURE 1-24 Unipolar versus bipolar depression history. Patterns of past symptoms as well as treatment-response history may aid in distinguishing between unipolar and bipolar illness. As shown here, although Patients A and B both present with major depressive episodes, they have divergent histories that suggest a unipolar illness for Patient A and a bipolar illness for Patient B.

Pattern of past symptoms can also give a hint as to whether a patient has a bipolar spectrum depression rather than a unipolar depression, as discussed above and as shown in Figure 1-24. Thus, prior response to antidepressants, prior hyperthymia or hypomania, can be hints from past symptoms to help distinguish unipolar from bipolar spectrum depression. Some hints, but not sufficient for diagnostic certainty, can even come from current symptoms to suggest a bipolar spectrum depression, such as more time sleeping, overeating, comorbid anxiety, motor retardation, mood lability, or psychotic or suicidal thoughts (Figure 1-25). Hints that the depression may be in the bipolar spectrum can come from the course of the untreated illness prior to the current symptoms, such as early age of onset, high frequency of depressive symptoms, high proportion of time spent ill, and acute abatement or onset of symptoms (Figure 1-26). Prior responses to antidepressants that suggest bipolar depression can be multiple antidepressant failures, rapid recovery, and the activation of side effects such as insomnia, agitation, and anxiety (Figure 1-27).

Although none of these features can discriminate bipolar depression from unipolar depression with certainty, the point is to be vigilant to the possibility that what looks like a unipolar depression might actually be a bipolar spectrum depression when investigated more carefully, and when response to treatment is monitored.

Are mood disorders progressive?

One of the major unanswered questions about the natural history of depressive illnesses is whether they are progressive (Figures 1-28 and 1-29). Specifically, it appears that many more patients in mental health practices have bipolar spectrum illnesses than unipolar illnesses, especially compared to a few decades ago. Is this merely the product of

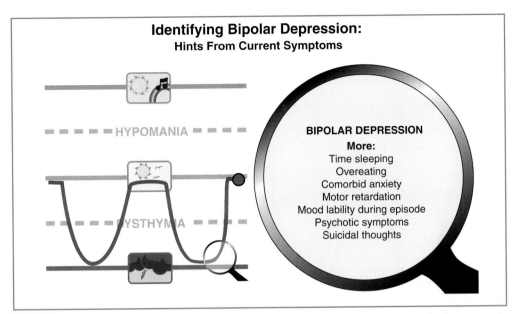

Identifying Bipolar Depression:
Hints From Current Symptoms

HYPOMANIA

DYSTHYMIA

BIPOLAR DEPRESSION
More:
Time sleeping
Overeating
Comorbid anxiety
Motor retardation
Mood lability during episode
Psychotic symptoms
Suicidal thoughts

FIGURE 1-25 Bipolar depression symptoms. Although all symptoms of a major depressive episode can occur in either unipolar or bipolar depression, some symptoms may present more often in bipolar versus unipolar depression, providing hints if not diagnostic certainty that the patient has a bipolar spectrum disorder. These symptoms include increased time sleeping, overeating, comorbid anxiety, psychomotor retardation, mood lability during episodes, psychotic symptoms, and suicidal thoughts.

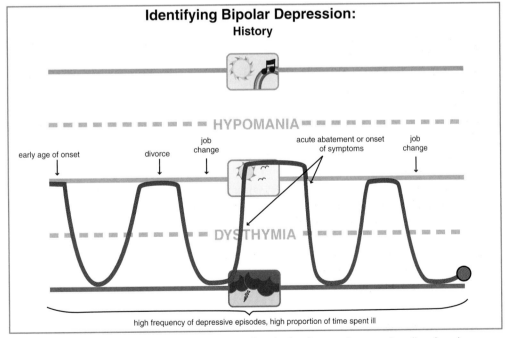

Identifying Bipolar Depression:
History

HYPOMANIA

early age of onset   divorce   job change   acute abatement or onset of symptoms   job change

DYSTHYMIA

high frequency of depressive episodes, high proportion of time spent ill

FIGURE 1-26 Identifying bipolar depression: history. Even in the absence of any previous (hypo)manic episodes, there are often specific hints in the untreated course of illness that suggest depression as part of the bipolar spectrum. These include early age of onset, high frequency of depressive episodes, high proportion of time spent ill, acute onset or abatement of symptoms, and behavioral symptoms such as frequent job or relationship changes.

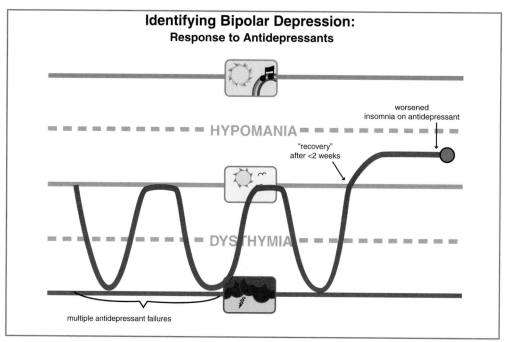

FIGURE 1-27 Identifying bipolar depression: response to antidepressants. Treatment-response history, particularly prior response to antidepressants, may provide insight into whether depression is unipolar or bipolar. Prior responses that suggest bipolar depression may include multiple antidepressant failures, rapid response to an antidepressant, and activating side effects such as insomnia, agitation, and anxiety.

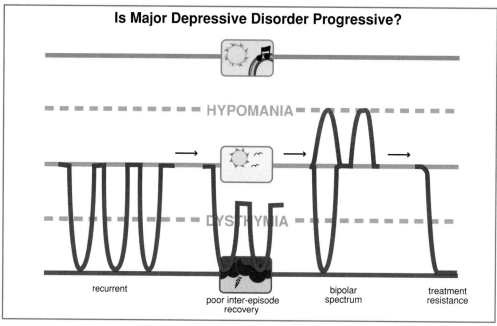

FIGURE 1-28 Is major depressive disorder progressive? A currently unanswered question is whether mood disorders are progressive. Does undertreatment of unipolar depression, in which residual symptoms persist and relapses occur, lead to progressive worsening of illness, such as more frequent recurrences and poor inter-episode recovery? And can this ultimately progress to a bipolar spectrum condition and finally treatment resistance?

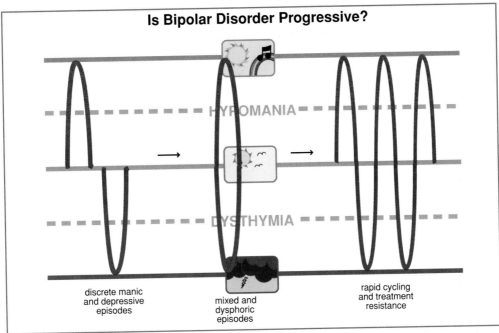

FIGURE 1-29 Is bipolar disorder progressive? There is some concern that undertreatment of discrete manic and depressive episodes may progress to mixed and dysphoric episodes and finally to rapid cycling and treatment resistance.

changing diagnostic criteria, or does unipolar depression progress to bipolar depression (Figure 1-28)?

A corollary of this question is whether chronic and widespread undertreatment of unipolar depression, allowing residual symptoms to persist and relapses and recurrences to occur, results first in more rapidly recurring episodes of major depression, then in poor inter-episode recovery, then progression to a bipolar spectrum condition, and finally to treatment resistance (Figure 1-28). Many treatment-resistant mood disorders in psychiatric practices have elements of bipolar spectrum disorder that can be identified, and many of these patients require treatment with more than antidepressants or with mood stabilizers and atypical antipsychotics instead of antidepressants. This is discussed in detail in Chapter 2, which covers antidepressants, and in Chapter 3, which covers mood stabilizers.

For patients already diagnosed with bipolar disorder, there is similar concern that the disorder may be progressive, especially without adequate treatment. Thus, discrete manic and depressive episodes may progress to mixed and dysphoric episodes and finally to rapid-cycling instability and treatment resistance (Figure 1-29). The hope is that recognition and treatment of both unipolar and bipolar depressions, causing all symptoms to remit for long periods of time, might prevent progression to more difficult states. This is not proved but is a major hypothesis in the field at present.

In the meantime, practitioners must decide whether to commit "sins of omission" and be conservative with the diagnosis of bipolar spectrum disorder, thus erring on the side of undertreatment, or "sins of commission," thus overdiagnosing and overtreating symptoms in the hope that this will prevent disease progression and "diabolical learning" in brain circuits.

Neurotransmitters and circuits in mood disorders

Three principle neurotransmitters have long been implicated in both the pathophysiology and treatment of mood disorders. They are norepinephrine, dopamine, and serotonin and comprise what is sometimes called the "trimonoaminergic" neurotransmitter system. These three monoamines often work in concert. Many of the symptoms of mood disorders are hypothesized to involve dysfunction of various combinations of these three systems. Essentially all known treatments for mood disorders act on one or more of these three systems.

Here we introduce both the norepinephrine system and also some interactions among these three monoaminergic neurotransmitter systems, showing how they interregulate one another. Although other neurotransmitter systems are undoubtedly involved in mood disorders, most is known about the links between trimonoaminergic neurotransmitters and mood disorders, so these neurotransmitters are emphasized here.

Noradrenergic neurons

The noradrenergic neuron utilizes norepinephrine (noradrenaline) as its neurotransmitter. Norepinephrine is synthesized, or produced, from the precursor amino acid tyrosine, which is transported into the nervous system from the blood by means of an active transport pump (Figure 1-30). Once inside the neuron, the tyrosine is acted on by three enzymes in sequence: first, tyrosine hydroxylase (TOH), the rate-limiting and most important enzyme in the regulation of NE synthesis. Tyrosine hydroxylase converts the amino acid tyrosine into dopa. The second enzyme then acts, namely, dopa decarboxylase (DDC), which converts dopa into dopamine (DA). DA itself is a neurotransmitter in dopamine neurons. However, for NE neurons, DA is just a precursor of NE. In fact the third and final NE synthetic enzyme, dopamine beta hydroxylase (DBH), converts DA into NE. NE is then stored in synaptic packages called vesicles until it is released by a nerve impulse (Figure 1-30).

NE action is terminated by two principal destructive or catabolic enzymes that turn NE into inactive metabolites. The first is monoamine oxidase (MAO) A or B, which is located in mitochondria in the presynaptic neuron and elsewhere (Figure 1-31). The second is catechol-O-methyl-transferase (COMT), which is thought to be located largely outside of the presynaptic nerve terminal (Figure 1-31).

The action of NE can be terminated not only by enzymes that destroy NE but also by a transport pump for NE that prevents NE from acting in the synapse without destroying it (Figure 1-31). In fact, such inactivated NE can be restored for reuse in a later neurotransmitting nerve impulse. The transport pump that terminates synaptic action of NE is sometimes called the "NE transporter" or "NET" and sometimes the "NE reuptake pump." This NE reuptake pump is located on the presynaptic noradrenergic nerve terminal as part of the presynaptic machinery of the neuron, where it acts like a vacuum cleaner, whisking NE out of the synapse, off the synaptic receptors, and stopping its synaptic actions. Once inside the presynaptic nerve terminal, NE can either be stored again for subsequent reuse when another nerve impulse arrives or it can be destroyed by NE-destroying enzymes (Figure 1-31).

The noradrenergic neuron is regulated by a multiplicity of receptors for NE (Figure 1-32). The norepinephrine transporter or NET is one type of receptor, as is the vesicular monoamine transporter (VMAT2), which transports NE in the cytoplasm of the presynaptic

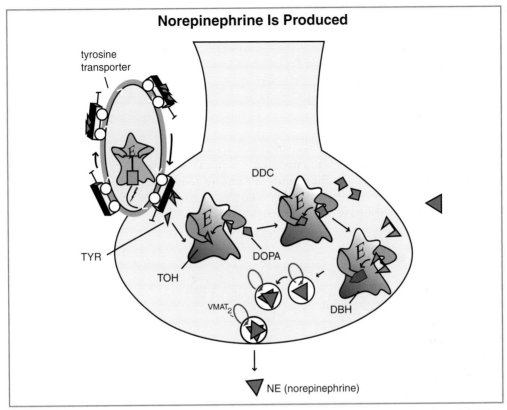

Norepinephrine Is Produced

tyrosine
transporter

DDC

TYR

TOH

DOPA

VMAT₂

DBH

↓

NE (norepinephrine)

FIGURE 1-30 Norepinephrine is produced. Tyrosine, a precursor to norepinephrine (NE), is taken up into NE nerve terminals via a tyrosine transporter and converted into dopa by the enzyme tyrosine hydroxylase (TOH). Dopa is then converted into dopamine (DA) by the enzyme dopa decarboxylase (DDC). Finally, DA is converted into NE by dopamine beta hydroxylase (DBH). After synthesis, NE is packaged into synaptic vesicles via the vesicular monoamine transporter (VMAT2) and stored there until its release into the synapse during neurotransmission.

neuron into storage vesicles (Figure 1-32). NE receptors are classified as alpha 1A, 1B, 1C or alpha 2A, 2B, or 2C, or as beta 1, beta 2, or beta 3. All can be postsynaptic, but only alpha 2 receptors can act as presynaptic autoreceptors (Figures 1-32 through 1-34). Postsynaptic receptors convert their occupancy by norepinephrine at alpha 1A, B, or C; alpha 2A, B, or C; or beta 1, 2, or 3 receptors into physiological functions and ultimately into changes in signal transduction and gene expression in the postsynaptic neuron (Figure 1-32).

Presynaptic alpha 2 receptors regulate norepinephrine release, so they are called "autoreceptors" (Figures 1-32 and 1-33). Presynaptic alpha 2 autoreceptors are located both on the axon terminal (i.e., terminal alpha 2 receptors; Figures 1-32 and 1-33) and at the cell body (soma) and nearby dendrites; thus, these latter alpha 2 presynaptic receptors are called somatodendritic alpha 2 receptors (Figure 1-34). Presynaptic alpha 2 receptors are important because both the terminal and somatodendritic alpha 2 receptors are autoreceptors. That is, when presynaptic alpha 2 receptors recognize NE, they turn off further release of NE (Figures 1-33 and 1-34). Thus, presynaptic alpha 2 autoreceptors act as a brake

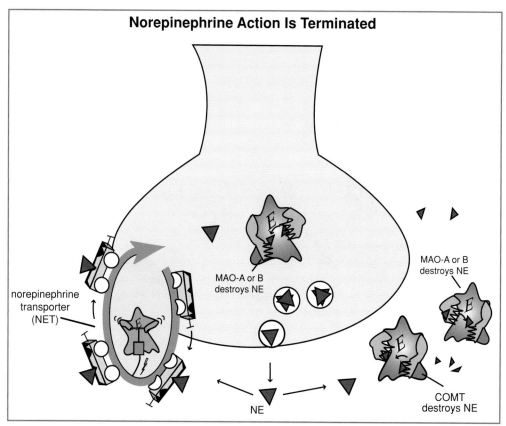

Norepinephrine Action Is Terminated

norepinephrine transporter (NET)

MAO-A or B destroys NE

MAO-A or B destroys NE

COMT destroys NE

NE

FIGURE 1-31 Norepinephrine's action is terminated. Norepinephrine's action can be terminated through multiple mechanisms. Dopamine can be transported out of the synaptic cleft and back into the presynaptic neuron via the norepinephrine transporter (NET), where it may be repackaged for future use. Alternatively, norepinephrine may be broken down extracellularly via the enzyme catechol-O-methyl-transferase (COMT). Other enzymes that break down norepinephrine are monoamine oxidase A (MAO-A) and monoamine oxidase B (MAO-B), which are present in mitochondria both within the presynaptic neuron and in other cells, including neurons and glia.

for the NE neuron and also cause what is known as a negative feedback regulatory signal. Stimulating this receptor (i.e., stepping on the brake) stops the neuron from firing. This probably occurs physiologically to prevent overfiring of the NE neuron, since it can shut itself off once the firing rate gets too high and the autoreceptor becomes stimulated. It is worthy of note that drugs can not only mimic the natural functioning of the NE neuron by stimulating the presynaptic alpha 2 neuron but that those which antagonize this same receptor will have the effect of cutting the brake cable, thus enhancing release of NE.

Monoamine interactions: NE regulation of 5HT release

We have shown above that norepinephrine regulates norepinephrine neurons (Figures 1-33 and 1-34). 5HT Serotonin also regulates 5HT neurons. In both cases, the regulation is that of negative feedback inhibition: both neurotransmitters inhibit their own release.

We now show that NE regulates 5HT neurons and reciprocally, that 5HT also regulates NE neurons. In the case of NE regulation of 5HT (Figures 1-35 through 1-38), there is not only negative feedback inhibition of NE on 5HT release at alpha 2 receptors on axon

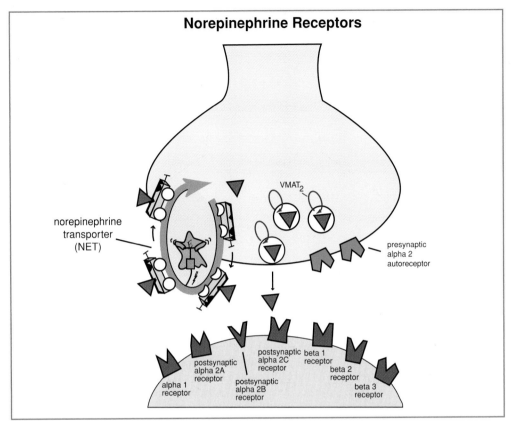

FIGURE 1-32 Norepinephrine receptors. Shown here are receptors for norepinephrine that regulate its neurotransmission. The norepinephrine transporter (NET) exists presynaptically and is responsible for clearing excess norepinephrine out of the synapse. The vesicular monoamine transporter (VMAT2) takes norepinephrine up into synaptic vesicles and stores it for future neurotransmission. There is also a presynaptic alpha 2 autoreceptor, which regulates release of norepinephrine from the presynaptic neuron. In addition, there are several postsynaptic receptors. These include alpha 1, alpha 2A, alpha 2B, alpha 2C, beta 1, beta 2, and beta 3 receptors.

terminals, thus acting as a brake on 5HT release (Figures 1-35 and 1-36), but also positive feedback at alpha 1 receptors at the somatodendritic area, thus acting as an accelerator of 5HT release (Figures 1-35 and 1-37). Thus, NE has bidirectional control of 5HT release, depending on whether input to the axon terminal alpha 2 heteroreceptor or to the somatodendritic alpha 1 receptor predominates (Figure 1-38).

Monoamine interactions: 5HT regulation of NE and DA release

In the other direction, 5HT also regulates NE release, but only as negative feedback at either 5HT2A or 5HT2C receptors, thus inhibiting NE release (Figures 1-39 and 1-40). This same serotonergic negative feedback regulation occurs for dopamine release. Here we show the simultaneous negative feedback regulation of 5HT on both NE and DA release in the prefrontal cortex due to the actions of 5HT in the brainstem on 5HT2A receptors (Figure 1-39) or on 5HT2C receptors (Figure 1-40). In both cases, 5HT blocks release of both NE and DA in the prefrontal cortex. In truth, the regulation of DA release by 5HT at 5HT2A receptors is more complicated than this, but our discussion here is

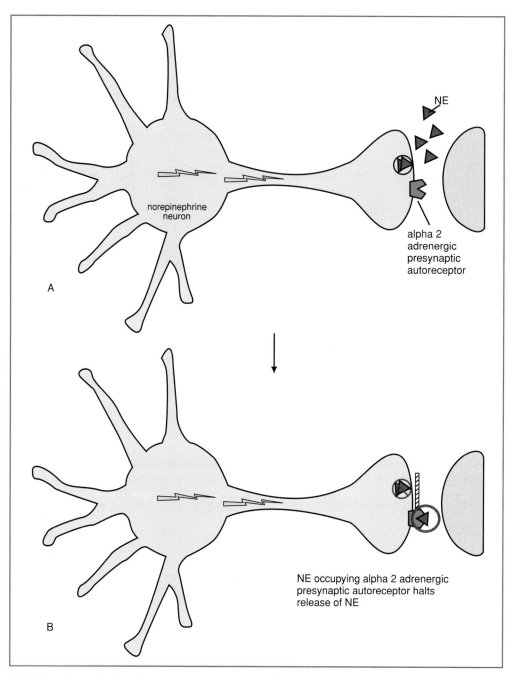

FIGURE 1-33A and B Alpha 2 receptors on axon terminal. Shown here are presynaptic alpha 2 adrenergic autoreceptors located on the axon terminal of the norepinephrine neuron. These autoreceptors are "gatekeepers" for norepinephrine. That is, when they are not bound by norepinephrine, they are open, allowing norepinephrine release (**A**). However, when norepinephrine binds to the gatekeeping receptors, they close the molecular gate and prevent norepinephrine from being released (**B**).

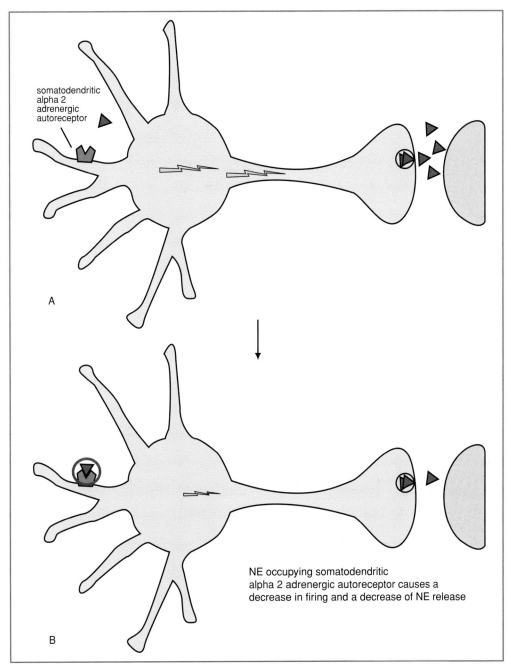

FIGURE 1-34 Somatodendritic alpha 2 receptors. Presynaptic alpha 2 adrenergic autoreceptors are also located in the somatodendritic area of the norepinephrine neuron, as shown here. When norepinephrine binds to these alpha 2 receptors, it shuts off neuronal impulse flow in the norepinephrine neuron (see loss of lightning bolts in the neuron in the lower figure), and this stops further norepinephrine release.

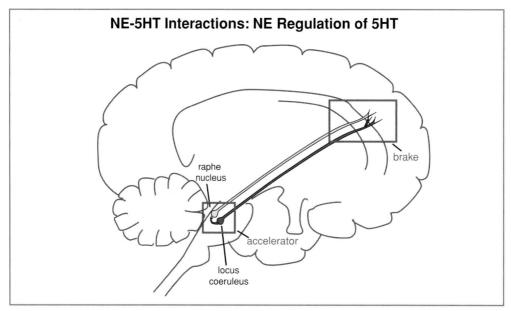

NE-5HT Interactions: NE Regulation of 5HT

raphe
nucleus

brake

accelerator

locus
coeruleus

FIGURE 1-35 Norepinephrine regulation of serotonin. Norepinephrine regulates serotonin release. It does this by acting as a brake on serotonin release at alpha 2 receptors on axon terminals and as an accelerator of serotonin release at alpha 1 receptors at the somatodendritic area.

aimed at providing a background for understanding the actions of atypical antipsychotics in mood disorders; this is not meant to be a comprehensive review of all aspects of 5HT2A receptor regulation of DA release. Other evidence suggests that some 5HT2A receptors in some brain areas under certain circumstances can actually facilitate DA release.

A separate circuit also regulates 5HT2C inhibition of DA release in the nucleus accumbens (Figure 1-41). In this case, 5HT acts upon GABA neurons in the brainstem, one of which inhibits the mesolimbic dopamine projection when 5HT2C receptors are occupied (Figure 1-41). 5HT actions on a second GABA neuron that projects to prefrontal cortex result in inhibition of a descending excitatory glutamate projection to the dopamine neuron, further inhibiting dopamine release in the nucleus accumbens (Figure 1-41).

In summary, there are numerous known interregulatory pathways and receptor interactions among the trimonoaminergic neurontransmitter systems so that they can influence each other and change the release not only of their own neurotransmitters but also of others within this system.

The monoamine hypothesis of depression

The classic theory about the biological etiology of depression hypothesizes that depression is due to a deficiency of monoamine neurotransmitters. At first, there was a great argument about whether norepinephrine (NE) or serotonin (5-hydroxytryptamine; 5HT) was the more important deficiency, and dopamine was relatively neglected. Now the monoamine theory suggests that the entire trimonoaminergic neurotransmitter system may be malfunctioning in various brain circuits, with different neurotransmitters involved depending on the patient's symptom profile.

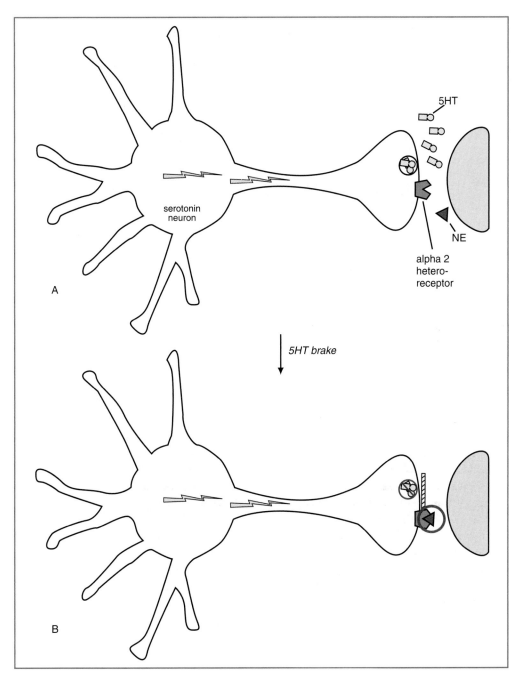

FIGURE 1-36A and B Norepinephrine as a brake on serotonin release. Alpha 2 adrenergic heteroreceptors are located on the axon terminals of serotonin neurons. When these receptors are unoccupied by norepinephrine, serotonin is released from the serotonin neuron (**A**). However, when norepinephrine binds to the alpha 2 receptor this closes the molecular gate and prevents serotonin from being released (**B**).

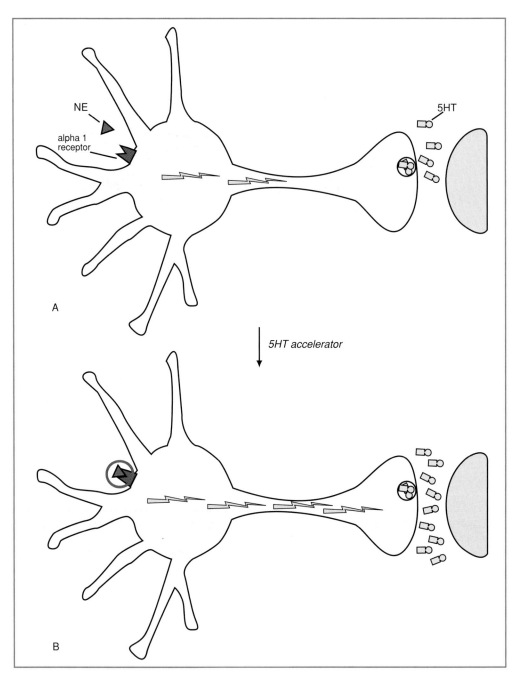

FIGURE 1-37A and B Norepinephrine as an accelerator of serotonin release. Alpha 1 adrenergic receptors are located in the somatodendritic regions of serotonin neurons. When these receptors are unoccupied by norepinephrine, some serotonin is released from the serotonin neuron (**A**). However, when norepinephrine binds to the alpha 1 receptor this stimulates the serotonin neuron, accelerating release of serotonin (**B**).

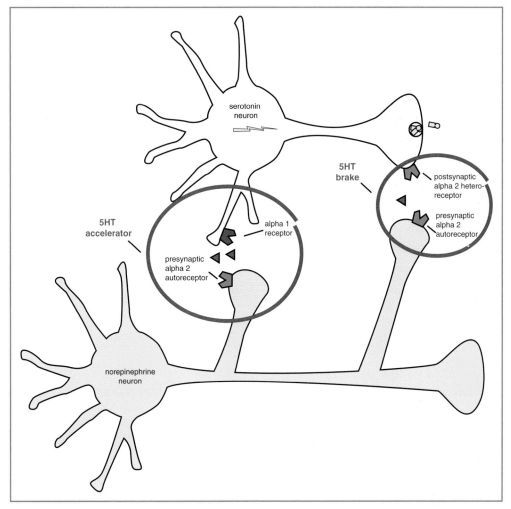

FIGURE 1-38 Norepinephrine bidirectional control of serotonin. Norepinephrine can act as a brake on serotonin release when it binds to alpha 2 receptors at the axon terminal and as an accelerator of serotonin release when it binds to alpha 1 receptors at somatodendritic regions. Thus norepinephrine has bidirectional control of serotonin release.

The original conceptualization was rather simplistic and based on observations that certain drugs which depleted these neurotransmitters could induce depression, and, further, that all effective antidepressants act by boosting one or more of these three monoamine neurotransmitters. Thus the idea was that the "normal" quantity of monoamine neurotransmitters (Figure 1-42A) somehow became depleted – perhaps by an unknown disease process, stress, or drugs (Figure 1-42B) – leading to the symptoms of depression.

Direct evidence for the monoamine hypothesis is still largely lacking. A good deal of effort was expended, especially in the 1960s and 1970s, to identify the theoretically predicted deficiencies of the monoamine neurotransmitters. This effort to date has unfortunately yielded mixed and sometimes confusing results. Some studies suggest that NE metabolites are deficient in some patients with depression, but this has not been uniformly observed. Other studies suggest that the 5HT metabolite 5HIAA (5-hydroxy-indole acetic acid) is

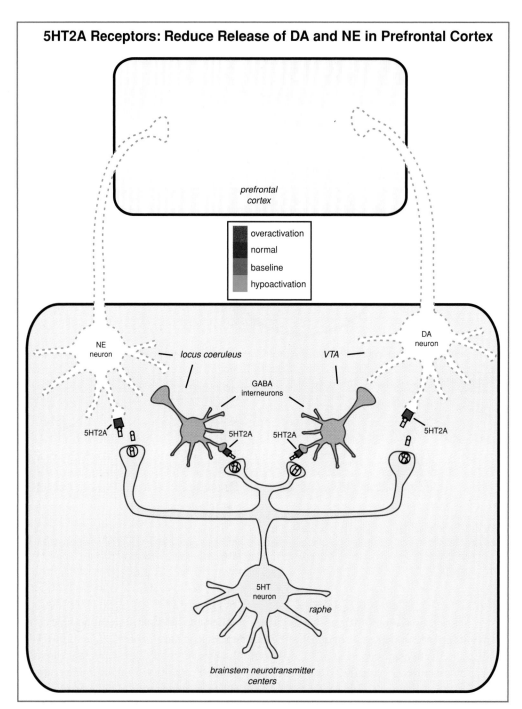

FIGURE 1-39 5HT2A receptors regulate norepinephrine and dopamine. Serotonin (5HT) regulates release of norepinephrine (NE) and dopamine (DA) in the prefrontal cortex via 5HT2A receptors located at the somatodendritic ends of NE, DA, and gamma-aminobutyric acid (GABA) neurons. Binding of 5HT at 5HT2A receptors on some NE and DA neurons in the brainstem directly inhibits release of these neurotransmitters into the prefrontal cortex. In addition, binding of 5HT at 5HT2A receptors on some GABA interneurons in the brainstem *increases* GABA release, which then inhibits NE and DA release.

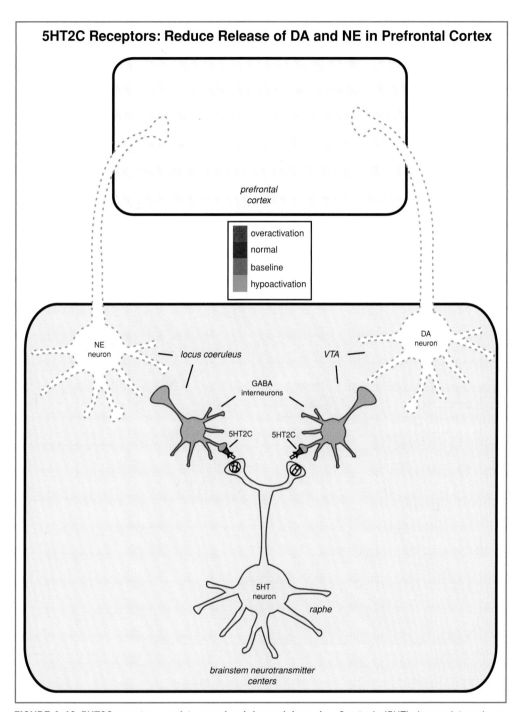

FIGURE 1-40 5HT2C receptors regulate norepinephrine and dopamine. Serotonin (5HT) also regulates release of norepinephrine (NE) and dopamine (DA) in the prefrontal cortex via 5HT2C receptors located on gamma-aminobutyric acid (GABA) interneurons in the brainstem. Binding of 5HT at 5HT2C receptors on these GABA interneurons *increases* GABA release, which then inhibits NE and DA release from their respective neurons.

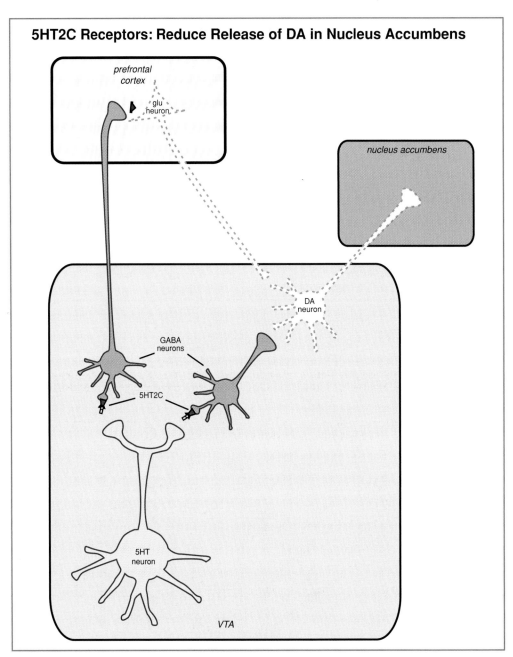

5HT2C Receptors: Reduce Release of DA in Nucleus Accumbens

prefrontal cortex

glu neuron

nucleus accumbens

DA neuron

GABA neurons

5HT2C

5HT neuron

VTA

FIGURE 1-41 5HT2C receptors regulate dopamine in nucleus accumbens. Serotonin (5HT) also regulates release of dopamine (DA) in the nucleus accumbens via 5HT2C receptors on two types of gamma-aminobutyric acid (GABA) neurons. First, stimulation of 5HT2C receptors on GABA interneurons within the brainstem (on the right) causes release of GABA there, which in turn inhibits activity of ascending mesolimbic dopamine projections. This results in reduced DA release in the nucleus accumbens. Second, stimulation of 5HT2C receptors on GABA neurons that project out of the brainstem and into the prefrontal cortex (on the left) leads to inhibition of descending glutamate projections to brainstem dopamine neurons. This, in turn, also leads to reduced DA in the nucleus accumbens.

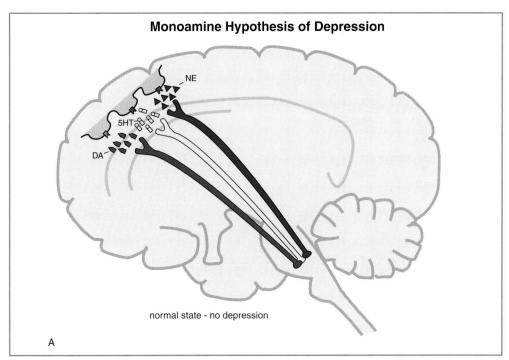

FIGURE 1-42A Classic monoamine hypothesis of depression, part 1. According to the classic monoamine hypothesis of depression, when there is a "normal" amount of monoamine neurotransmitter activity, there is no depression present.

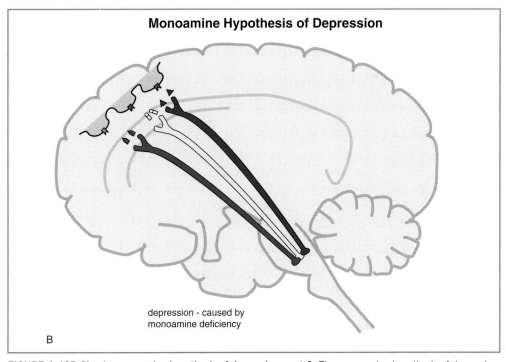

FIGURE 1-42B Classic monoamine hypothesis of depression, part 2. The monoamine hypothesis of depression posits that if the "normal" amount of monoamine neurotransmitter activity becomes reduced, depleted, or dysfunctional for some reason, depression may ensue.

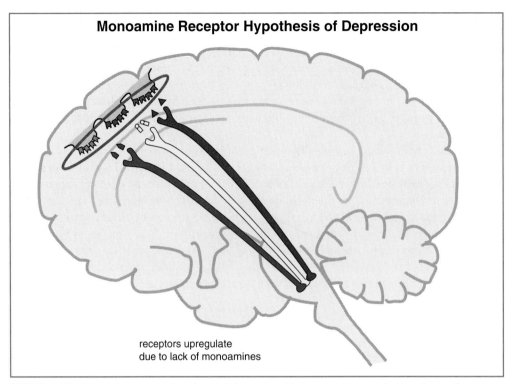

Monoamine Receptor Hypothesis of Depression

receptors upregulate
due to lack of monoamines

FIGURE 1-43 **Monoamine receptor hypothesis of depression.** The monoamine receptor hypothesis of depression extends the classic monoamine hypothesis of depression, positing that deficient activity of monoamine neurotransmitters causes upregulation of postsynaptic monoamine neurotransmitter receptors, and that this leads to depression.

reduced in the cerebrospinal fluid of depressed patients. On closer examination, however, it has been found that only some of the depressed patients have low CSF 5HIAA, and they tend to be those with impulsive behaviors, such as suicide attempts of a violent nature. Subsequently, it was also reported that CSF 5HIAA is decreased in other populations noted to be subject to violent outbursts or poor impulse control but who were not depressed – namely, patients with antisocial personality disorder who were arsonists and those with borderline personality disorder who engaged in self-destructive acts. Thus, low CSF 5HIAA may be linked more closely with impulse-control problems rather than with depression.

The monoamine hypothesis, monoamine receptors, and gene expression

Because of these and other difficulties with the monoamine hypothesis of depression, the focus of hypotheses for the etiology of depression has shifted from the monoamine neurotransmitters themselves to their receptors and the downstream molecular events that these receptors trigger, including the regulation of gene expression. For example, the neurotransmitter receptor hypothesis of depression posits that an abnormality in the receptors for monoamine neurotransmitters leads to depression (Figure 1-43). Thus, if depletion of monoamine neurotransmitters is the central theme of the monoamine hypothesis of depression (Figure 1-42B), the neurotransmitter receptor hypothesis of depression takes this theme one step further: namely, that the depletion of neurotransmitter causes compensatory upregulation of postsynaptic neurotransmitter receptors (Figure 1-43).

Direct evidence for this is also generally lacking. Postmortem studies do consistently show increased numbers of serotonin 2 receptors in the frontal cortex of patients who commit suicide. Also, some neuroimaging studies have identified abnormalities in serotonin receptors of depressed patients, but this approach has not yet been successful in identifying consistent and replicable molecular lesions in receptors for monoamines in depression.

Thus, there is no clear and convincing evidence that monoamine deficiency accounts for depression; that is, there is no "real" monoamine deficit. Likewise, there is no clear and convincing evidence that abnormalities in monoamine receptors account for depression. Emphasis is now turning to the possibility that in depression there may be a deficiency in downstream signal transduction of the monoamine neurotransmitter and its postsynaptic neuron that is occurring in the presence of normal amounts of neurotransmitter and receptor. Thus the hypothesized molecular problem in depression could lie within the molecular events distal to the receptor, in the signal transduction cascade system and in appropriate gene expression. This is the subject of much current research into the potential molecular basis of affective disorders.

One candidate mechanism that has been proposed as the site of a possible flaw in signal transduction from monoamine receptors is the target gene for brain-derived neurotrophic factor (BDNF). Normally, BDNF sustains the viability of brain neurons; but under stress, the gene for BDNF may be repressed, leading to the atrophy and possible apoptosis of vulnerable neurons in the hippocampus when their neurotrophic factor BDNF is cut off. The idea is that this, in turn, leads to depression and to the consequences of repeated depressive episodes; namely, more and more episodes and less and less responsiveness to treatment. This possibility that hippocampal neurons are decreased in size and impaired in function during depression and anxiety disorders is supported by recent clinical imaging studies showing decreased brain volume of related structures.

This provides a molecular and cellular hypothesis of depression consistent with a mechanism distal to the neurotransmitter receptor and involving an abnormality in gene expression. Thus, stress-induced vulnerability decreases the expression of genes that make neurotrophic factors such as BDNF, which are critical to the survival and function of key neurons. A corollary to this hypothesis is that antidepressants act by reversing this by causing the genes for neurotrophic factors to be activated.

Although the monoamine hypothesis is obviously an overly simplified notion about depression, it has been very valuable in focusing attention on the three monoamine neurotransmitter systems: norepinephrine, dopamine, and serotonin. This has led to a much better understanding of the physiological functioning of these three neurotransmitters and especially the various mechanisms by which all known antidepressants act to boost neurotransmission at one or more of these three monoamine neurotransmitter systems.

Symptoms and circuits in depression

The monoamine hypothesis of depression is now being applied to elucidating how the trimonoaminergic neurotransmitter system regulates the efficiency of information processing in a wide variety of neuronal circuits that may be responsible for mediating the various symptoms of depression. Obviously numerous symptoms are required for the diagnosis of a major depressive episode (Figure 1-44). Each symptom is hypothetically associated

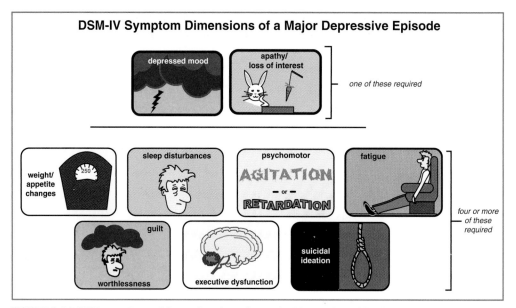

FIGURE 1-44 DSM- symptoms of depression. According to the *Diagnostic and Statistical Manual of Mental Disorders*, fourth edition (DSM-), a major depressive episode consists of either depressed mood or loss of interest and at least four of the following: weight/appetite changes, insomnia or hypersomnia, psychomotor agitation or retardation, fatigue, feelings of guilt or worthlessness, executive dysfunction, and suicidal ideation.

with inefficient information processing in various brain circuits, with different symptoms topographically localized to specific brain regions (Figure 1-45).

Not only can each of the nine symptoms listed for the diagnosis of a major depressive episode be mapped onto brain circuits that theoretically mediate these symptoms (Figure 1-45), but the hypothetical trimonoaminergic regulation of each of these brain areas can also be mapped onto each brain region they innervate (Figures 1-46 to 1-54). This creates a set of monoamine neurotransmitters that regulate each specific hypothetically malfunctioning brain region. Targeting each region with drugs that act on the relevant neurotransmitters within the trimonoaminergic neurotransmitter system could potentially lead to reduction of each individual symptom experienced by a specific patient by enhancing the efficiency of information processing in malfunctioning circuits for each specific symptom. If successful, this targeting of monoamines in specific brain areas could eliminate symptoms and cause a major depressive episode to go into remission (Figures 1-46 through 1-54).

Generally, the monoaminergic functioning in these circuits in major depressive disorder are represented as being blue, or reduced, consistent with the monoamine hypothesis. However, the more accurate portrayal may be "out of tune" rather than simply deficient. Some brain regions in depression, in fact, have enhanced neuronal activation, and others have reduced neuronal activation. Nevertheless, trimonoaminergic treatments available today for depression all generally boost one or more of the monoamines.

For example, the core symptom of a major depressive episode is depressed mood, thought to be linked to inefficient information processing in the amygdala and in "emotional" areas of the prefrontal cortex, especially the ventromedial prefrontal cortex (VMPFC) and the nearby subgenual area of the anterior cingulate cortex (Figure 1-46). Each of the three monoamine neurotransmitters of the trimonoaminergic neurotransmitter system

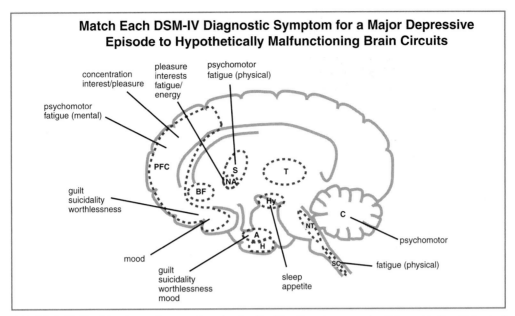

Match Each DSM-IV Diagnostic Symptom for a Major Depressive Episode to Hypothetically Malfunctioning Brain Circuits

FIGURE 1-45 Matching depression symptoms to circuits. Alterations in neuronal activity and in the efficiency of information processing within each of the eleven brain regions shown here can lead to symptoms of a major depressive episode. Functionality in each brain region is hypothetically associated with a different constellation of symptoms. PFC, prefrontal cortex; BF, basal forebrain; S, striatum; NA, nucleus accumbens; T, thalamus; HY, hypothalamus; A, amygdala; H, hippocampus; NT, brainstem neurotransmitter centers; SC, spinal cord; C, cerebellum.

innervates these areas; it is therefore not surprising that antidepressants that boost any of these neurotransmitters can improve mood in depression (Figure 1-46).

Apathy or loss of interest is another key symptom of depression and may be more common in elderly patients with depression, even in the absence of depressed mood. How can someone have apathy without depressed mood? The answer is because these symptoms may involve different brain circuits and different neurotransmitters. That is, apathy may involve the prefrontal cortex diffusely, including not only VMPFC but also especially dorsolateral prefrontal cortex as well as the hypothalamic "drive" centers and the nucleus accumbens "pleasure" or interest center (Figure 1-47). Furthermore, whereas deficient dopamine and norepinephrine may regulate these areas and boosting them with antidepressants may help relieve such symptoms associated with these areas, boosting serotonin may actually act to reduce both of these neurotransmitters and make symptoms worse. The mechanisms by which serotonin reduces them are discussed earlier in this chapter and illustrated in Figures 1-39 to 1-41. Thus only NE and DA are shown in Figure 1-47.

Sleep disturbances may be diffusely represented in several brain areas, especially hypothalamus, thalamus, basal forebrain, and diffusely throughout prefrontal cortex, with regulatory input by all three monoamines (Figure 1-48). Fatigue or loss of energy is linked to deficient functioning of NE and DA in prefrontal cortex, especially for mental fatigue, as well as in striatum and nucleus accumbens, especially for physical fatigue (Figure 1-49). Executive dysfunction is fairly well characterized as having localization in the dorsolateral prefrontal cortex (DLPFC) and being regulated mostly by DA and NE (Figure 1-50). Psychomotor symptoms, either agitation or retardation, are linked to motor circuits, especially in the striatum but also in the prefrontal cortex and secondarily perhaps in the cerebellum

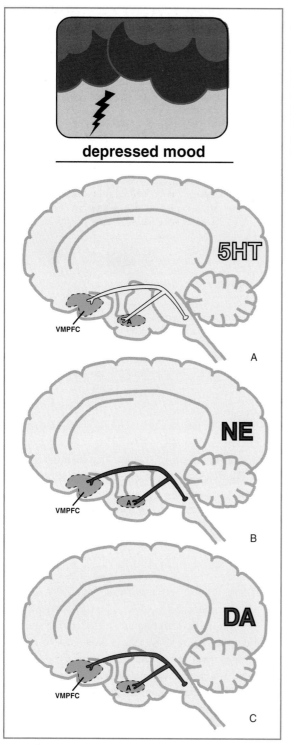

depressed mood

FIGURE 1-46A, B, and C Depressed mood circuits. Depressed mood is believed to be linked to inefficient information processing in the amygdala (A) and the ventromedial prefrontal cortex (VMPFC), both of which are innervated by serotonergic (**A**), noradrenergic (**B**), and dopaminergic (**C**) projections from brainstem nuclei. Reduced, dysfunctional, and inefficient monoaminergic functioning in these regions is depicted here as hypoactive (blue color).

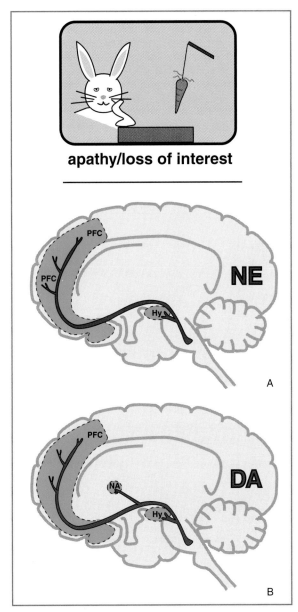

apathy/loss of interest

FIGURE 1-47A and B Apathy circuits. Although apathy and depressed mood are often considered similar symptoms, they are hypothetically regulated by different brain circuits. Apathy is believed to be related to inefficient information processing (depicted here as blue or hypoactive) diffusely through the prefrontal cortex (PFC) as well as in hypothalamic centers (Hy) and the nucleus accumbens (NA). These functions within the prefrontal cortex and hypothalamus are thought to be regulated in part by noradrenergic neurons that project there (**A**), while within prefrontal cortex, hypothalamus, and nucleus accumbens these functions are also thought to be regulated by dopaminergic projections (**B**).

as well (Figure 1-51). Changes in weight and appetite, either increased or decreased, have important hypothalamic and serotonergic components to their regulation (Figure 1-52). Suicidal ideation (Figure 1-53) as well as feelings of guilt and worthlessness (Figure 1-54) all have profound connections to serotonin and to circuits connecting to amygdala and emotional regulatory areas of the prefrontal cortex, including the ventromedial prefrontal cortex and perhaps the orbitofrontal cortex.

Many of the mood-related symptoms of depression can be categorized as having either too little positive affect or too much negative affect (Figure 1-55). This idea is linked to the fact that there are diffuse anatomic connections of the trimonoaminergic neurotransmitter system throughout the brain, with diffuse dopamine dysfunction in this system

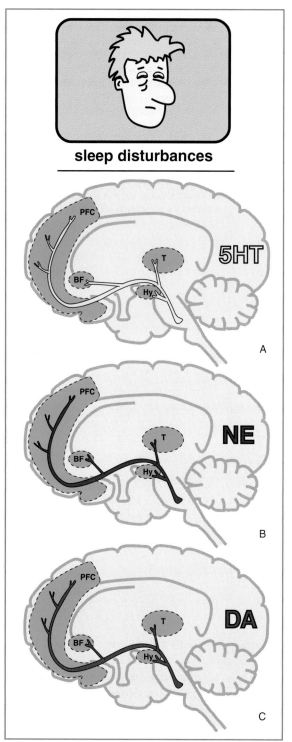

sleep disturbances

FIGURE 1-48A, B, and C Sleep circuits.
Sleep disturbances are believed to be linked to inefficient information processing in the hypothalamus (Hy), thalamus (T), basal forebrain (BF), and diffusely in the prefrontal cortex (PFC), depicted here by the blue color representing hypoactivity. All of these brain regions are regulated by serotonergic (**A**), noradrenergic (**B**), and dopaminergic (**C**) projections from brainstem nuclei.

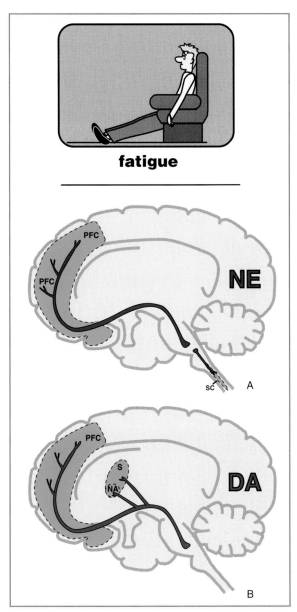

fatigue

FIGURE 1-49A and B Fatigue circuits.
Fatigue or loss of energy is linked to inefficient information processing in several brain regions as well as in the spinal cord, shown here as hypoactivity (blue color). Specifically, mental fatigue is related to deficient noradrenergic functioning in the prefrontal cortex (PFC), while physical fatigue is related to deficient noradrenergic functioning in descending spinal cord (SC) projections (**A**). Dopamine also plays a role in fatigue, with deficient dopaminergic functioning in the PFC related to mental fatigue and deficient dopaminergic functioning in the striatum (S), nucleus accumbens (NA), hypothalamus (Hy), and SC related to physical fatigue (**B**).

driving predominantly the reduction of positive affect, with diffuse serotonin dysfunction driving predominantly the increase in negative affect, and with norepinephrine dysfunction being involved in both. Thus reduced positive affect includes such symptoms as depressed mood but also loss of happiness, joy, interest, pleasure, alertness, energy, enthusiasm, and self-confidence (Figure 1-55, on the left). Enhancing dopamine function and possibly also norepinephrine function may improve information processing in the circuits mediating this cluster of symptoms. On the other hand, increased negative affect includes not only depressed mood but also guilt, disgust, fear, anxiety, hostility, irritability, and loneliness (Figure 1-55, on the right). The enhancement of serotonin function and possibly also norepinephrine function may improve information processing in the circuits that

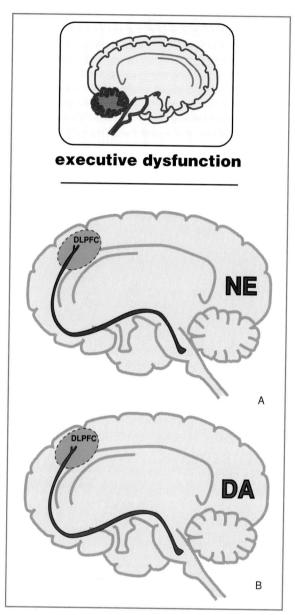

executive dysfunction

FIGURE 1-50A and B Executive dysfunction circuits. Executive dysfunction is associated with inefficient information processing (depicted here as blue or hypoactive), specifically in the dorsolateral prefrontal cortex (DLPFC), which receives important regulatory projections from both noradrenergic (**A**) and dopaminergic (**B**) neurons.

hypothetically mediate this cluster of symptoms. Patients with symptoms of both clusters may require triple-action treatments that boost all three of the trimonoamine neurotransmitters.

Symptoms and circuits in mania

The same general paradigm of trimonoaminergic neurotransmitter system regulation of the efficiency of information processing in specific brain circuits can be applied to mania as well as depression, although this is frequently thought to be in the opposite direction and in some overlapping but some different brain regions compared to depression. The numerous

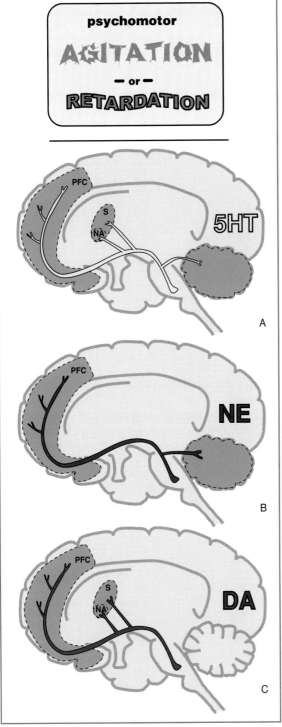

FIGURE 1-51A, B, and C Psychomotor symptom circuits. Psychomotor agitation or retardation may be related to inefficient information processing in multiple brain regions innervated by serotonergic (**A**), noradrenergic (**B**), and/or dopaminergic (**C**) projections. These regions include the cerebellum, which receives serotonergic and noradrenergic projections, the striatum and nucleus accumbens, which receive serotonergic and dopaminergic projections, and the prefrontal cortex (PFC), which receives projections from all three monoamines. In this figure, the monoaminergic functioning is depicted as hypoactive (blue color).

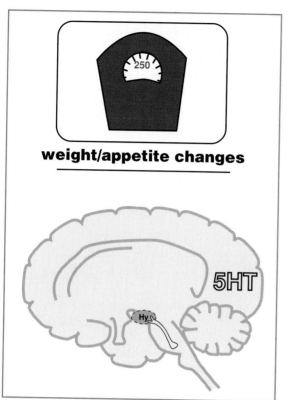

FIGURE 1-52 Weight and appetite circuit.
Appetite and weight are mediated in large part by the hypothalamus (Hy), which receives serotonergic projections. Thus, any changes in weight or appetite as a symptom of depression may be related in part to serotonergic control of the hypothalamus (shown here as blue to denote hypoactivity).

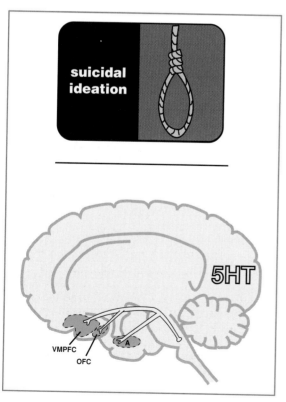

FIGURE 1-53 Suicide circuit. Suicidal ideation is believed to be regulated by inefficient information processing (shown here in blue for hypoactivity) in brain regions associated with emotionality, such as the amygdala (A), ventromedial prefrontal cortex (VMPFC), and orbital frontal cortex (OFC). These brain regions receive important regulatory control for suicidality from serotonergic projections.

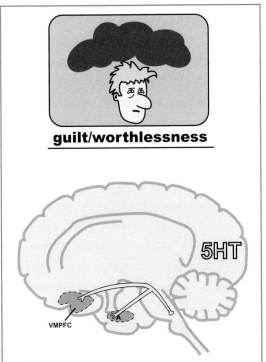

guilt/worthlessness

FIGURE 1-54 Guilt/worthlessness circuit. As with suicidal ideation, feelings of guilt or worthlessness are regulated by "emotional" brain regions such as the amygdala (A) and ventromedial prefrontal cortex (VMPFC), which are innervated by important serotonergic regulatory projections. Inefficient information processing in these regions (depicted here as blue or hypoactive) may cause these symptoms to occur.

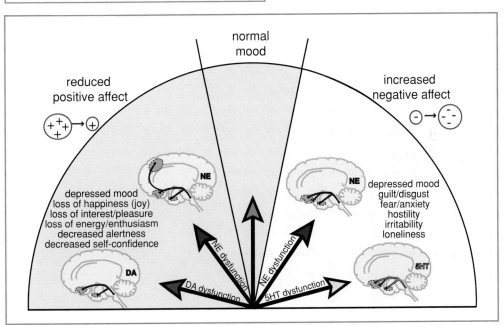

FIGURE 1-55 Positive and negative affect. Mood-related symptoms of depression can be characterized by their affective expression – that is, whether they cause a reduction in positive affect or an increase in negative affect. Symptoms related to reduced positive affect include depressed mood; loss of happiness, interest, or pleasure; loss of energy or enthusiasm; decreased alertness; and decreased self-confidence. Reduced positive affect may be hypothetically related to dopaminergic dysfunction, with a possible role of noradrenergic dysfunction as well. Symptoms associated with increased negative affect include depressed mood, guilt, disgust, fear, anxiety, hostility, irritability, and loneliness. Increased negative affect may be linked hypothetically to serotonergic dysfunction and perhaps also noradrenergic dysfunction.

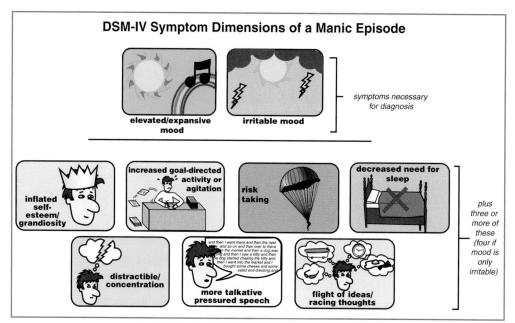

FIGURE 1-56 DSM- symptoms of mania. According to the *Diagnostic and Statistical Manual of Mental Disorders*, fourth edition (DSM-), a manic episode consists of either elevated/expansive mood or irritable mood. In addition, at least three of the following must be present (four if mood is irritable): inflated self-esteem/grandiosity, increased goal-directed activity or agitation, risk taking, decreased need for sleep, distractibility, pressured speech, and racing thoughts.

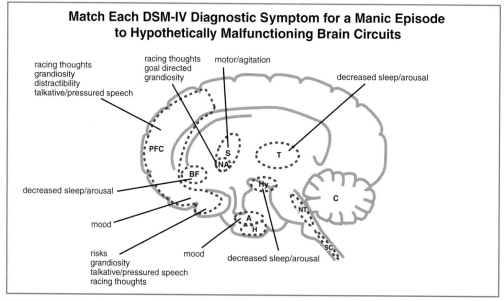

FIGURE 1-57 Matching mania symptoms to circuits. Alterations in neurotransmission within each of the eleven brain regions shown here can be hypothetically linked to the various symptoms of a manic episode. Functionality in each brain region may be associated with a different constellation of symptoms. PFC, prefrontal cortex; BF, basal forebrain; S, striatum; NA, nucleus accumbens; T, thalamus; HY, hypothalamus; A, amygdala; H, hippocampus; NT, brainstem neurotransmitter centers; SC, spinal cord; C, cerebellum.

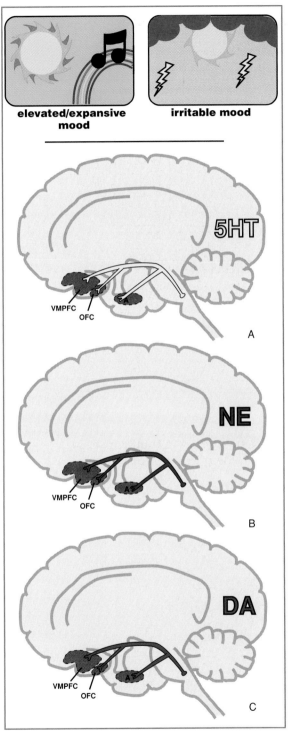

elevated/expansive mood

irritable mood

FIGURE 1-58A, B, and C Elevated/irritable mood circuits. Elevated/expansive or irritable mood may be hypothetically linked to inefficient information processing (depicted here in red to denote hyperactivity) in the amygdala (A), ventromedial prefrontal cortex (VMPFC), and orbital frontal cortex (OFC), all of which are innervated by serotonergic (**A**), noradrenergic (**B**), and dopaminergic (**C**) projections from brainstem nuclei.

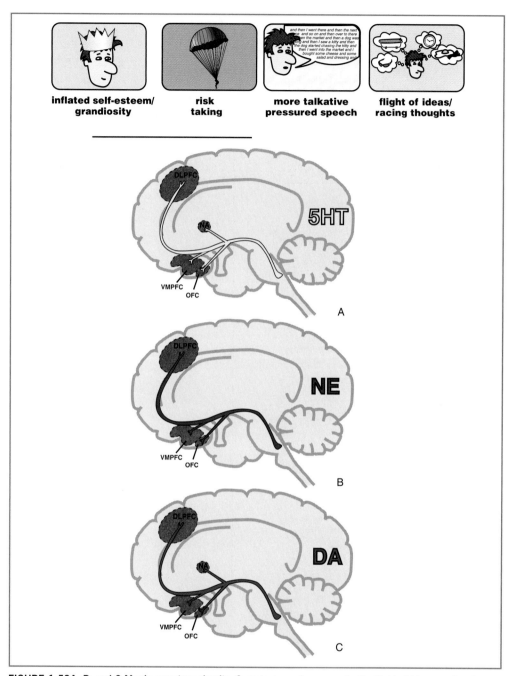

inflated self-esteem/ grandiosity

risk taking

more talkative pressured speech

flight of ideas/ racing thoughts

FIGURE 1-59A, B, and C Mania symptom circuits. Symptoms such as grandiosity, flight of ideas, and racing thoughts may be hypothetically linked to inefficient information processing (depicted here in red as hyperactivity) in the same brain regions associated with positive symptoms of psychosis [i.e., nucleus accumbens (NA)]. Other manic symptoms, such as risk taking and pressured speech, may be manifestations of poor impulse control and thus regulated by the orbital frontal cortex (OFC). Other areas of the prefrontal cortex, such as the dorsolateral prefrontal cortex (DLPFC) and ventromedial prefrontal cortex (VMPFC), may also be involved in these symptoms. Regulation of these areas of presumed inefficient information processing in prefrontal cortex include serotonergic (**A**), noradrenergic (**B**), and dopaminergic (**C**) projections, while the nucleus accumbens is innervated by serotonergic (**A**) and dopaminergic (**C**) projections.

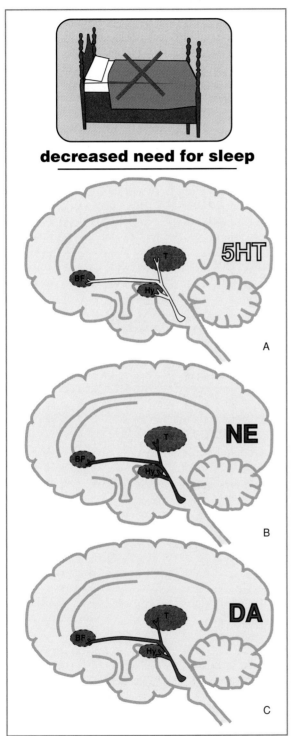

decreased need for sleep

FIGURE 1-60A, B, and C Sleep circuits. Although sleep disturbances manifest themselves differently in a major depressive versus a manic episode (i.e., insomnia or hypersomnia versus decreased subjective need for sleep), they may still be regulated by many of the same brain regions. Thus decreased need for sleep may be linked to inefficient information processing in the hypothalamus (Hy), thalamus (T), and basal forebrain (BF), depicted here by the red color representing hyperactivity. All of these brain regions are innervated by serotonergic (**A**), noradrenergic (**B**), and dopaminergic (**C**) projections from brainstem nuclei.

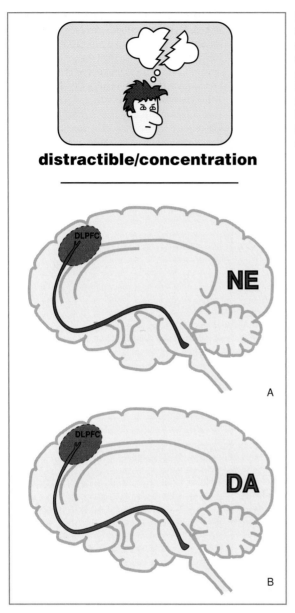

distractible/concentration

FIGURE 1-61A and B Distractibility circuit. Cognitive problems in mania, such as distractibility or poor concentration, may be associated with aberrant information processing (depicted here as red or hyperactive) specifically in the dorsolateral prefrontal cortex (DLPFC), which receives important regulatory projections from both noradrenergic (**A**) and dopaminergic (**B**) neurons.

symptoms required for the diagnosis of a manic episode are shown in Figure 1-56. As in the case of major depression, each symptom of mania is also hypothetically associated with inefficient information processing in various brain circuits, with different symptoms topographically localized to specific brain regions (Figure 1-57).

Generally, the monoaminergic functioning in these circuits in mania is represented as being red, or hyperactive, and thus essentially the opposite of the malfunctioning hypothesized for depression (see Figures 1-46 through 1-54). As for depression, however, the more accurate portrayal may be "out of tune" rather than simply excessive, especially since some patients can simultaneously have both manic and depressed symptoms. Generally,

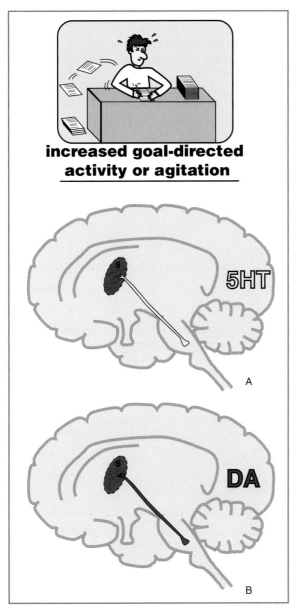

increased goal-directed
activity or agitation

FIGURE 1-62A and B Goal-directed activity circuit. Increased goal-directed activity or agitation in mania may be associated with inefficient information processing in the striatum, perhaps related to hyperactivity of serotonergic (**A**) and dopaminergic (**B**) projections (depicted as red).

however, treatments of mania either reduce or stabilize trimonoaminergic regulation of circuits associated with symptoms of mania.

Just as shown for depression, each of the nine symptoms listed for the diagnosis of mania (Figure 1-56) can also be mapped onto brain circuits that theoretically mediate these symptoms (Figure 1-57), and the hypothetical trimonoaminergic regulation of each of these brain areas can be mapped onto each of the brain regions they innervate as well (Figures 1-58 through 1-62). Targeting each affected region with drugs that act on the relevant neurotransmitters within the trimonoaminergic neurotransmitter system could potentially lead to reduction of each individual manic symptom experienced by a specific patient by enhancing

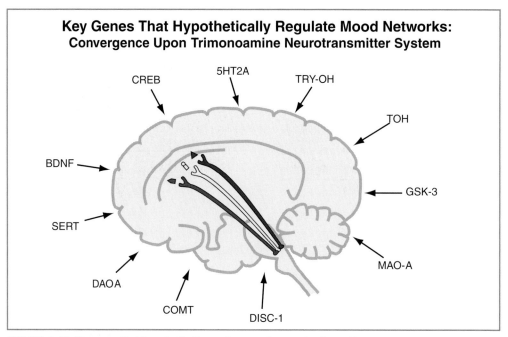

Key Genes That Hypothetically Regulate Mood Networks: Convergence Upon Trimonoamine Neurotransmitter System

FIGURE 1-63 Key genes that hypothetically regulate mood networks. Several key genes that code for proteins that regulate mood networks are shown here. Many of these genes converge on the trimonoaminergic neurotransmitter system, supporting the role of these three neurotransmitters – serotonin, norepinephrine, and dopamine – in both the symptoms and treatments of mood disorders.

the efficiency of information processing in malfunctioning circuits for each specific symptom. If successful, this targeting of monoamines in specific brain areas could eliminate manic symptoms and cause a manic episode to remit (Figures 1-58 through 1-62).

For example, the core symptoms of a manic episode are elevated, expansive, or irritable mood (Figure 1-58). Thus, patients may have some elements of enhanced negative affect, such as irritability and dysphoria, as experienced by some depressed patients (Figure 1-55). As is the case for depressed mood, these other moods are hypothetically linked to the amygdala, ventromedial prefrontal cortex, and orbitofrontal cortex, with regulation by all three monoamine neurotransmitters (Figure 1-58).

On the other hand, symptoms of inflated self-esteem, grandiosity, flight of ideas, and racing thoughts may be linked to psychotic symptoms and thus to limbic areas such as nucleus accumbens, with risk taking and pressured speech linked to poor impulse control and perhaps therefore to orbitofrontal cortex (Figure 1-59). Sleep disturbance as a symptom of a manic episode (Figure 1-60) may be linked to many of the same areas as sleep disturbance as a symptom of depression (Figure 1-48), although the symptom in mania is not really insomnia but rather a decreased subjective need for sleep. Similarly, distractibility and problems concentrating as symptoms of a manic episode (Figure 1-61) are likely associated with the same brain area as that associated with executive dysfunction such as problems concentrating in a major depressive episode (Figure 1-50) – namely, the dorsolateral prefrontal cortex. Increased goal-directed activity or agitation may be linked to the striatum in mania (Figure 1-62).

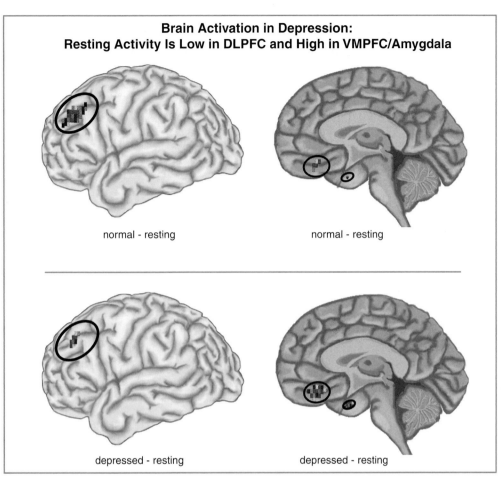

FIGURE 1-64 Neuroimaging of brain activation in depression. Neuroimaging studies of brain activation suggest that resting activity in the dorsolateral prefrontal cortex (DLPFC) of depressed patients is low compared to that in nondepressed individuals (left, top and bottom), whereas resting activity in the amygdala and ventromedial prefrontal cortex (VMPFC) of depressed patients is high compared to that in nondepressed individuals (right, top and bottom).

As the reader can see, there is considerable overlap between mania and depression, and common symptoms are hypothetically mediated by the same circuits. Obviously this is a simplistic and reductionistic approach to mapping symptoms of mania and depression; many brain areas are involved, since each brain area is linked to many others. Nevertheless, this idea of constructing a diagnosis, then deconstructing it into its symptom components, and then matching each symptom to a hypothetically malfunctioning brain circuit can be useful in choosing treatments for individual patients. This approach is sometimes called symptom-based treatment selection and combination and is discussed in much further detail in Chapter 2, on antidepressants, and in Chapter 3, on mood stabilizers.

Genes and neuroimaging in mood disorders

Many of the issues in identifying gene abnormalities in mood disorders are the same as those for identifying gene abnormalities in schizophrenia. In fact, many of the same genetic abnormalities associated with schizophrenia may apply in part to mood disorders,

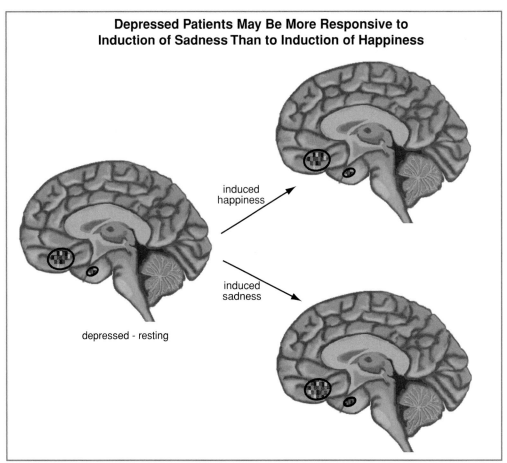

Depressed Patients May Be More Responsive to Induction of Sadness Than to Induction of Happiness

induced happiness

induced sadness

depressed - resting

FIGURE 1-65 Depressed patient's neuronal response to induced sadness versus happiness. Emotional symptoms such as sadness or happiness are regulated by the ventromedial prefrontal cortex (VMPFC) and the amygdala, two regions in which activity is high in the resting state of depressed patients (left). Interestingly, provocative tests in which these emotions are induced show that neuronal activity in the amygdala is overreactive to induced sadness (bottom right) but underreactive to induced happiness (top right).

especially bipolar disorder; the confluence of genetic risk plus environmental stressors is thought to be the same general paradigm. Several of the key genes that hypothetically regulate mood networks not surprisingly all converge on the trimonoamine neurotransmitter system (Figure 1-63). How these genes influence neurodevelopment, synaptic plasticity, neuronal connectivity, and the efficiency of neuronal information processing in mood disorders is currently under intense investigation.

In terms of neuroimaging mood disorders, there is general agreement that in depression, the dorsolateral prefrontal cortex, associated with cognitive symptoms, may have reduced activity, and the amygdala and ventromedial prefrontal cortex, associated with various emotional symptoms including depressed mood, may have increased activity (Figure 1-64). Furthermore, provocative testing of patients with mood disorders may provide some insight into the malfunctioning of brain circuits that are exposed to environmental input and required to process it. For example, some studies of depressed patients show

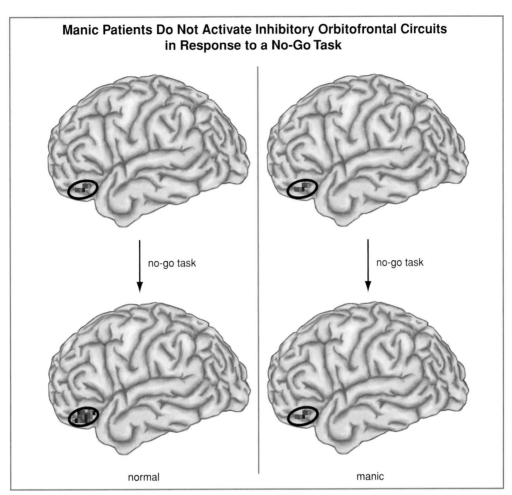

Manic Patients Do Not Activate Inhibitory Orbitofrontal Circuits in Response to a No-Go Task

no-go task

no-go task

normal

manic

FIGURE 1-66 Manic patient's neuronal response to no-go task. Impulsive symptoms of mania, such as risk taking and pressured speech, are related to activity in the orbital frontal cortex (OFC). Neuroimaging data show that this brain region is hypoactive in manic (bottom right) versus normal (bottom left) individuals during the no-go task, which is designed to test response inhibition.

that their neuronal circuits at the level of the amygdala and ventromedial prefrontal cortex are overly reactive to induced sadness but underreactive to induced happiness (Figure 1-65). On the other hand, imaging the orbitofrontal cortex of manic patients shows that they fail to appropriately activate this brain region in a test that requires them to suppress a response, suggesting problems with impulsivity associated with mania and with this specific brain region (Figure 1-66). In general, these neuroimaging findings support the mapping of symptoms to brain regions discussed earlier in this chapter, but much further work is currently in progress and must be completed before the results of neuroimaging can be applied to diagnostic or therapeutic decision making in clinical practice.

Summary

This chapter has described the mood disorders, including those across the bipolar spectrum. For prognostic and treatment purposes, it is increasingly important to be able to distinguish unipolar depression from bipolar spectrum depression. Although mood disorders are indeed disorders of mood, they are much more, and several different symptoms in addition to a mood symptom are required to make a diagnosis of a major depressive episode or a manic episode. Each symptom can be matched to a hypothetically malfunctioning neuronal circuit. The monoamine hypothesis of depression suggests that dysfunction – generally due to underactivity – of one or more of the three monoamines DA, NE, or 5HT of the trimonoaminergic neurotransmitter system may be linked to symptoms in major depression. Boosting one or more of the monoamines in specific brain regions may improve the efficiency of information processing there and reduce the symptom caused by that area's malfunctioning. Other brain areas associated with the symptoms of a manic episode can similarly be mapped to various hypothetically malfunctioning brain circuits. Understanding the localization of symptoms in circuits – as well as the neurotransmitters that regulate these circuits in different brain regions – can set the stage for choosing and combining treatments for each individual symptom of a mood disorder, with the goal being to reduce all symptoms and bring about remission.

Antidepressants

This chapter reviews the pharmacological concepts underlying the use of antide-pressant drugs. There are many different classes of antidepressants and dozens of individual drugs. The goal of this chapter is to acquaint the reader with current ideas about how the various antidepressants work. It explains the mechanisms of action of these drugs by building upon general pharmacological concepts. It also discusses concepts about how to use these drugs in clinical practice, including strategies for what to do if initial treatments fail and how to rationally combine one antidepressant with another or with a modulating agent. Finally, the reader is introduced to several new antidepressants in clinical development.

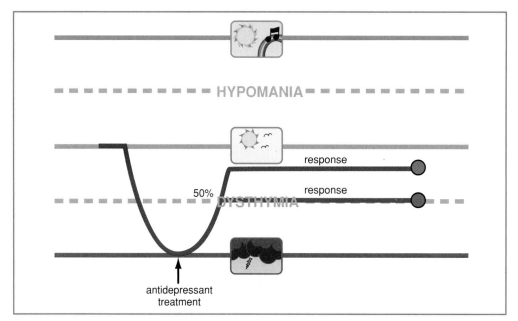

FIGURE 2-1 Response. When treatment of depression results in at least 50% improvement in symptoms, it is called a response. Such patients are better but not well. Previously, this was considered the goal of depression treatment.

The treatment of antidepressants in this chapter is at the conceptual level, not at the pragmatic level. The reader should consult standard drug handbooks (such as the companion *Essential Psychopharmacology: Prescriber's Guide*) for details of doses, side effects, drug interactions, and other issues relevant to the prescribing of these drugs in clinical practice.

General principles of antidepressant action

Patients undergoing a major depressive episode who receive treatment with any antidepressant often experience improvement in their symptoms; when this improvement reaches the level of reducing symptoms by 50% or more, it is called a response (Figure 2-1). This used to be the goal of treatment with antidepressants: namely, to reduce symptoms substantially, at least by 50%. However, the paradigm for antidepressant treatment has shifted dramatically in recent years, so that now the goal of treatment is complete remission of symptoms (Figure 2-2) and maintaining that level of improvement, so that the patient's major depressive episode does not relapse shortly after remission and the patient will not have a recurrent episode in the future (Figure 2-3). Given the known limits to the efficacy of available antidepressants, especially when multiple antidepressant treatment options are not deployed aggressively, this goal of treatment can be difficult to reach. In fact, the goal of remission (Figure 2-3) is not usually reached with the first antidepressant treatment administered.

There are various strategies for putting together an antidepressant treatment portfolio for each patient. This is often accomplished by utilizing multiple pharmacological mechanisms and that increasingly requires treatment with more than one drug in order to generate numerous therapeutic options for reaching the important if sometimes difficult goal of remission. This treatment strategy for depression is very different from that for schizophrenia, where the expected improvement in symptomatology may be only a

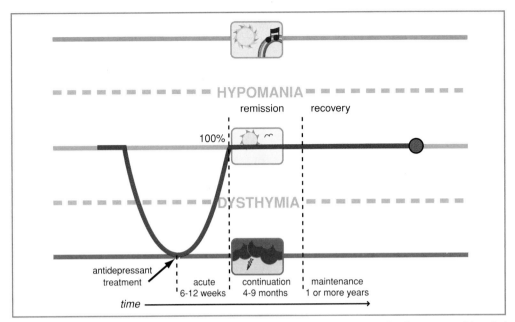

FIGURE 2-2 Remission. When treatment of depression results in removal of essentially all symptoms, it is called remission for the first several months and then recovery if it is sustained for longer than six to twelve months. Such patients are not just better – they are well. However, they are not cured, since depression can still recur. Remission and recovery are now the goals when treating patients with depression.

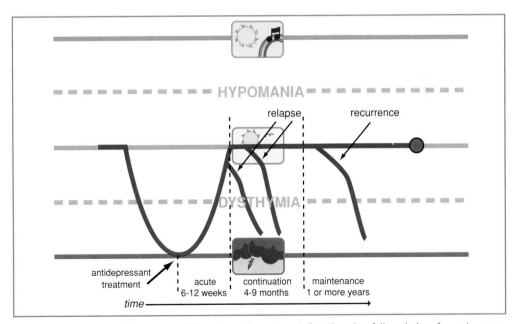

FIGURE 2-3 Relapse and recurrence. When depression returns before there is a full remission of symptoms or within the first several months following remission of symptoms, it is called a relapse. When depression returns after a patient has recovered, it is called a recurrence.

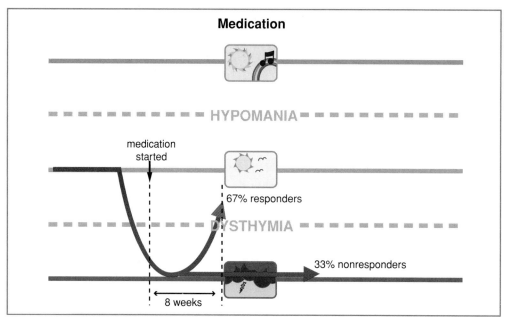

FIGURE 2-4 Antidepressant response rates. Virtually every known antidepressant has the same response rate: 67% of depressed patients respond to any given medication and 33% fail to respond.

20% to 30% reduction of symptoms, and few if any patients become truly asymptomatic or go into remission. Thus the attainment of a genuine state of asymptomatic remission in major depression is the current challenge for those who treat this disorder; this is the reason for learning the mechanisms of action of so many drugs, the complex biological rationale for combining specific sets of drugs, and the practical tactics for tailoring a unique drug treatment portfolio to fit the needs of an individual patient.

All known antidepressants studied in clinical trials designed for marketing approval cause about two-thirds of patients to respond within 8 weeks of initiating treatment (Figure 2-4), whereas placebo causes only about one-third of patients to respond within 8 weeks (Figure 2-5). In addition, patients who respond to an antidepressant and continue it (Figure 2-6) have a much lower relapse rate than those who are switched to placebo (Figure 2-7). These are classic statements but belie the fact that it is becoming more and more difficult to prove that antidepressants – even well-established antidepressants – actually work any better than placebo in clinical trials. This problem of translating results from clinical trials into clinical practice may be due to fluctuating placebo response rates, which occasionally are as high as drug response rates in clinical trial settings, as well as to many other complex factors, such as the highly structured treatment environment of the clinical trial setting, where some are receiving placebo, payments are being made to investigators and sometimes to patients, and patients with comorbid conditions as well as those who are severely ill, suicidal, or treatment-resistant are excluded from trials.

Further complicating the translation of clinical trial findings to the clinical practice setting is the fact that up to one-third of patients in clinical practice never fill their first antidepressant prescription; of those who do, perhaps less than half get a second month of treatment and maybe less than one-fourth get an adequate trial of 3 months or longer. One thing is for sure about antidepressants, and that is that they don't work if you don't take them. Thus, the effectiveness of antidepressants in clinical practice settings is reduced by

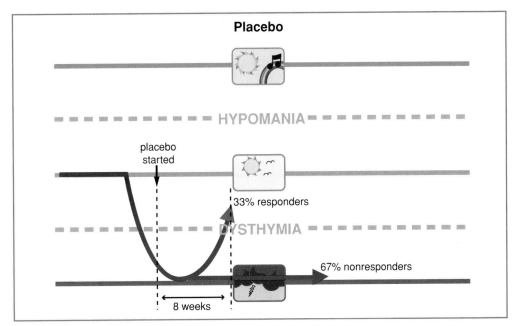

FIGURE 2-5 Placebo response rates. In controlled clinical trials, 33% of patients respond to placebo treatment and 67% fail to respond.

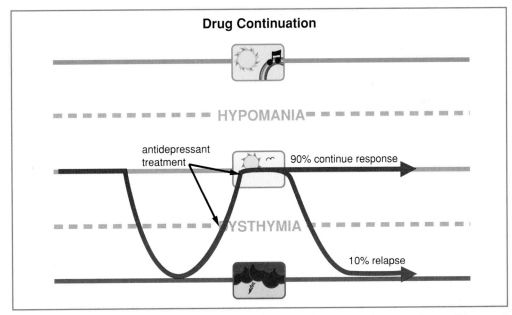

FIGURE 2-6 Drug continuation. Depressed patients who have an initial treatment response to an antidepressant will relapse at a rate only of about 10% to 20% if their medication is continued for six months to a year following recovery.

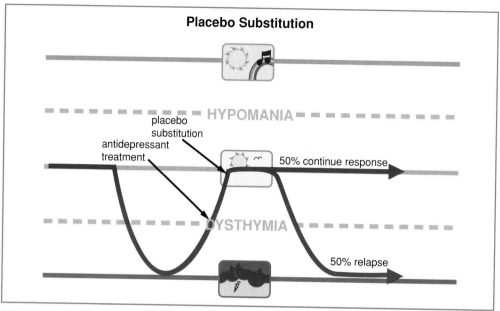

FIGURE 2-7 Placebo substitution. Depressed patients who have an initial treatment response to an antidepressant will relapse at the rate of 50% within six to twelve months if their medication is withdrawn and a placebo is substituted.

this failure of "persistency" of treatment for a long enough period of time to give the drug a chance to work.

"Real world" trials of antidepressants test them in clinical practice settings that include patients normally excluded from marketing trials, such as the STAR-D (Sequenced Treatment Alternatives to Relieve Depression) trial of antidepressants. These trials have recently provided sobering results. Only one-third of such patients remit on their first antidepressant treatment; even after a year of treatment with a sequence of four different antidepressants given for twelve weeks each, only about two-thirds of depressed patients achieve remission (Figure 2-8).

What are the most common symptoms that persist after antidepressant treatment, causing this disorder not to go into remission? The answer is shown in Figure 2-9, and the symptoms include insomnia, fatigue, multiple painful physical complaints (even though these are not part of the formal diagnostic criteria for depression), as well as problems concentrating and lack of interest or motivation. Antidepressants appear to work fairly well in improving depressed mood, suicidal ideation, and psychomotor retardation (Figure 2-9).

Why should we care whether a patient is in remission from major depression or has just a few persistent symptoms? The answer can be found in Figure 2-10, which shows both good news and bad news about antidepressant treatment over the long run. The good news is that if an antidepressant gets your patient into remission, that patient has a significantly lower relapse rate. The bad news is that there are still very frequent relapses in the remitters, and these relapse rates get worse the more treatments the patient needs to take in order to get into remission (Figure 2-10).

Data like these have galvanized researchers and clinicians alike to treat patients to the point of remission of all symptoms whenever possible and to try to intervene as early as

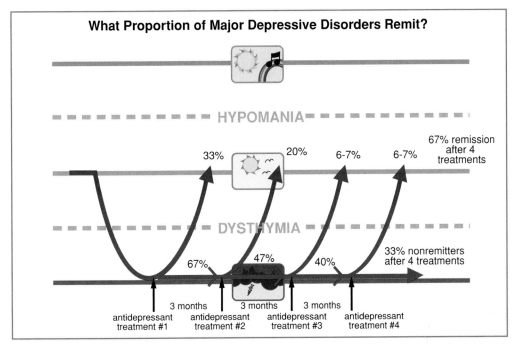

FIGURE 2-8 Remission rates in MDD. Approximately one-third of depressed patients will remit during treatment with any antidepressant initially. Unfortunately, for those who fail to remit, the likelihood of remission with another antidepressant monotherapy goes down with each successive trial. Thus, after a year of treatment with four sequential antidepressants taken for twelve weeks each, only two-thirds of patients will have achieved remission.

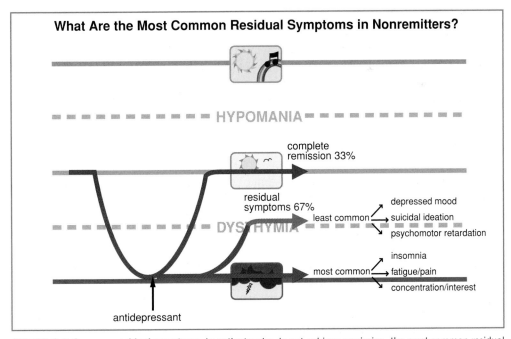

FIGURE 2-9 Common residual symptoms. In patients who do not achieve remission, the most common residual symptoms are insomnia, fatigue, painful physical complaints, problems concentrating, and lack of interest. The least common residual symptoms are depressed mood, suicidal ideation, and psychomotor retardation.

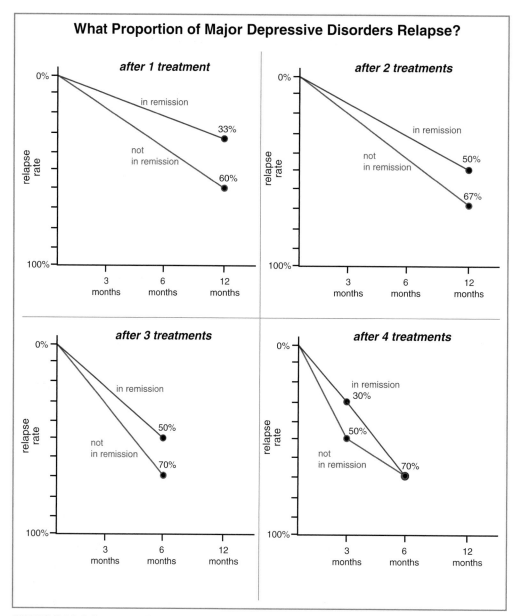

FIGURE 2-10 Relapse rates. The rate of relapse of major depression is significantly less for patients who achieve remission. However, there is still risk of relapse even in remitters, and the likelihood increases with the number of treatments it takes to get the patient to remit. Thus the relapse rate for patients who do not remit ranges from 60% at twelve months after one treatment to 70% at six months after four treatments; but for those who do remit, it ranges from only 33% at twelve months after one treatment all the way to 70% at six months after four treatments. In other words, the protective nature of remission virtually disappears once it takes four treatments to achieve remission.

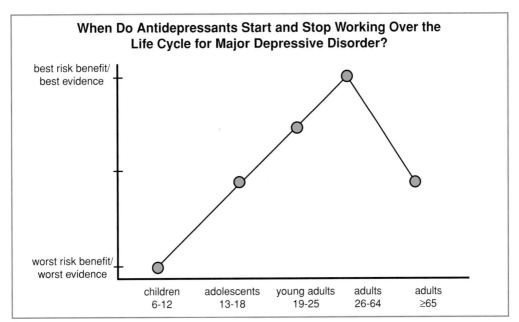

FIGURE 2-11 Antidepressants over the life cycle. The efficacy, tolerability, and safety of antidepressants have been studied mostly in individuals between the ages of 25 to 64. Existing data across all age groups suggest that the risk/benefit ratio is most favorable for adults between the ages of 25 to 64 and somewhat less so for adults between the ages of 19 to 25 due to a possibly increased risk of suicidality in younger adults. Limited data in children and adolescents also suggest increased risk of suicidality; this, coupled with a lack of data demonstrating clear antidepressant efficacy, gives children between the ages of 6 to 12 the worst risk/benefit ratio, with adolescents intermediate between young adults and children. Elderly patients 65 years of age and older may not respond as well or as quickly to antidepressants as other adults and may also experience more side effects than younger adults.

possible in major depression, not only to be merciful in trying to relieve current suffering from depressive symptoms but also because of the possibility that aggressive treatment may prevent disease progression. The concept of disease progression in major depression is controversial, unproven, and provocative, but it makes a good deal of sense intuitively for many clinicians and investigators. It is being vigorously researched at the present time. This concept of disease progression is also discussed in Chapter 1 and illustrated in Figures 1-28 and 1-29. The idea is that chronicity of major depression, development of treatment resistance, and likelihood of relapse could all be reduced with aggressive treatment of major depressive episodes that leads to remission of all symptoms, thus potentially modifying the course of illness. This may pose an especially difficult challenge for the treatment of younger patients, where antidepressant efficacy and safety are currently being debated.

Do antidepressants work in the same way over the entire life cycle? The answer seems to be no. Adults between the ages of 25 and 65 might have the best chance of getting a good response and having good tolerability to an antidepressant (Figure 2-11). However, adults above age 65 may not respond as quickly or as robustly to antidepressants, especially if their first episode starts at this age and their presenting symptoms are lack of interest and cognitive dysfunction rather than depressed mood.

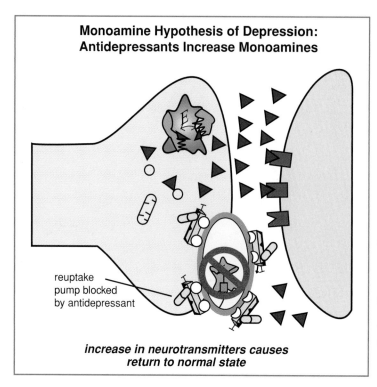

Monoamine Hypothesis of Depression: Antidepressants Increase Monoamines

reuptake pump blocked by antidepressant

increase in neurotransmitters causes return to normal state

FIGURE 2-12

Antidepressants increase monoamines. According to the monoamine hypothesis of depression, a deficiency in serotonin, norepinephrine, and/or dopamine leads to depression. Thus an increase in these neurotransmitters should cause a return to a normal state. In general, all antidepressants boost the synaptic action of one or more of the monoamines, in most cases by blocking presynaptic transporters. In this figure, an antidepressant is blocking the norepinephrine transporter (NET), thus increasing synaptic availability of norepinephrine and theoretically reducing symptoms of depression.

At the other end of the adult age range, those between the ages of 18 and 24 may benefit from antidepressant efficacy. However, there is now concern that the risk of antidepressants inducing suicidality may be greater in these young adults than in adults above age 25 (Figure 2-11). Thus there is possibly more risk in treating these patients with antidepressants. Finally, the younger the patient, the less evidence there is for antidepressant efficacy and the more evidence for the induction of suicidality. That is, children show the highest risk and least proven benefit from antidepressants, whereas adolescents rank intermediate in benefit and risk of suicidality between children and young adults (Figure 2-11). These findings are an important part of the consideration of whether, when, and how to treat a patient with antidepressants throughout the life cycle.

Antidepressant classes

Although the details of individual antidepressants' mechanisms of action are complex and are described in detail throughout the rest of this chapter, the general principle is actually quite simple: namely, all effective antidepressants boost the synaptic action of one or more of the three monoamines – dopamine, norepinephrine, and serotonin (Figure 2-12). This is often but not exclusively done by acutely blocking one or more of the presynaptic transporters for these monoamines, namely the dopamine transporter (DAT), the norepinephrine transporter (NET) (see Figure 1-31), and/or the serotonin transporter (SERT).

This pharmacological action at monoamine transporters is entirely consistent with the monoamine hypothesis of depression, which states that monoamines are somehow depleted (Figure 1-42) and, when boosted with effective antidepressants (Figure 2-12), relieve depression. One problem for the monoamine hypothesis, however, is that the action

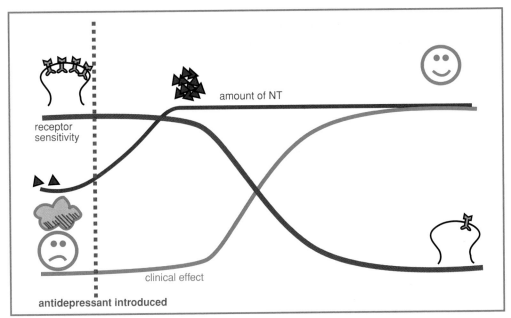

FIGURE 2-13 Time course of antidepressant effects. This figure depicts the different time courses for three effects of antidepressant drugs – namely, clinical changes, neurotransmitter (NT) changes, and receptor sensitivity changes. Specifically, the amount of NT changes relatively rapidly after an antidepressant is introduced. However, the clinical effect is delayed, as is the desensitization, or downregulation, of neurotransmitter receptors. This temporal correlation of clinical effects with changes in receptor sensitivity has given rise to the hypothesis that changes in neurotransmitter receptor sensitivity may actually mediate the clinical effects of antidepressant drugs. These clinical effects include not only antidepressant and anxiolytic actions but also the development of tolerance to the acute side effects of antidepressant drugs.

of antidepressants at monoamine transporters can raise monoamine levels quite rapidly in some brain areas, and certainly sooner than the antidepressant clinical effects occur in patients weeks later (Figure 2-13). How could immediate changes in neurotransmitter levels caused by antidepressants be linked to clinical actions seen much later in time? The answer may be that the acute increases in neurotransmitter levels cause adaptive changes in neurotransmitter **receptor sensitivity** in a delayed time course consistent with the onset of clinical antidepressant actions (Figure 2-13). Specifically, acutely enhanced synaptic levels of neurotransmitter (Figure 2-14A) could lead to adaptive downregulation and desensitization of postsynaptic neurotransmitter receptors over time (Figure 2-14B).

This concept of antidepressants causing changes in neurotransmitter receptor sensitivity is also consistent with the neurotransmitter receptor hypothesis of depression causing upregulation of neurotransmitter receptors in the first place (Figures 1-43). Thus antidepressants theoretically reverse this pathological upregulation of receptors over time (Figure 2-14B). Furthermore, the time course of receptor adaptation fits both with the onset of therapeutic effects and with the onset of tolerance to many side effects. Different receptors likely mediate these different actions, but both the onset of therapeutic action and the onset of tolerance to side effects may occur with the same delayed time course.

Adaptive changes in receptor number or sensitivity are likely the result of alterations in gene expression (Figure 2-15). This may include not only turning off the synthesis of neurotransmitter receptors but also increasing the synthesis of various neurotrophic factors

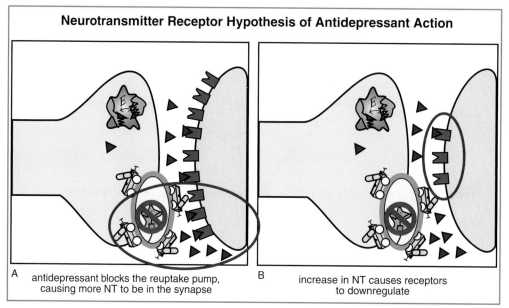

Neurotransmitter Receptor Hypothesis of Antidepressant Action

A antidepressant blocks the reuptake pump, causing more NT to be in the synapse

B increase in NT causes receptors to downregulate

FIGURE 2-14A and B Neurotransmitter receptor hypothesis of antidepressant action. Although antidepressants cause an immediate increase in monoamines, they do not have immediate therapeutic effects. This may be explained by the monoamine receptor hypothesis of depression, which states that depression is caused by upregulation of monoamine receptors; thus antidepressant efficacy would be related to downregulation of those receptors, as shown here. (**A**) When an antidepressant blocks a monoamine reuptake pump, this causes more neurotransmitter (NT) (in this case, norepinephrine) to accumulate in the synapse. (**B**) The increased availability of NT ultimately causes receptors to downregulate. The time course of receptor adaptation is consistent both with the delayed clinical effects of antidepressants and with development of tolerance to antidepressant side effects.

such as brain-derived neurotrophic factor (BDNF) (Figure 2-15). Such mechanisms may apply broadly to all effective antidepressants and may provide a final common pathway for the action of antidepressants.

Serotonin selective reuptake inhibitors (SSRIs)

Rarely has a class of drugs transformed a field as dramatically as the SSRIs have transformed clinical psychopharmacology (Table 2-1). Introduced in the late 1980s, most are now off patent, but not before becoming so widely prescribed within psychiatry, mental health, and primary care that up to six prescriptions per second, around the clock and around the year, are said to be written for these agents. Clinical indications for the use of SSRIs range far beyond major depressive disorder to premenstrual dysphoric disorder, many different anxiety disorders, eating disorders, and beyond. There are six principal agents in this group (Table 2-1). All six of these drugs share the common property of serotonin reuptake inhibition; thus they all belong to the same drug class, known as SSRIs (Figure 2-16). However, each of these six drugs also has unique pharmacological properties that allow it to be distinguished from the others. First, what these six drugs share in common is discussed, and then their distinctive individual properties are explored – properties that allow sophisticated prescribers to match specific drug profiles to individual patient symptom profiles.

TABLE 2-1 Serotonin selective reuptake inhibitors

fluoxetine (Prozac)
sertraline (Zoloft)
paroxetine (Paxil, Aropax, Seroxat)
fluvoxamine (Luvox, Faverin)
citalopram (Celexa, Cipramil)
escitalopram (Lexapro, Cipralex)

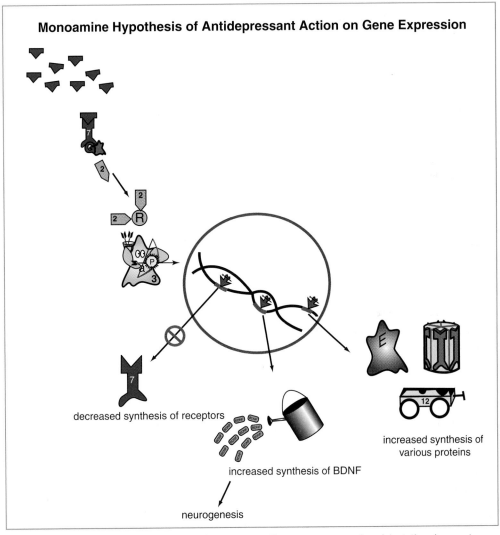

Monoamine Hypothesis of Antidepressant Action on Gene Expression

decreased synthesis of receptors

increased synthesis of BDNF

increased synthesis of various proteins

neurogenesis

FIGURE 2-15 Monoamine hypothesis of antidepressant action on gene expression. Adaptations in receptor number or sensitivity are likely due to alterations in gene expression, as shown here. The neurotransmitter at the top is presumably increased by an antidepressant. The cascading consequence of this is ultimately to change the expression of critical genes in order to effect an antidepressant response. This includes downregulating some genes so that there is decreased synthesis of receptors as well as upregulating other genes so that there is increased synthesis of critical proteins, such as brain-derived neurotrophic factor (BDNF).

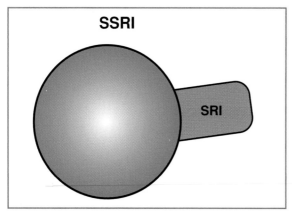

FIGURE 2-16 Serotonin selective reuptake inhibitors. Shown here is an icon depicting the core feature of serotonin selective reuptake inhibitors (SSRIs), namely serotonin reuptake inhibition. Although the six agents in this class have unique pharmacological profiles, they all share the common property of serotonin transporter (SERT) inhibition.

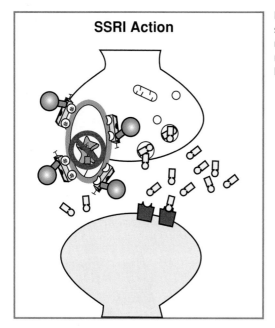

FIGURE 2-17 SSRI action. In this figure, the serotonin reuptake inhibitor (SRI) portion of the SSRI molecule is shown inserted into the serotonin reuptake pump (the serotonin transporter, or SERT), blocking it and causing an antidepressant effect.

What the six SSRIs have in common

These drugs include fluoxetine, sertraline, paroxetine, fluvoxamine, citalopram, and escitalopram (Table 2-1). All share a single major pharmacological feature: selective and potent inhibition of serotonin reuptake, also known as inhibition of the serotonin transporter, or SERT. This concept is shown in Figure 2-17.

Pharmacological and molecular mechanism of action of the SSRIs

Although the action of SSRIs at the **presynaptic axon terminal** has classically been emphasized (Figure 2-17), it now appears that events occurring at the **somatodendritic end** of the serotonin neuron (near the cell body) may be more important in explaining the therapeutic actions of the SSRIs (Figures 2-18 through 2-22). That is, in the depressed state, the monoamine hypothesis of depression states that serotonin may be deficient, both at

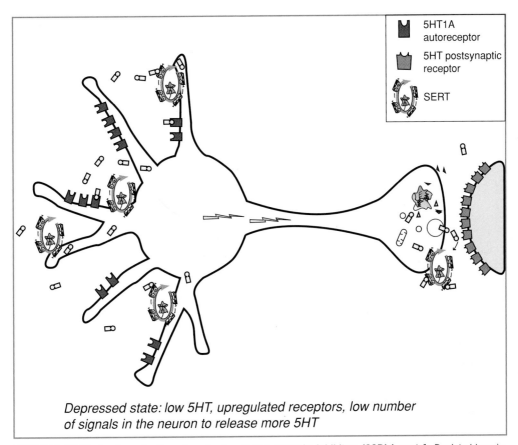

Depressed state: low 5HT, upregulated receptors, low number of signals in the neuron to release more 5HT

FIGURE 2-18 Mechanism of action of serotonin selective reuptake inhibitors (SSRIs), part 1. Depicted here is a serotonin (5HT) neuron in a depressed patient. In depression, the 5HT neuron is conceptualized as having a relative deficiency of the neurotransmitter 5HT. Also, the number of 5HT receptors is upregulated, including presynaptic 5HT1A autoreceptors as well as postsynaptic 5HT receptors.

presynaptic somatodendritic areas near the cell body (on the left in Figure 2-18) and in the synapse itself near the axon terminal (on the right in Figure 2-18). This is discussed in Chapter 1 and illustrated in Figure 1-42.

Furthermore, the neurotransmitter receptor hypothesis states that pre- and postsynaptic receptors may be upregulated; this is also discussed in Chapter 1 and illustrated in Figure 1-43. Both of these elements are shown for the serotonin neuron in Figure 2-18, which represents the depressed state before treatment. Neuronal firing rates for this neuron may also be dysregulated in depression, contributing to regional abnormalities in information processing and the development of specific symptoms, depending on the region affected, as discussed in Chapter 1 and shown in Figures 1-45 to 1-55.

When an SSRI is given acutely, it is well known that 5HT rises due to blockade of SERT. What is somewhat surprising, however, is that blocking the presynaptic SERT does *not* immediately lead to a great deal of serotonin in many synapses. In fact, when SSRI treatment is initiated, 5HT rises much more at the somatodendritic area located in the midbrain raphe (on the left in Figure 2-19), due to blockade of SERTs there, rather than in the areas of the brain where the axons terminate (on the right in Figure 2-19).

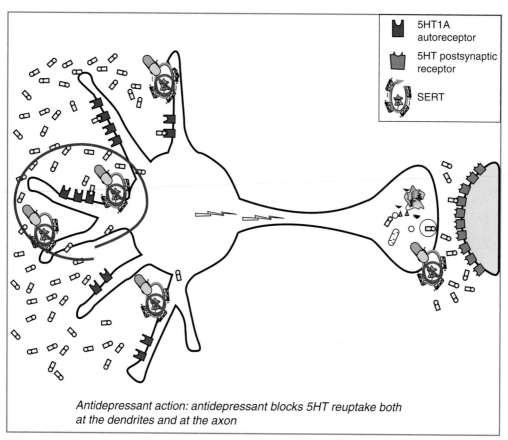

Antidepressant action: antidepressant blocks 5HT reuptake both at the dendrites and at the axon

FIGURE 2-19 Mechanism of action of serotonin selective reuptake inhibitors (SSRIs), part 2. When an SSRI is administered, it immediately blocks the serotonin reuptake pump [see icon of an SSRI drug capsule blocking the reuptake pump, or serotonin transporter (SERT)]. However, this causes serotonin to increase initially only in the somatodendritic area of the serotonin neuron (left) and not very much in the axon terminals (right).

The somatodendritic area of the serotonin neuron is therefore where 5HT increases first (on the left in Figure 2-19). Serotonin receptors in this brain area have 5HT1A pharmacology. When serotonin levels rise in the somatodendritic area, they stimulate nearby 5HT1A autoreceptors (also on the left in Figure 2-19). These immediate pharmacological actions obviously cannot explain the delayed therapeutic actions of the SSRIs. However, they may explain the side effects caused by the SSRIs when treatment is initiated.

Over time, the increased 5HT levels acting at the somatodendritic 5HT1A autoreceptors cause them to downregulate and become desensitized (on the left in Figure 2-20). This desensitization occurs because the increase in serotonin is recognized by these presynaptic 5HT1A receptors, and this information is sent to the cell nucleus of the serotonin neuron. The genome's reaction to this information is to issue instructions that cause these same receptors to become desensitized over time. The time course of this desensitization correlates with the onset of therapeutic actions of the SSRIs.

Once the 5HT1A somatodendritic autoreceptors are desensitized, 5HT can no longer effectively turn off its own release. Since 5HT is no longer inhibiting its own release, the serotonin neuron is therefore disinhibited (Figure 2-21). This results in a flurry of 5HT

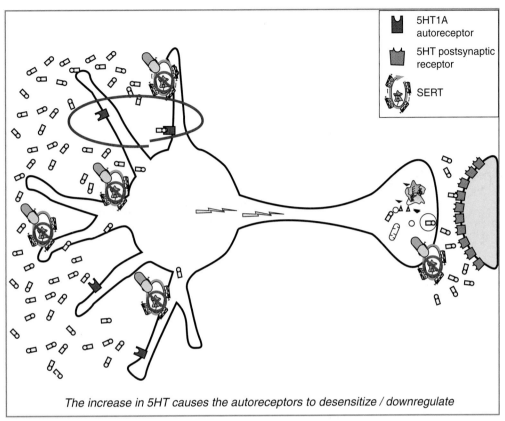

The increase in 5HT causes the autoreceptors to desensitize / downregulate

FIGURE 2-20 Mechanism of action of serotonin selective reuptake inhibitors (SSRIs), part 3. The consequence of serotonin increasing in the somatodendritic area of the serotonin (5HT) neuron, as depicted in Figure 2-19, is that the somatodendritic 5HT1A autoreceptors desensitize or downregulate (red circle).

release from axons and an increase in neuronal impulse flow (shown as lightning in Figure 2-21 and release of serotonin from the axon terminal on the right). This is just another way of saying that the serotonin release is "turned on" at the axon terminals. The serotonin that now pours out of the various projections of serotonin pathways in the brain is what theoretically mediates the various therapeutic actions of the SSRIs.

While the presynaptic somatodendritic 5HT1A autoreceptors are desensitizing (Figure 2-20), serotonin builds up in synapses (Figure 2-21) and causes the postsynaptic serotonin receptors to desensitize as well (on the right in Figure 2-22). This happens because the increase in synaptic serotonin is recognized by postsynaptic serotonin 2A, 2C, 3, and many other serotonin receptors there. These various postsynaptic serotonin receptors, in turn, send information to the cell nucleus of the **postsynaptic** neuron that serotonin is targeting (on the far right of Figure 2-22). The reaction of the genome in the postsynaptic neuron is also to issue instructions to downregulate or desensitize these receptors as well. The time course of this desensitization correlates with the onset of tolerance to the side effects of the SSRIs (Figure 2-22).

This theory suggests a pharmacological cascading mechanism whereby the SSRIs exert their therapeutic actions: namely, powerful but delayed disinhibition of serotonin release in key pathways throughout the brain. Furthermore, side effects are hypothetically caused

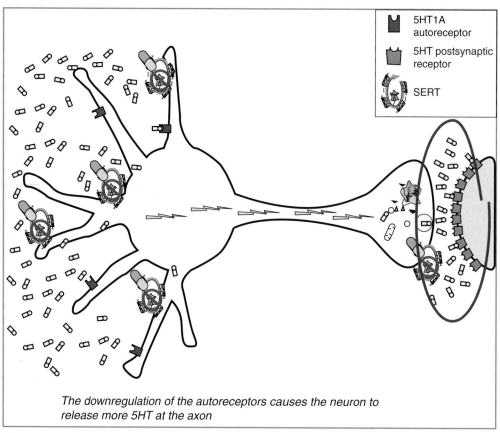

The downregulation of the autoreceptors causes the neuron to release more 5HT at the axon

FIGURE 2-21 Mechanism of action of serotonin selective reuptake inhibitors (SSRIs), part 4. Once the somatodendritic receptors downregulate, as depicted in Figure 2-21, there is no longer inhibition of impulse flow in the serotonin (5HT) neuron. Thus, neuronal impulse flow is turned on. The consequence of this is release of 5HT in the axon terminal (red circle). However, this increase is delayed as compared with the increase of 5HT in the somatodendritic areas of the 5HT neuron, depicted in Figure 2-20. This delay is the result of the time it takes for somatodendritic 5HT to downregulate the 5HT1A autoreceptors and turn on neuronal impulse flow in the 5HT neuron. This delay may explain why antidepressants do not relieve depression immediately. It is also the reason why the mechanism of action of antidepressants may be linked to increasing neuronal impulse flow in 5HT neurons, with 5HT levels increasing at axon terminals before an SSRI can exert its antidepressant effects.

by the acute actions of serotonin at undesirable receptors in undesirable pathways. Finally, side effects may attenuate over time by desensitization of the very receptors that mediate them.

There are potentially exciting corollaries to this hypothesis. First, if the ultimate increase in 5HT at critical synapses is required for therapeutic actions, then its failure to occur may explain why some patients respond to an SSRI and some do not. Also, if new drugs could be designed to increase 5HT at the right places at a faster rate or to a greater degree, it could result in a much needed rapid-acting antidepressant, an antidepressant with greater efficacy than an SSRI, or one that could be used to augment an SSRI. Such ideas are active research hypotheses at this time and are leading to many new approaches to modulating the serotonin system with new drugs, which are discussed in the final section of this chapter on future antidepressants.

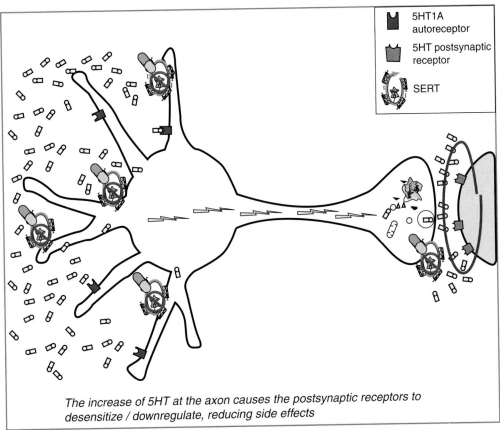

The increase of 5HT at the axon causes the postsynaptic receptors to desensitize / downregulate, reducing side effects

FIGURE 2-22 Mechanism of action of serotonin selective reuptake inhibitors (SSRIs), part 5. Finally, once the SSRIs have blocked the reuptake pump [or serotonin transporter (SERT) in Figure 2-19], increased somatodendritic serotonin (5HT) (Figure 2-19), desensitized somatodendritic 5HT1A autoreceptors (Figure 2-20), turned on neuronal impulse flow (Figure 2-21), and increased release of 5HT from axon terminals (Figure 2-21), the final step (shown here) may be the desensitization of postsynaptic 5HT receptors. This desensitization may mediate the reduction of side effects of SSRIs as tolerance develops.

Serotonin pathways and receptors that hypothetically mediate therapeutic actions and side effects of SSRIs

As mentioned above, the SSRIs cause both their therapeutic actions and their side effects by increasing serotonin at synapses where reuptake is blocked and serotonin release is disinhibited. In general, increasing serotonin in desirable pathways and at targeted receptor subtypes leads to the well-known therapeutic actions of these drugs. However, SSRIs increase serotonin in virtually every serotonin pathway and at virtually every serotonin receptor, and some of these actions are undesirable; these therefore account for the side effects. By understanding the functions of the various serotonin pathways and the distribution of the various serotonin receptor subtypes, it is possible to gain insight into both the therapeutic actions and the side effects that the SSRIs share as a class.

In terms of the potential therapeutic actions of boosting serotonin for the many symptoms of depression, Chapter 1 extensively discusses the various specific projections of serotonin neurons from the midbrain raphe as hypothetical regulators of various specific symptoms of depression (Figures 1-44 through 1-55).

Since serotonin does not influence all brain areas equally, it does not necessarily influence all the symptoms of depression equally. Furthermore, the therapeutic effects from boosting serotonin in the brain will not have the same clinical profile as the therapeutic effects that result from boosting other neurotransmitters, such as NE or DA, since there is not an identical overlap of all three monoamine inputs to all brain circuits. Specifically, a "serotonin deficiency syndrome" in major depression is linked to the concept of "increased negative affect" discussed in Chapter 1 and illustrated in Figure 1-55. SSRIs are often considered to have an excellent profile in such patients, who not only have depressed mood but also guilt, disgust, fear, anxiety, hostility, irritability, and loneliness (Figure 1-55).

On the other hand, because of the distribution of serotonin pathways in the brain, SSRIs often fail to target the other symptoms of major depression as robustly as they target the symptoms of increased negative affect. That is, SSRIs often fail to relieve symptoms of "reduced positive affect" or can even produce some of these symptoms as side effects, including loss of happiness, joy, interest, pleasure, energy, enthusiasm, alertness, and self-confidence (Figure 1-55). When symptoms of increased negative affect improve but symptoms of reduced positive affect persist or are induced by SSRI treatment, this can sometimes be called an "apathetic" recovery. For these latter symptoms to improve, it may require adding or switching to agents that act on NE and/or DA, as discussed below.

In terms of the potential side effects of SSRIs, acute stimulation of any of the plethora of serotonin receptor subtypes may be responsible for mediating these undesirable actions. This includes at least 5HT2A, 5HT2C, 5HT3, and 5HT4 postsynaptic receptors. Since many SSRI side effects are acute, starting from the first dose, and attenuate over time, it may be that a small but acute increase in synaptic serotonin is sufficient to mediate these side effects (Figure 2-19) but insufficient to mediate therapeutic effects until the much more robust disinhibition of the neuron "kicks in" once autoreceptors are downregulated (Figure 2-22). If the postsynaptic serotonin receptors that theoretically mediate side effects downregulate or desensitize, the side effects attenuate or go away (Figure 2-23). Presumably the signal of receptor occupancy of serotonin to the postsynaptic receptor is detected by the genome of the target neuron, and by changing the genetic expression of those receptors that mediate specific side effects, those side effects will go away.

The undesirable side effects of SSRIs seem not only to involve specific serotonin receptor subtypes but also the action of serotonin at these receptors in specific areas of the body, including brain, spinal cord, and gut. The topography of serotonin receptor subtypes in different serotonin pathways may thus help to explain how side effects are mediated. In fact, the same pathways that appear to mediate the delayed therapeutic effects of SSRIs may also mediate the acute side effects of SSRIs, acting at different receptors and in a different time course. Thus, acute stimulation of serotonin 2A and 2C receptors in the serotonin projection from raphe to amygdala and limbic cortex, such as ventromedial prefrontal cortex, may cause acute mental agitation, anxiety, or panic attacks, which can be observed with early dosing of an SSRI prior to anxiolytic actions kicking in (Figure 1-46). Acute stimulation of 5HT2A receptors in the basal ganglia may lead to acute changes in motor movements due to serotonin's inhibition of dopamine neurotransmission there. Thus, akathisia (restlessness), psychomotor retardation, or even mild parkinsonism and dystonic movements can result from acute SSRI administration. Stimulation of serotonin

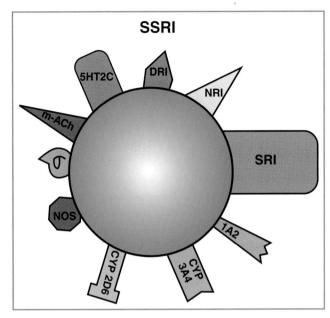

FIGURE 2-23 Secondary pharmacological properties of SSRIs. This icon depicts the various secondary pharmacological properties that may be associated with one or more of the six different serotonin selective reuptake inhibitors (SSRIs). These include not only serotonin reuptake inhibition (SRI) but also lesser degrees of actions at other neurotransmitters and enzymes, including norepinephrine reuptake inhibition (NRI), dopamine reuptake inhibition (DRI), serotonin 2C antagonist actions (5HT2C), muscarinic/cholinergic antagonist actions (M1), sigma 1 receptor actions (σ), inhibition of nitric oxide synthetase (NOS), and inhibition of CYP450 2D6, 3A4, and 1A2.

2A receptors in the brainstem sleep centers may contribute to the induction of rapid muscle movements, called myoclonus, during the night; it may also disrupt slow-wave sleep and cause nocturnal awakenings (Figure 1-48). Stimulation of serotonin 2A and 2C receptors in the spinal cord may inhibit the spinal reflexes of orgasm and ejaculation and cause sexual dysfunction. Stimulation of serotonin 2A receptors in mesocortical pleasure centers may reduce dopamine activity there and cause apathy or decreased libido (Figure 1-47). Thus, in a patient treated with an SSRI who has agitation, anxiety, sexual dysfunction, and apathy, it can be difficult to know whether this represents incomplete recovery from depression or drug-induced side effects! In either case, persistence of these symptoms will likely require adding or switching to a different pharmacological mechanism that boosts DA, NE, and/or GABA (gamma-aminobutyric acid). This strategy is discussed below, in the section on antidepressants in clinical practice.

Stimulation of serotonin 3 receptors in the hypothalamus or brainstem may cause nausea or vomiting after SSRI administration (Figure 1-52). Stimulation of serotonin 3 and/or serotonin 4 receptors in the GI tract may cause increased bowel motility, GI cramps, and diarrhea. Tolerance to these side effects usually develops rapidly.

Thus, virtually all side effects of the SSRIs can be understood as undesirable actions of serotonin in undesirable pathways at undesirable receptor subtypes. This appears to be the "cost of doing business," as it is not possible for a systemically administered SSRI to act only at the desirable receptors in the desirable places; it must act everywhere it is distributed, which means all over the brain and all over the body. Fortunately SSRI side effects are more of a nuisance than a danger, and they generally attenuate over time, although they can cause an important subset of patients to discontinue an SSRI prematurely due to intolerance or to lack of remission of all symptoms of depression.

The not-so-selective serotonin reuptake inhibitors: six unique drugs
or one class of six drugs?

Although the SSRIs clearly share the same mechanism of action, therapeutic profiles, and side effect profiles, individual patients often react very differently to one SSRI versus another. This is not generally observed in large clinical trials, where group differences between two SSRIs either in efficacy or side effects are very difficult to document. Rather, such differences are seen by prescribers treating patients one at a time, with some patients experiencing a therapeutic response to one SSRI and not another and other patients tolerating one SSRI and not another.

If blockade of SERT explains the shared clinical and pharmacological actions of SSRIs, what explains their differences? Although there is no generally accepted explanation that accounts for the commonly observed clinical phenomena of different efficacy and tolerability of various SSRIs in individual patients, it makes sense to consider those unique pharmacological characteristics of the six SSRIs that are not shared among them as candidates to explain the broad range of individual patient reactions to different SSRIs (Figure 2-23 and Table 2-1). Each SSRI has secondary pharmacological actions other than SERT blockade, and no two SSRIs have identical secondary pharmacological characteristics. These are depicted in Figure 2-23 for the class of SSRIs and include actions such as norepinephrine reuptake blockade, dopamine reuptake blockade, serotonin 2C antagonism, muscarinic cholinergic antagonism, sigma 1 receptor actions, inhibition of the enzyme nitric oxide synthetase, and inhibition of the various cytochrome P450 enzymes 1A2, 2D6, and 3A4. Whether these secondary binding profiles can account for the differences in efficacy and tolerability in individual patients remains to be proven. However, it does lead to provocative hypothesis generation and gives a rational basis for physicians not to be denied access to one or another of the SSRIs by payors claiming that "they are all the same." Sometimes only an empirical trial of different SSRIs will lead to the best match of drug to an individual patient.

Fluoxetine: an SSRI with 5HT2C antagonist and thus norepinephrine and dopamine
disinhibiting (NDDI) properties

This SSRI has 5HT2C antagonist actions, which may explain many of its unique clinical properties (Figure 2-24). This is a novel concept for antidepressant action (Table 2-2) and is now a recognized property of several known antidepressants (discussed in the sections on various antidepressants below) and atypical antipsychotics and is an important action of some novel antidepressants still in testing (discussed below in the section on future antidepressants).

Serotonin action at 5HT2C receptors normally *inhibits* both NE and DA release, as discussed in Chapter 1 and as illustrated in Figures 1-40 through 1-42. Drugs that *block* 5HT2C receptors have the opposite action and thus *disinhibit* both NE and DA release (Figure 2-25). Therefore fluoxetine, as a 5HT2C antagonist, is not only an SSRI but also a norepinephrine and dopamine disinhibitor, or NDDI. NDDI actions may lead to increases in DA and NE release in prefrontal cortex (Figure 2-25) and contribute to therapeutic actions in major depression.

The good news about this action is that it is generally activating and may be why many patients, even from the first dose, detect an energizing and fatigue-reducing effect of fluoxetine, with improvement in concentration and attention as well. This mechanism is perhaps best matched to depressed patients with reduced positive affect, hypersomnia, psychomotor retardation, apathy, and fatigue but perhaps least well matched to patients

TABLE 2-2 Putative antidepressant mechanisms

SSRI	Serotonin selective reuptake inhibitor
SNRI	Serotonin norepinephrine reuptake inhibitor
NDRI	Norepinephrine dopamine reuptake inhibitor
selective NRI	Selective norepinephrine reuptake inhibitor
A2A	Alpha 2 antagonist
SARI	Serotonin antagonist/reuptake inhibitor
MAOI	Monoamine oxidase inhibitor
TCA	Tricyclic antidepressant
5HT2C antagonist*	Serotonin 2C antagonist
SNDI*	Serotonin norepinephrine disinhibitor
NDDI*	Norepinephrine dopamine disinhibitor
TMM*	Trimonoamine modulator

*New concepts/mechanisms

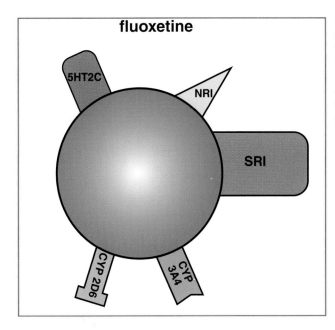

FIGURE 2-24 Icon of fluoxetine. In addition to serotonin reuptake inhibition, fluoxetine has norepinephrine reuptake inhibition (NRI), CYP450 2D6 and 3A4 inhibition, and serotonin 2C antagonist actions (5HT2C). Fluoxetine's activating effects may be due to its actions at serotonin 2C receptors. Norepinephrine reuptake inhibition may be clinically relevant only at very high doses.

with agitation, insomnia, and anxiety who may experience unwanted activation and even a panic attack if given an agent that further activates them.

5HT2C antagonism may also contribute to the anorexia and antibulimia therapeutic actions approved only for this SSRI and only at high doses. Finally, 5HT2C antagonism may explain fluoxetine's ability to boost the antidepressant actions of olanzapine in bipolar depression. Olanzapine also has 5HT2C antagonist actions. Adding together the 5HT2C antagonist actions of both drugs could theoretically lead to enhanced DA and NE release in cortex to mediate antidepressant actions in bipolar depression, since the combination of both drugs is approved for the treatment of bipolar depression, whereas neither of the individual drugs is approved as monotherapy for this indication.

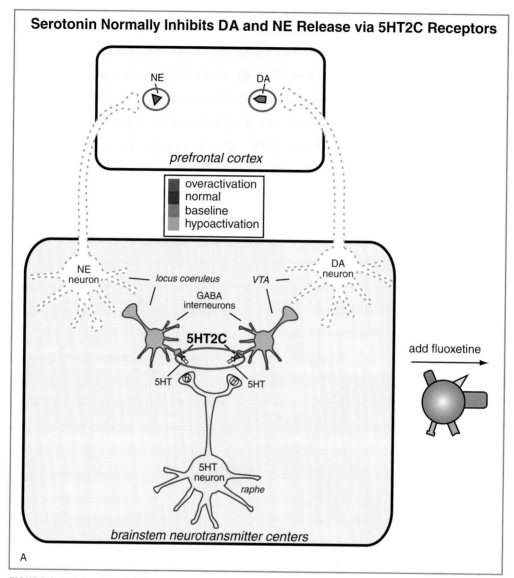

Serotonin Normally Inhibits DA and NE Release via 5HT2C Receptors

FIGURE 2-25A Serotonin inhibits norepinephrine and dopamine release. In addition to its direct pharmacological effects, fluoxetine can also indirectly increase norepinephrine and dopamine release via blockade of 5HT2C receptors. Normally, serotonin binding at 5HT2C receptors on gamma-aminobutyric acid (GABA) interneurons (bottom red circle) inhibits norepinephrine and dopamine release in the prefrontal cortex (top red circle).

Other unique properties of fluoxetine (Figure 2-24) are weak NE reuptake blocking properties, which may become clinically relevant at very high doses, and inhibition of CYP 2D6 and 3A4 by the parent compound and its active metabolite. Also, fluoxetine has a very long half-life (two to three days); its active metabolite has an even longer half-life (two weeks). This long half-life is advantageous in that it seems to reduce the withdrawal reactions characteristic of sudden discontinuation of some SSRIs, but it also means that it takes a long time to clear the drug and its active metabolite after discontinuing fluoxetine and prior to starting other agents, such as an MAO inhibitor. Fluoxetine is available not

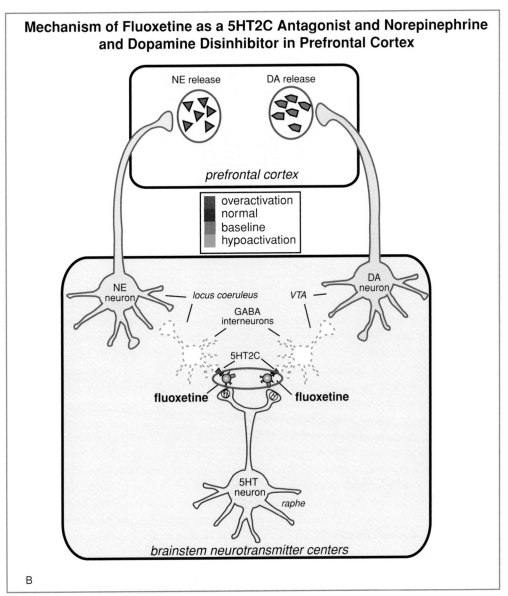

Mechanism of Fluoxetine as a 5HT2C Antagonist and Norepinephrine and Dopamine Disinhibitor in Prefrontal Cortex

NE release

DA release

prefrontal cortex

- overactivation
- normal
- baseline
- hypoactivation

NE neuron

locus coeruleus

VTA

GABA interneurons

5HT2C

fluoxetine　　　　**fluoxetine**

DA neuron

5HT neuron

raphe

brainstem neurotransmitter centers

B

FIGURE 2-25B Fluoxetine disinhibits norepinephrine and dopamine release. When fluoxetine binds to 5HT2C receptors on gamma-aminobutyric acid (GABA) interneurons (bottom red circle), it prevents serotonin from binding there and thus prevents inhibition of norepinephrine and dopamine release in the prefrontal cortex; in other words, it disinhibits their release (top red circle).

only as a once-daily formulation but also as a once-weekly oral dosage formulation; however, the weekly formulation has never become popular.

Sertraline: an SSRI with dopamine transporter (DAT) inhibition

This SSRI has two candidate mechanisms that distinguish it: dopamine transporter (DAT) inhibition and sigma 1 receptor binding (Figure 2-26). It may also have some weak CYP 2D6 inhibitory properties at high doses. The DAT inhibitory actions are controversial since they are weaker than the SERT inhibitory actions, thus leading some experts to suggest that

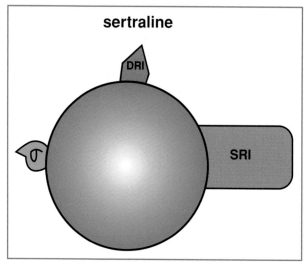

FIGURE 2-26 Icon of sertraline.
Sertraline has dopamine reuptake inhibition (DRI) and sigma 1 receptor binding in addition to serotonin reuptake inhibition (SRI). The clinical relevance of sertraline's DRI is unknown, although it may improve energy, motivation, and concentration. Its sigma properties may contribute to anxiolytic actions and may also be helpful in patients with psychotic depression.

there is not sufficient DAT occupancy by sertraline to be clinically relevant. However, as discussed later in the section on norepinephrine and dopamine reuptake inhibitors (NDRIs), it is not clear that high degrees of DAT occupancy are necessary or even desirable in order to contribute to antidepressant actions. That is, perhaps only a small amount of DAT inhibition is sufficient to cause improvement in energy, motivation, and concentration, especially when added to another action such as SERT inhibition. In fact, high-impact DAT inhibition is the property of reinforcing stimulants, including cocaine and methylphenidate, and would not generally be desired in an antidepressant.

Anecdotally, clinicians have observed the mild and desirable activating actions of sertraline in some patients with "atypical depression," improving symptoms of hypersomnia, low energy, and mood reactivity. A favorite combination of some clinicians for depressed patients is to add bupropion to sertraline (i.e., Wellbutrin to Zoloft, sometimes called "Welloft"), adding together the weak DAT inhibitory properties of each agent. Clinicians have also observed the overactivation of some patients with panic disorder by sertraline, thus requiring slower dose titration in some patients with anxiety symptoms. All of these actions of sertraline are consistent with the weak DAT inhibitory actions of sertraline contributing to its clinical portfolio of actions. Combination of the NDRI bupropion with SSRIs is discussed below in the section on NDRIs.

The sigma 1 actions of sertraline are not well understood but might contribute to its anxiolytic effects and especially to its effects in psychotic and delusional depression, where sertraline may have advantageous therapeutic effects compared to some other SSRIs. Sigma 1 actions could theoretically contribute both to anxiolytic actions and to antipsychotic actions as will be discussed further in the section on fluvoxamine below.

Paroxetine: an SSRI with muscarinic anticholinergic and norepinephrine transporter (NET) inhibitory actions

This SSRI is preferred by many clinicians for patients with anxiety symptoms. It tends to be more calming, even sedating, early in treatment compared to the more activating actions of both fluoxetine and sertraline discussed above. Perhaps the mild anticholinergic actions of paroxetine contribute to this clinical profile (Figure 2-27). Paroxetine also has weak NET inhibitory properties, which could contribute to efficacy in depression, especially at high

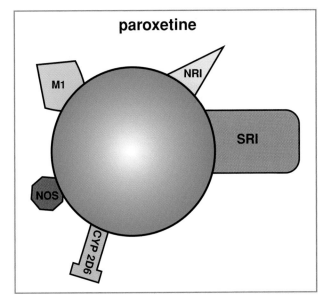

FIGURE 2-27 Icon of paroxetine. In addition to serotonin reuptake inhibition (SRI), paroxetine has mild anticholinergic actions (M1), which can be calming or possibly sedating, weak norepinephrine reuptake inhibition (NRI), which may contribute to further antidepressant actions, and inhibition of the enzyme nitric oxide synthetase (NOS), which may contribute to sexual dysfunction. Paroxetine is also a potent inhibitor of CYP450 2D6.

doses. The advantages of dual serotonin plus norepinephrine reuptake–inhibiting properties, or SNRI actions, are discussed below in the section on SNRIs. The possibility that weak to moderate NET inhibition may nevertheless contribute importantly to antidepressant actions is discussed below not only in the section on SNRIs but also in the section on NDRIs.

Paroxetine is a potent 2D6 inhibitor and also may inhibit the enzyme nitric oxide synthetase, which could theoretically contribute to sexual dysfunction, especially in men. Paroxetine is also notorious for causing withdrawal reactions upon sudden discontinuation, with symptoms such as akathisia, restlessness, gastrointestinal upset, dizziness, and tingling, especially when suddenly discontinued from long-term high-dose treatment. This is possibly due not only to SERT inhibition properties, since all SSRIs can cause discontinuation reactions, but with additional contributions from anticholinergic rebound when paroxetine is rapidly discontinued. Furthermore, paroxetine is both a substrate and an inhibitor for CYP 2D6, which leads to a very rapid decline in plasma drug levels when paroxetine is discontinued, possibly contributing to withdrawal symptoms. Paroxetine is available in a controlled-release formulation, which may mitigate some of its side effects, including discontinuation reactions, but this form of the drug is not widely used in clinical practice.

Fluvoxamine: an SSRI with sigma 1 receptor binding properties

This SSRI was among the first to be launched for the treatment of depression worldwide but was never officially approved for depression in the United States, where it has been considered more of an agent for the treatment of obsessive compulsive disorder and anxiety. A secondary binding property of fluvoxamine, like sertraline, is its interaction at sigma 1 sites, but this action is more potent for fluvoxamine than for sertraline (Figure 2-28). The physiological function of sigma 1 sites is still a mystery, sometimes called the "sigma enigma," but has been linked both to anxiety and psychosis. Although it is not entirely clear how to define an agonist or antagonist at sigma 1 sites, recent studies suggest that fluvoxamine may be an agonist at sigma 1 receptors and that this property may contribute

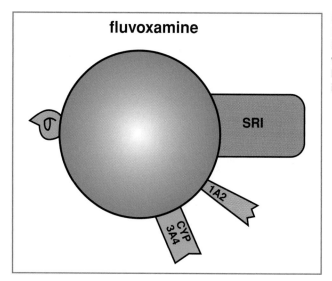

fluvoxamine

FIGURE 2-28 Icon of fluvoxamine.
Fluvoxamine's secondary properties include actions at sigma 1 receptors, which may be anxiolytic as well as beneficial for psychotic depression, and inhibition of CYP450 1A2 and 3A4.

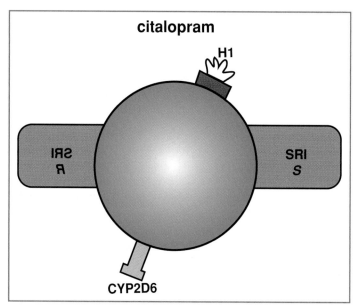

citalopram

FIGURE 2-29 Icon of citalopram. Citalopram consists of two enantiomers, R and S. The R enantiomer has weak antihistamine properties and is a weak inhibitor of CYP450 2D6.

an additional pharmacological action to help explain fluvoxamine's well-known anxiolytic properties. Fluvoxamine has also shown therapeutic activity in both psychotic and delusional depression, where it, like sertraline, may have advantages over other SSRIs.

Fluvoxamine is now available as a controlled-release formulation, which makes once-a-day administration possible, unlike immediate-release fluvoxamine, whose shorter half-life often requires twice-daily administration. In addition, recent trials of controlled-release fluvoxamine show impressive remission rates in both obsessive compulsive disorder and social anxiety disorder as well as possibly less peak-dose sedation.

Citalopram: an SSRI with a "good" and a "bad" enantiomer

This SSRI (Figure 2-29) comprises two enantiomers, R and S, one of which is the mirror image of the other (Figure 2-30). The mixture of these enantiomers is known as racemic

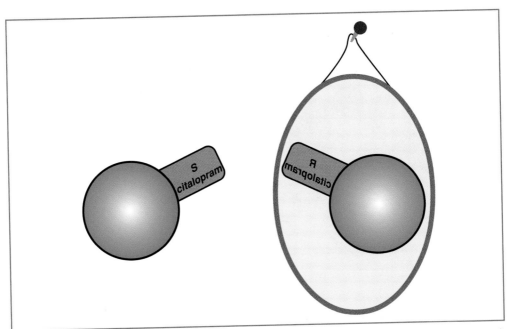

FIGURE 2-30 R and S enantiomers of citalopram. The R and S enantiomers of citalopram are mirror images of each other but have slightly different clinical properties. The R enantiomer is the one with weak antihistamine properties and weak inhibition of CYP450 2D6, while the S enantiomer does not have these properties. The R and S enantiomers may also differ in their effects at the serotonin transporter, as shown in Figure 2-31.

citalopram, or commonly just as citalopram, and has mild antihistamine properties and mild inhibition of CYP450 2D6, with both of these properties residing in the R enantiomer (Figure 2-29). Racemic citalopram is generally one of the better tolerated SSRIs and has favorable findings in the treatment of depression in the elderly. However, it has a somewhat inconsistent therapeutic action at the lowest dose, often requiring dose increases to optimize treatment. This may be due to a recent finding suggesting that the R enantiomer may be pharmacologically active at SERT in a manner that does not inhibit SERT but actually interferes with the ability of the active S enantiomer to inhibit SERT. This could lead to reduced inhibition of SERT, reduced synaptic 5HT, and possibly reduced net therapeutic actions, especially at low doses (Figure 2-31).

Escitalopram: the quintessential SSRI

The solution to improving the properties of racemic citalopram (which is still a very safe and effective SSRI) is to remove the unwanted R enantiomer. The resulting drug is known as escitalopram, as it is made up of only the pure active S enantiomer (Figure 2-32). This maneuver appears to remove the antihistaminic and CYP450 2D6 inhibitory properties (compare Figures 2-29 and 2-32). In addition, removal of the potentially interfering R isomer makes the lowest dose of escitalopram more predictably efficacious (Figure 2-31). Escitalopram is therefore the SSRI for which pure SERT inhibition is most likely to explain almost all of its pharmacological actions. Escitalopram is considered perhaps the best-tolerated SSRI, with the fewest CYP450-mediated drug interactions, although it is still an expensive agent in many countries, since it is not yet available as a generic.

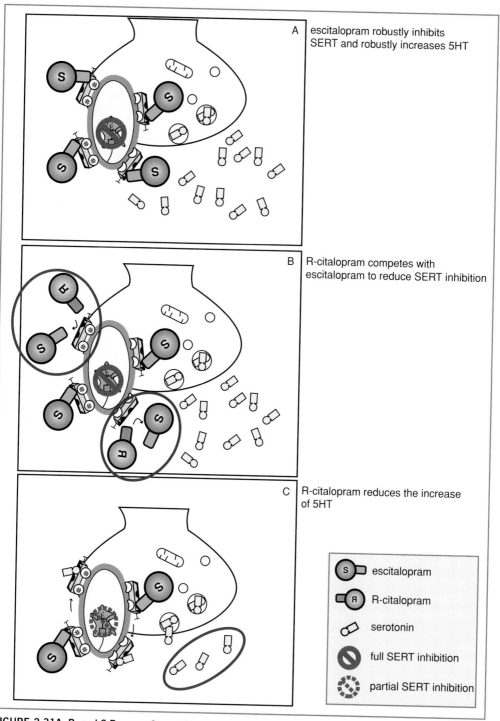

A | escitalopram robustly inhibits SERT and robustly increases 5HT

B | R-citalopram competes with escitalopram to reduce SERT inhibition

C | R-citalopram reduces the increase of 5HT

- ⬤S⬛ escitalopram
- ⬛Я⬤ R-citalopram
- serotonin
- 🚫 full SERT inhibition
- partial SERT inhibition

FIGURE 2-31A, B, and C R versus S enantiomer at the serotonin transporter. (A) The S enantiomer of citalopram (escitalopram) robustly inhibits the serotonin transporter (SERT) and robustly increases serotonin (5HT) **(A)**. The R enantiomer of citalopram (R-citalopram) binds to SERT but does not inhibit it **(B)**. Thus it competes with escitalopram to reduce SERT inhibition **(B)**, which reduces the ability of the S enantiomer to increase 5HT **(C)**.

TABLE 2-3 Serotonin norepinephrine reuptake inhibitors

venlafaxine XR (Effexor XR; Efexor XR)
desvenlafaxine XR (Pristiq)
duloxetine (Cymbalta, Xeristar)
milnacipran (Ixel, Toledomin)

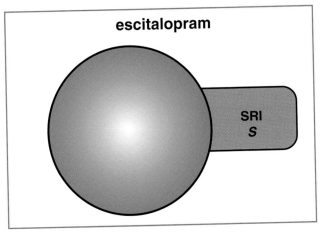

FIGURE 2-32 Icon of escitalopram.
The S enantiomer of citalopram has been developed and marketed as the antidepressant escitalopram. This agent is the most selective of the serotonin selective reuptake inhibitors (SSRIs).

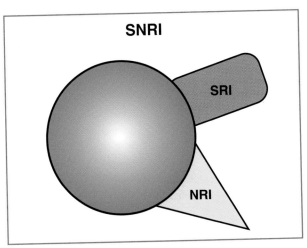

FIGURE 2-33 Icon of a serotonin norepinephrine reuptake inhibitor (SNRI).
Dual reuptake inhibitors of serotonin and norepinephrine by definition combine the actions of both a serotonin reuptake inhibitor (SRI) and a norepinephrine reuptake inhibitor (NRI).

Serotonin norepinephrine reuptake inhibitors (SNRIs)

Antidepressants that block the reuptake of both serotonin and norepinephrine – known as SNRIs – have rapidly become among the most frequently prescribed classes of antidepressants, particularly in mental health practices (Table 2-3). These agents combine the robust SERT inhibition of the SSRIs with various degrees of inhibition of the norepinephrine transporter (or NET) (Figure 2-33). This has led to this highly debated question: Are two mechanisms better than one (Figure 2-34)?

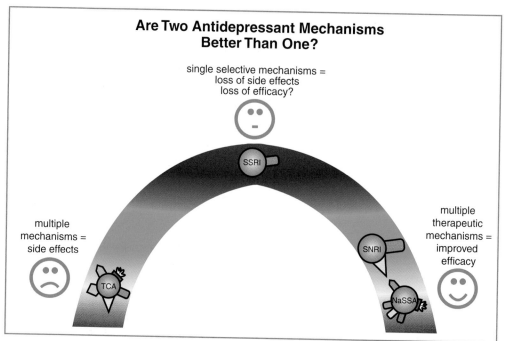

FIGURE 2-34 Are two antidepressant mechanisms better than one? Originally, multiple pharmacological mechanisms were synonymous with "dirty drugs," because they implied unwanted side effects. This is shown as tricyclic antidepressants on the left, with serotonin and norepinephrine reuptake inhibition but also anticholinergic, antihistaminic, and antiadrenergic actions. The trend to develop selective drugs (center) led to the removal of unwanted side effects and to the inclusion of only a single therapeutic action. More recently, the trend has again been to add multiple therapeutic actions together so as to improve tolerability and enhance efficacy. Enhanced efficacy from synergistic pharmacological mechanisms may increase response in some patients, especially those resistant to single-mechanism agents.

Are two antidepressant mechanisms better than one?

The original tricyclic antidepressants (TCAs) had multiple pharmacological mechanisms and were termed "dirty drugs" because many of these mechanisms were undesirable, as they caused side effects (Figure 2-34). The idea was then to "clean up" these agents by making them selective; thus, the SSRI era was born. Indeed, the development of such selective agents made them devoid of pharmacological properties mediating the *side effects* of the first generation tricyclic antidepressants, such as anticholinergic, antihistaminic, and anti-adrenergic side effects (tricyclic antidepressants are discussed below). However, selectivity may be less desired when that means loss of multiple *therapeutic* mechanisms (Figure 2-34). In practice, many difficult, severe, or treatment-resistant cases require multiple therapeutic mechanisms before an adequate therapeutic effect is attained, and serotonergic action alone is frequently not enough for such patients.

Thus psychotropic drug development is trending back to incorporating multiple pharmacological mechanisms in the hope that this will exploit potential synergies among two or more independent therapeutic mechanisms. For antidepressants, this has led to the development of drugs that exhibit "intramolecular polypharmacy," such as the dual action of the SNRIs discussed here (Figure 2-35). It has also led to the increasing use of two antidepressants together for treatment-resistant cases, combining two or more synergistic therapeutic mechanisms, as discussed below in the section on antidepressants in clinical practice.

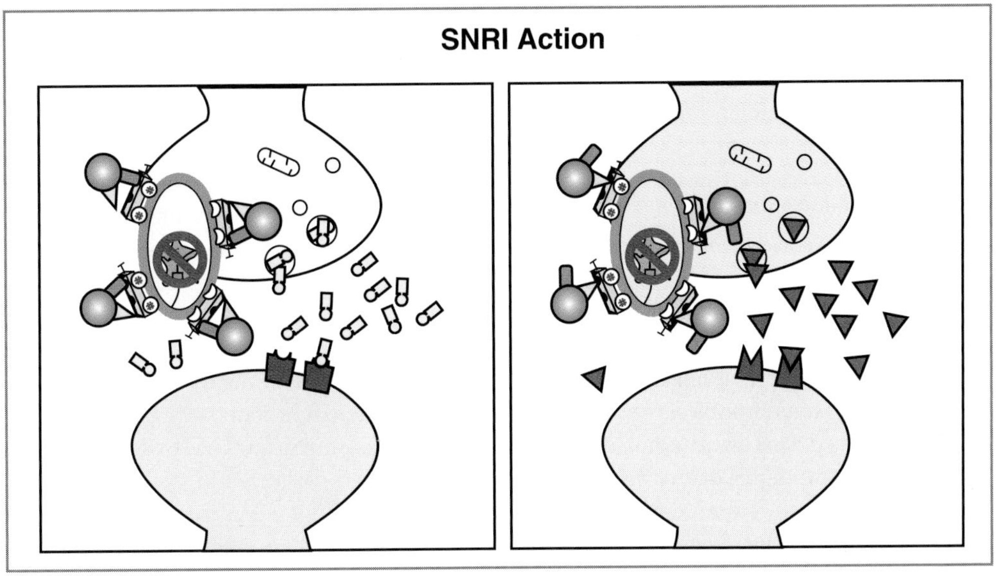

SNRI Action

FIGURE 2-35 SNRI actions. In this figure, the dual actions of the serotonin norepinephrine reuptake inhibitors (SNRIs) are shown. Both the serotonin reuptake inhibitor (SRI) portion of the SNRI molecule (left panel) and the norepinephrine reuptake inhibitor (NRI) portion of the SNRI molecule (right panel) are inserted into their respective reuptake pumps. Consequently, both pumps are blocked, and the drug mediates an antidepressant effect.

Of course there is "no free lunch," meaning that adding more mechanisms almost always means adding more mechanism-related side effects. Nevertheless, the hallmark of the current era of antidepressant treatment is to aim for sustained remission of all symptoms, and it frequently takes more than one mechanism to get this degree of therapeutic efficacy. In fact, the field is now moving to the use of as many mechanisms as necessary to gain remission, whether that means utilizing one drug with several different mechanisms or utilizing several drugs, each with a different mechanism.

Clinicians and experts currently debate whether remission rates are higher with SNRIs compared to SSRIs or whether SNRIs are more helpful in patients who fail to respond to SSRIs than are other options. The data may lean in favor of higher remission rates for SNRIs compared to SSRIs, but that is not really the point. The important thing to keep in mind is the need to attain remission in any patient, and to do this in any way that works. SSRI treatment frequently results in remission. When it does not, certainly a dual-action SNRI could be considered. However, when treatment with any antidepressant does not result in remission, the point is to do something else, generally substituting or adding an additional pharmacological mechanism until remission is achieved. This is discussed in detail in the section below on antidepressants in clinical practice.

Theoretically, there should be some therapeutic advantage of adding NET inhibition to SERT inhibition, since one mechanism may add efficacy to the other by widening the reach of the trimonoamine neurotransmitter system throughout more brain regions (Figures 1-46 through 1-55). A practical indication that dual monoamine mechanisms may lead to more efficacy is the finding that the SNRI venlafaxine frequently seems to have greater efficacy as the dose increases, theoretically due to the recruitment of more and more NET inhibition as the dose is raised (i.e., the noradrenergic "boost").

NET inhibition increases DA in prefrontal cortex

Although SNRIs are commonly called "dual action" serotonin-norepinephrine agents, they actually have a third action on dopamine in the prefrontal cortex but not elsewhere in the brain. Thus they are not "full" triple-action agents, since they do not inhibit the dopamine transporter (DAT); but SNRIs can perhaps be considered to have "two and a half actions" (Figure 2-36) and not just two (Figure 2-35). That is, SNRIs boost not only serotonin and norepinephrine throughout the brain (Figure 2-35) but also dopamine specifically in prefrontal cortex (Figure 2-36). This third mechanism of boosting dopamine in an important area of the brain associated with several symptoms of depression should add another theoretical advantage to the pharmacology of SNRIs and to their efficacy in the treatment of major depression.

How does NET inhibition boost DA in prefrontal cortex? The answer is illustrated in Figure 2-36. In prefrontal cortex, SERTs and NETs are present in abundance on serotonin and norepinephrine nerve terminals, respectively, but there are very few DATs on dopamine nerve terminals in this part of the brain (Figure 2-36). The consequence of this is that once DA is released, it is free to cruise away from the synapse (Figure 2-36A). The diffusion radius of DA is thus wider (Figure 2-36A) than that of NE in prefrontal cortex (Figure 2-36B), since there is NET at the NE synapse (Figure 2-36B) but no DAT at the DA synapse (Figure 2-36A). This arrangement may enhance the regulatory importance of dopamine in prefrontal cortex functioning, since DA in this part of the brain can interact with DA receptors not only at its own synapse but also at a distance, perhaps enhancing the ability of DA to regulate cognition in an entire area within its diffusion radius, not just at a single synapse.

Dopamine action is therefore not terminated by DAT in prefrontal cortex but by two other mechanisms. That is, DA diffuses away from the DA synapse until it either encounters the enzyme COMT (catechol-O-methyl transferase), which degrades it, or it encounters a norepinephrine reuptake pump or NET that transports it into the NE neuron (Figure 2-36A). NETs, in fact, have a greater affinity for DA than they do for NE, so they will pump DA as well as NE into NE nerve terminals, halting the action of either.

It is interesting what happens when NET is inhibited in prefrontal cortex. As expected, NET inhibition enhances synaptic NE levels and increases the diffusion radius of NE (Figure 2-36B). Somewhat surprising may be the fact that NET inhibition also enhances DA levels and increases DA's diffusion radius (Figure 2-36C). The bottom line is that NET inhibition increases both NE and DA in prefrontal cortex. Thus, SNRIs have "two and a half" mechanisms: boosting serotonin throughout the brain, boosting norepinephrine throughout the brain, and boosting dopamine in prefrontal cortex (but not in other DA projection areas).

Serotonergic, noradrenergic, and dopaminergic pathways and receptors as mediators of therapeutic actions and side effects of SNRIs

The role of serotonin receptors and pathways in the therapeutic actions and side effects of SSRIs is discussed above, and this discussion applies to the serotonergic aspect of SNRI actions as well. In addition, SNRIs have additional considerations due to their NET inhibitory actions. For a full understanding of the mechanism of therapeutic actions and side effects of SNRIs, we must therefore add a discussion of the role of norepinephrine pathways and receptors and, in prefrontal cortex, the role of dopamine pathways and receptors.

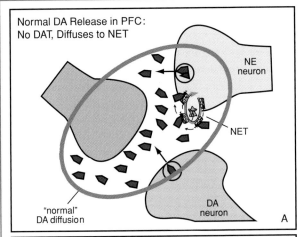

Normal DA Release in PFC:
No DAT, Diffuses to NET

NE
neuron

NET

"normal"
DA diffusion

DA
neuron

A

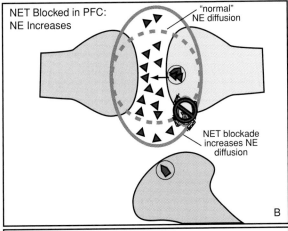

NET Blocked in PFC:
NE Increases

"normal"
NE diffusion

NET blockade
increases NE
diffusion

B

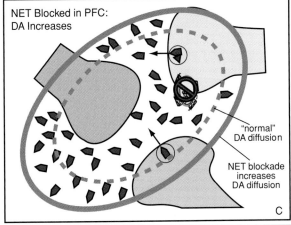

NET Blocked in PFC:
DA Increases

"normal"
DA diffusion

NET blockade
increases
DA diffusion

C

FIGURE 2-36A, B, and C
Norepinephrine transporter blockade
and dopamine in the prefrontal cortex.
(**A**) Although there are abundant
serotonin transporters (SERTs) and
norepinephrine transporters (NETs) in
the prefrontal cortex, there are very few
dopamine transporters (DATs). This
means that dopamine can diffuse away
from the synapse and therefore exert its
actions within a larger radius.
Dopamine's actions are terminated at
norepinephrine axon terminals, because
DA is taken up by NET. (**B**) NET
blockade in the prefrontal cortex leads to
an increase in synaptic norepinephrine,
thus increasing norepinephrine's
diffusion radius. (**C**) Because NET takes
up dopamine as well as norepinephrine,
NET blockade also leads to an increase
in synaptic dopamine, further increasing
its diffusion radius. Thus, agents that
block NET increase norepinephrine
throughout the brain and both
norepinephrine and dopamine in the
prefrontal cortex.

That is, increasing norepinephrine and/or dopamine at desirable synapses and desirable noradrenergic or dopaminergic receptors would theoretically lead to the therapeutic properties of SNRIs. However, increasing norepinephrine or dopamine at undesirable places would theoretically lead to side effects as the "cost of doing business" owing to NET inhibition, thus increasing norepinephrine in virtually every noradrenergic pathway and at virtually every noradrenergic receptor. As has been discussed, NET inhibition also increases DA in some dopamine pathways and at some dopamine receptors in prefrontal cortex. By understanding the functions of the various norepinephrine and prefrontal dopamine pathways and the distribution of the various noradrenergic and dopamine receptor subtypes, it is possible to gain insight into both the therapeutic actions and side effects that can be attributed to the NET inhibitory actions of SNRIs.

In terms of therapeutic actions of NET inhibition, Chapter 1 extensively discusses the various specific projections of noradrenergic neurons from the midbrain locus coeruleus and of dopamine neurons from midbrain dopamine centers as hypothetical regulators of various specific symptoms of depression (Figures 1-44 through 1-55).

Since norepinephrine does not influence all brain areas equally, it does not necessarily influence all the symptoms of depression equally. Furthermore, the therapeutic effects from boosting norepinephrine or dopamine in the brain will not have the same clinical profile as the therapeutic effects that result from boosting other neurotransmitters such as 5HT, since there is not an identical overlap of all three monoamine inputs to all brain circuits. Specifically, a "norepinephrine deficiency syndrome" in major depression is linked to the concept of "reduced positive affect" (Figure 1-55), although this concept may fit even better with the idea of a "dopamine deficiency syndrome" (discussed below in the section on NDRIs and MAO inhibitors). Norepinephrine, in fact, may be linked across the affective spectrum, including both "reduced positive affect" as well as "increased negative affect," and it certainly has a wider theoretical clinical spectrum than serotonin (see Figure 1-55). This may be the reason why a larger portfolio of symptoms is relieved by SNRIs than by SSRIs in some patients. Add to this the regional boosting of DA in prefrontal cortex, and there is a broad set of pharmacological targets within the trimonoaminergic neurotransmitter system that are linked to the therapeutic mechanism of action of SNRIs.

Nevertheless, like SSRIs, SNRIs not infrequently fail to relieve all symptoms of reduced positive affect or may even produce some of these symptoms as side effects, including loss of happiness, joy, interest, pleasure, energy, enthusiasm, alertness, and self-confidence (Figure 1-55). It has already been mentioned that when symptoms of increased negative affect improve but symptoms of reduced positive affect persist or are induced by either SSRI or SNRI treatment, this can sometimes be called an "apathetic" recovery. For such symptoms to improve, it may be necessary to raise the dose of the SNRI or to add or switch to agents that act more robustly on DA, particularly in brain regions outside of the prefrontal cortex, as discussed below.

In terms of potential side effects of NET inhibition by SNRIs, these can hypothetically be linked to acute stimulation of several clinically important noradrenergic receptor subtypes in various parts of the brain and body: alpha 1, alpha 2, and/or beta 1 adrenergic receptors. The undesirable side effects linked to NET inhibition seem to involve not only specific norepinephrine receptor subtypes but also the action of NE at receptors in specific areas of the body, including the brain, spinal cord, peripheral autonomic nervous system, heart, and bladder. The topography of NE receptor subtypes in different NE pathways and peripheral tissues may thus help to explain how side effects are mediated.

Thus, acute stimulation of beta 1 and/or beta 2 receptors in the cerebellum or peripheral sympathetic nervous system may cause motor activation or tremor (Figure 1-51). Acute stimulation of noradrenergic receptors in the amygdala or limbic cortex, such as ventromedial prefrontal cortex, may cause agitation (Figure 1-46). Acute stimulation of noradrenergic receptors in the brainstem cardiovascular centers and descending into the spinal cord may alter blood pressure. This can be a particularly troubling side effect in some patients taking SNRIs, especially at high doses. Stimulation of beta 1 receptors in the heart may cause changes in heart rate.

Stimulation of noradrenergic receptors in the sympathetic nervous system may also cause a net reduction of parasympathetic cholinergic tone, since these systems often have reciprocal roles in peripheral organs and tissues. Thus increased norepinephrine activity at alpha 1 receptors may produce symptoms reminiscent of "anticholinergic" side effects. This is not due to direct blockade of muscarinic cholinergic receptors but to indirect reduction of net parasympathetic tone due to increased sympathetic tone. Thus, a "pseudo-anticholinergic" syndrome of dry mouth, constipation, and urinary retention may be caused by high degrees of NET inhibition, even though SNRIs have no direct actions on muscarinic cholinergic receptors. Usually, however, the indirect reduction of cholinergic tone yields milder symptoms than does direct blockade of muscarinic cholinergic receptors.

Thus, virtually all side effects of the selective NET inhibition can be understood as undesirable actions of norepinephrine in undesirable pathways at undesirable receptor subtypes. Just as for the SSRIs, this occurs because it is not possible for a systemically administered drug to act only at the desirable receptors in the desirable places; it must act everywhere it is distributed, which means all over the brain and all over the body. Fortunately, side effects from NET inhibition are more of a nuisance than a danger and they generally attenuate over time, although they can cause an important subset of patients to discontinue treatment.

Venlafaxine

Venlafaxine is the first SNRI marketed in the United States (Figure 2-37 and Table 2-3). It has now become generally the most frequently prescribed individual antidepressant by most mental health professionals and by many primary care physicians in many countries. Depending on the dose, venlafaxine has different degrees of inhibition of 5HT reuptake (most potent and present even at low doses) versus NE reuptake (moderate potency and present at higher doses) (Figure 2-37). However, there are no significant actions on other receptors.

Venlafaxine has pioneered the concept that multiple pharmacological mechanisms in a single agent may be linked to greater efficacy than single pharmacological mechanisms, either in terms of enhanced remission rates, more robust sustained remission over long-term treatment, or greater efficacy for treatment-resistant depression. Recent long-term recurrence prevention studies with venlafaxine show very low recurrence rates not only over the first year but surprisingly over the second year of maintenance treatment. It is not clear whether these recurrence rates are lower than for single mechanism SSRIs, but they do appear to be lower than those reported in the STAR-D study with a variety of antidepressants (Figure 2-10). However, the study populations in these different studies may not be comparable. Although this concept of greater efficacy with multiple mechanisms is widely embraced as a strategy for achieving and maintaining remission in depression, it

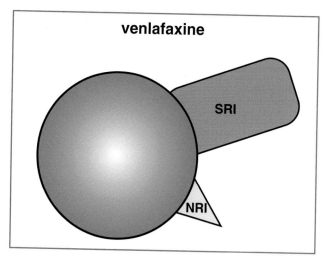

venlafaxine

FIGURE 2-37 Icon of venlafaxine.
Venlafaxine inhibits reuptake of both
serotonin (SRI) and norepinephrine
(NRI), thus combining two therapeutic
mechanisms in one agent. Venlafaxine's
serotonergic actions are present at low
doses, while its noradrenergic actions
are progressively enhanced as dose
increases.

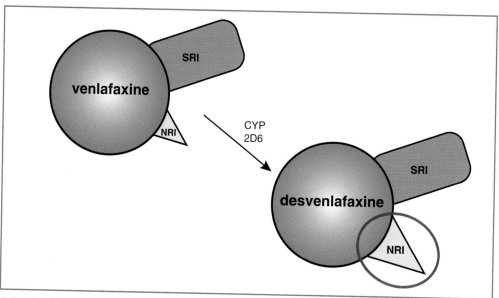

FIGURE 2-38 Venlafaxine conversion to desvenlafaxine. Venlafaxine is converted to its active metabolite
desvenlafaxine by CYP450 2D6. Like venlafaxine, desvenlafaxine inhibits reuptake of serotonin (SRI) and
norepinephrine (NRI), but its NRI actions are greater relative to its SRI actions compared to venlafaxine.
Venlafaxine administration usually results in plasma levels of venlafaxine that are about half those of
desvenlafaxine; however, this can vary depending on genetic polymorphisms of CYP450 2D6 and if patients are
taking drugs that are inhibitors or inducers of CYP450 2D6. Thus the degree of NET inhibition with venlafaxine
administration may be unpredictable.

remains controversial whether the specific mixing of SERT and NET inhibition by venlafaxine itself is consistently and robustly more efficacious than SERT inhibition by SSRIs
alone for the treatment of depression.

Venlafaxine is a substrate for CYP450 2D6, which converts it to the active metabolite desvenlafaxine (Figure 2-38). Desvenlafaxine has greater NET inhibition relative
to SERT inhibition compared to venlafaxine (Figures 2-37 to 2-39). After venlafaxine

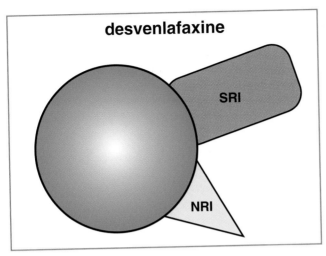

desvenlafaxine

SRI

NRI

FIGURE 2-39 Icon of desvenlafaxine.
Desvenlafaxine, the active metabolite of venlafaxine, has now been developed as a separate drug. It has relatively greater norepinephrine reuptake inhibition (NRI) than venlafaxine but is still more potent at the serotonin transporter.

administration, the plasma levels of venlafaxine are normally about half of those for desvenlafaxine. However, this is highly variable, depending on whether the patient is taking another drug that is a CYP450 2D6 inhibitor, which shifts the plasma levels toward more venlafaxine and less desvenlafaxine, also reducing the relative amount of NET inhibition. Variability in plasma levels of venlafaxine versus desvenlafaxine is also due to genetic polymorphisms for CYP450 2D6, such that poor metabolizers will shift the ratio of these two drugs toward more parent venlafaxine and away from the active metabolite desvenlafaxine and thus reduce the relative amount of NET inhibition. As a result of these considerations, how much NET inhibition a given dose of venlafaxine will have in a given patient at a given time can be somewhat unpredictable. Expert clinicians have learned to solve this problem with skilled dose titration, but the recent development of desvenlafaxine as a separate drug may also solve this problem with less need for dose titration and more consistent NET inhibition at a given dose across all patients.

Venlafaxine is available as an extended-release formulation (venlafaxine XR), which not only allows for once daily administration but also significantly reduces side effects, especially nausea. In contrast to several other psychotropic drugs available in controlled-release formulations, venlafaxine XR is a considerable improvement over the immediate-release formulation, which has fallen into little or no use because of unacceptable nausea and other side effects associated with the immediate-release formulation, especially when started or stopped. However, venlafaxine even in controlled-release formulation can cause withdrawal reactions, sometimes quite bothersome, especially after sudden discontinuation from high-dose long-term treatment. Nevertheless, the controlled-release formulation is highly preferred because of enhanced tolerability.

Venlafaxine is also approved and widely used for several anxiety disorders.

Desvenlafaxine

This is the active metabolite of venlafaxine (Figure 2-38); it has relatively greater NET inhibition than venlafaxine but still has less potent actions on NET than on SERT (Figure 2-39). It is not a substrate of CYP450 enzymes, including 2D6, so its plasma drug concentrations are not influenced by 2D6 inhibitors or by genetic polymorphisms in 2D6, as

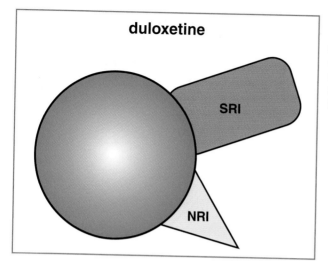

FIGURE 2-40 Icon of duloxetine. Duloxetine inhibits reuptake of both serotonin (SRI) and norepinephrine (NRI). Its noradrenergic actions may contribute to efficacy for painful physical symptoms. Duloxetine is also an inhibitor of CYP450 2D6.

those of venlafaxine are. The bottom line is that the plasma levels of desvenlafaxine should be more consistent than those of venlafaxine and that the relative amount of NET versus SERT should generally be more consistent and greater at comparable doses.

Whether this will lead to any advantages in the treatment of depression remains to be seen, although it might prove to be easier to dose and be more predictable than venlafaxine. What is perhaps more interesting is that owing to its relatively more robust and predictable NET inhibition, desvenlafaxine has been tested in two novel indications: vasomotor symptoms and fibromyalgia, both theoretically thought to require robust NET inhibition as well as SERT inhibition. Many perimenopausal women develop hot flushes and other vasomotor symptoms, including night sweats, insomnia, and even depression, but do not wish to take estrogen replacement therapy. Desvenlafaxine appears to have robust efficacy in reducing vasomotor symptoms in such women and provides an alternative to estrogen replacement therapy. Other considerations, such as the treatment of perimenopausal women who have both vasomotor symptoms and either depression or risk of depression are discussed later in this chapter in the section on trimonoamine modulators and estrogen.

Desvenlafaxine, like the other SNRIs milnacipran and duloxetine, is also being tested with promising results for the treatment of fibromyalgia.

Duloxetine

This is an SNRI (Figure 2-40 and Table 2-3) that not only is indicated for the treatment of depression and for anxiety disorders but is also the first SNRI approved as a treatment for painful neuropathy associated with diabetes. It is worth noting that duloxetine has established efficacy not only in depression and chronic pain but also in patients with chronic painful physical symptoms of depression. These symptoms are frequently ignored or missed by patients and clinicians alike. Until recently, the link of these symptoms to major depression was not well appreciated, in part because painful physical symptoms are not included in the list of symptoms for the formal diagnostic criteria for depression. Nevertheless, it is now widely appreciated that painful physical symptoms are frequently associated with a major depressive episode and are also among the leading residual symptoms after treatment

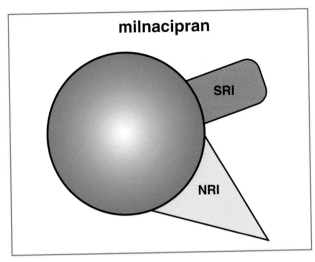

FIGURE 2-41 Icon of milnacipran.
Milnacipran inhibits reuptake of both serotonin (SRI) and norepinephrine (NRI) but is a more potent inhibitor of the norepinephrine transporter (NET) than the serotonin transporter (SERT). Its robust NET inhibition may contribute to efficacy for painful physical symptoms.

with an antidepressant (Figure 2-9). It appears that the dual SNRI actions of duloxetine and other SNRIs may be superior to the selective serotonergic actions of SSRIs for treating conditions such as the neuropathic pain of diabetes and chronic painful physical symptoms associated with depression. Duloxetine also appears to be effective in the treatment of fibromyalgia.

Duloxetine has shown efficacy in the treatment of the cognitive symptoms of depression prominent in geriatric depression, possibly exploiting the NET inhibition of the SNRI mechanism in the prefrontal cortex (see Figure 2-36).

Duloxetine can supposedly be given once a day, but this is usually a good idea only after the patient has had a chance to become tolerant to it after initiating it at twice-daily dosing, especially during titration to the higher doses often used in psychiatry and in the treatment of painful conditions. Duloxetine may need to be given in some difficult-to-treat patients at doses higher than the normal prescribing range; in this case, twice-daily dosing may be preferred. Duloxetine may be associated with a lower incidence of hypertension and milder withdrawal reactions than venlafaxine. Duloxetine is a CYP450 2D6 inhibitor, which may cause some drug interactions (see section on antidepressant pharmacokinetics, below).

Milnacipran

Milnacipran is the first SNRI marketed in Japan and many European countries such as France, where it is currently marketed as an antidepressant. As of this writing, milnacipran is not yet marketed in the United States (Table 2-3).

Milnacipran is a somewhat atypical SNRI in that it is a more potent NET than SERT inhibitor (Figure 2-41) whereas the others are more potent SERT than NET inhibitors (Figures 2-37 to 2-40). This unique pharmacological profile may explain milnacipran's somewhat different clinical profile compared to other SNRIs. Since noradrenergic actions may be equally or more important for the treatment of pain-related conditions compared to serotonergic actions, the robust NET inhibition of milnacipran suggests that it may be particularly useful in conditions ranging from the painful physical symptoms associated with depression to chronic neuropathic pain to fibromyalgia. Among these conditions, milnacipran is probably best studied in fibromyalgia, where it shows positive evidence of efficacy and is in the late stages of testing in the United States and other countries.

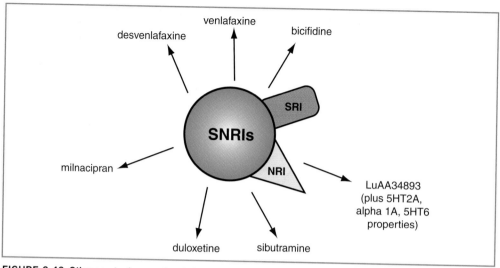

FIGURE 2-42 Other serotonin norepinephrine reuptake inhibitors (SNRIs). SNRIs in addition to venlafaxine, desvenlafaxine, duloxetine, and milnacipran include sibutramine, which is marketed as an appetite suppressant; bicifidine, which is in testing for painful conditions and depression; and LuAA34893, which, in addition to SNRI actions, is an antagonist at serotonin 2A, alpha 1A, and serotonin 6 receptors.

Milnacipran's potent NET inhibition also suggests a potentially favorable pharmacological profile for the treatment of cognitive symptoms, including cognitive symptoms of depression as well as those frequently associated with fibromyalgia, sometimes called "fibrofog."

Other clinical observations possibly linked to milnacipran's robust NET inhibition are that it can be more energizing and activating than other SNRIs while perhaps also causing more sweating and urinary hesitancy. For patients with urinary hesitancy, generally due theoretically to robust pro-noradrenergic actions at bladder alpha 1 receptors, an alpha 1 antagonist can be helpful. Milnacipran must generally be given twice daily due to its relatively short half-life.

Other SNRIs (Figure 2-42)

Sibutramine is marketed as an appetite suppressant but also has SNRI pharmacological properties, yet it is not approved for the treatment of depression. Bicifidine is an agent in clinical testing for back pain, other painful conditions, and depression. LuAA34893 is an early-stage compound with "SNRI plus" properties, namely SNRI actions plus 5HT2A, alpha 1A, and 5HT6 antagonist actions.

Norepinephrine and dopamine reuptake inhibitors (NDRIs)

Bupropion is the prototypical agent of this group (Figure 2-43 and Table 2-2). For many years, the mechanism of action of bupropion has been unclear, and it still remains somewhat controversial. Bupropion itself has only weak reuptake blocking properties for dopamine (DAT inhibition) and for norepinephrine (NET inhibition) (Figure 2-44). No other specific or potent pharmacologic actions have been consistently identified for this agent. Bupropion's actions both as an antidepressant and upon norepinephrine and dopamine neurotransmission, however, have always appeared to be more powerful than these weak properties could

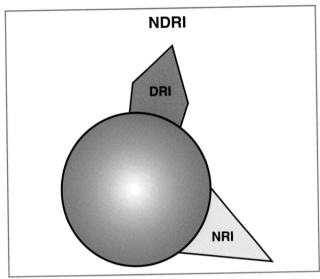

NDRI

DRI

NRI

FIGURE 2-43 Icon of a norepinephrine and dopamine reuptake inhibitor (NDRI). Another class of antidepressant consists of norepinephrine and dopamine reuptake inhibitors (NDRIs), for which the prototypical agent is bupropion. Bupropion has weak reuptake blocking properties for dopamine (DRI) and norepinephrine (NRI) but is an efficacious antidepressant, which may be explained in part by the more potent inhibitory properties of its metabolites.

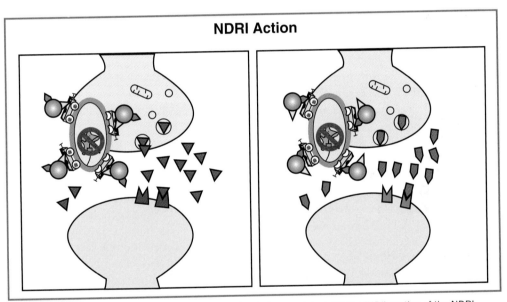

NDRI Action

FIGURE 2-44 NDRI actions. In this figure the norepinephrine reuptake inhibitor (NRI) portion of the NDRI molecule (left panel) and the dopamine reuptake inhibitor (DRI) portion of the NDRI molecule (right panel) are inserted into their respective reuptake pumps. Consequently both pumps are blocked, and the drug mediates an antidepressant effect.

explain, leading to the proposal that bupropion acts rather vaguely as an adrenergic modulator of some type.

More recently, it has been found that bupropion is metabolized to a number of active metabolites, some of which are not only more potent NET inhibitors than bupropion itself (and equally potent DAT inhibitors) but are also concentrated in the brain. In some ways, therefore, bupropion is both an active drug and a precursor for other active drugs (i.e., a

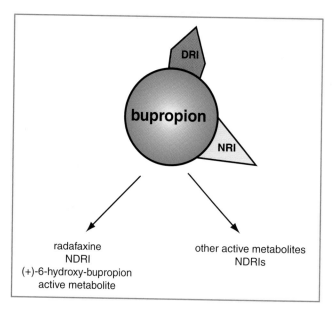

FIGURE 2-45 **Bupropion conversion to its metabolites.** Bupropion is converted to multiple active metabolites, the most potent of which is (+)-6-hydroxy-bupropion, also called radafaxine.

radafaxine
NDRI
(+)-6-hydroxy-bupropion
active metabolite

other active metabolites
NDRIs

prodrug for multiple active metabolites) (Figure 2-45). The most potent of these is the + enantiomer of the 6-hydroxy metabolite of bupropion, also known as radafaxine (Figure 2-45). Radafaxine is also a weak NDRI (Figure 2-44).

Can the net effects of bupropion on NET (Figure 2-46A and 2-46B) and DAT (Figure 2-46C) account for its clinical actions in depressed patients at therapeutic doses? If one believes that 90% transporter occupancy of DAT and NET are required for antidepressant actions, the answer would be no. Human positron emission tomography (PET) scans suggest that as little as 10% to 15% and perhaps no more than 20% to 30% of striatal DATs may be occupied at therapeutic doses of bupropion. NET occupancy would be expected to be in this same range. Is this enough to explain bupropion's antidepressant actions?

Whereas it is clear from many research studies that SSRIs must be dosed to occupy a substantial fraction of SERT, perhaps up to 80% or 90% of these transporters in order to be effective antidepressants, this is far less clear for NET or DAT occupancy, particularly in the case of drugs with an additional pharmacological mechanism that may be synergistic with NET or DAT inhibition. That is, when most SNRIs are given in doses that occupy 80% to 90% of SERT, substantially fewer NETs are occupied, yet there is evidence of both additional therapeutic actions and NE-mediated side effects of these agents with perhaps as little as 50% NET occupancy.

Furthermore, there appears to be such a thing as "too much DAT occupancy." That is, when 50% or more of DATs are occupied rapidly and briefly, this can lead to unwanted clinical actions, such as euphoria and reinforcement. In fact, a rapid, short-lasting, high degree of DAT occupancy is the pharmacological characteristic of abusable stimulants such as cocaine. When 50% or more of DATs are occupied more slowly and in a more lasting manner, especially with controlled-release formulations, stimulants are less abusable and more useful for attention deficit hyperactivity disorder (ADHD). The issue to be considered here is whether a low level of slow-onset and long-lasting DAT occupancy is

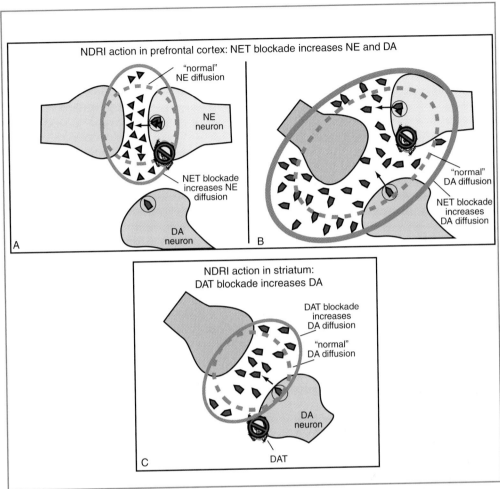

FIGURE 2-46A, B and C NDRI actions in prefrontal cortex and striatum. Norepinephrine and dopamine reuptake inhibitors (NDRIs) block the transporters for both norepinephrine (NET) and dopamine (DAT). (**A**) NET blockade in the prefrontal cortex leads to an increase in synaptic norepinephrine, thus increasing norepinephrine's diffusion radius. (**B**) Because the prefrontal cortex lacks DATs, and NETs transport dopamine as well as norepinephrine, NET blockade also leads to an increase in synaptic dopamine as well as NE in the prefrontal cortex, further increasing DA's diffusion radius. Thus, despite the absence of DAT in the prefrontal cortex, NDRIs still increase dopamine in the prefrontal cortex. (**C**) DAT is present in the striatum, and thus DAT inhibition increases dopamine diffusion there.

the "goldilocks" solution for this mechanism to be useful as an antidepressant: thus, not "too hot" and therefore abusable; not "too cold" and therefore ineffective; but "just right" – namely an antidepressant? This issue is also mentioned below in the section on future antidepressants in relation to the new triple reuptake inhibitors in clinical development, which are currently determining the optimal amount of DAT inhibition to add to SERT and NET inhibition.

The fact that bupropion is not known to be particularly abusable, is not a scheduled substance, yet is proven effective for treating nicotine addiction is consistent with the possibility that it is occupying DATs in the striatum and nucleus accumbens in a manner

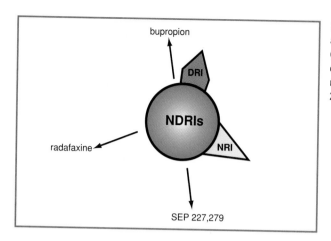

FIGURE 2-47 Other norepinephrine and dopamine reuptake inhibitors (NDRIs). There are at least two NDRIs in clinical testing: radafaxine (the active metabolite of bupropion) and SEP 227,279.

sufficient to mitigate craving but not sufficient to cause abuse (Figure 2-46C). Perhaps this is also how bupropion works in depression, combined with an equal action on NETs (Figure 2-46A and 2-46B). Clinical observations of depressed patients are also consistent with DAT and NET inhibition as bupropion's mechanism of action (Figure 2-46A, B, and C), since this agent appears especially useful in targeting the symptoms of "reduced positive affect" within the affective spectrum (see Figure 1-55), including improvement in the symptoms of loss of happiness, joy, interest, pleasure, energy, enthusiasm, alertness, and self-confidence.

Bupropion was originally marketed only in the United States as an immediate-release dosage formulation for thrice-daily administration as an antidepressant. Development of a twice-daily formulation (bupropion SR) and more recently a once-daily formulation (bupropion XL) has not only reduced the frequency of seizures at peak plasma drug levels, which are reduced with these formulations, but also increased convenience and enhanced compliance. Thus, the use of immediate-release bupropion has been all but abandoned in favor of once- or twice-daily administration.

Bupropion is generally activating or even stimulating. Interestingly, bupropion does not appear to cause the bothersome sexual dysfunction that frequently occurs with antidepressants acting by SERT inhibition, probably because bupropion lacks a significant serotonergic component to its mechanism of action. Thus, bupropion has proven to be a useful antidepressant not only for patients who cannot tolerate the serotonergic side effects of SSRIs but also for those whose depression does not respond to serotonergic boosting by SSRIs. As discussed above, given its pharmacological profile, bupropion is especially targeted at the symptoms of the "dopamine-deficiency syndrome" and "reduced positive affect" (Figure 1-55). Almost every active clinician knows that patients who have residual symptoms of reduced positive affect following treatment with an SSRI or an SNRI or who develop these symptoms as a side effect of an SSRI or SNRI frequently benefit from switching to bupropion or from augmenting their SSRI or SNRI treatment with bupropion. The combination of bupropion with an SSRI or an SNRI has a theoretical rationale as a strategy for covering the entire symptom portfolio from symptoms of reduced positive affect to symptoms of increased negative affect (Figure 1-55).

Other NDRIs

At least two other NDRIs have entered clinical testing, including not only the active metabolite of bupropion, radafaxine, but also SEP 227,279 (Figure 2-47).

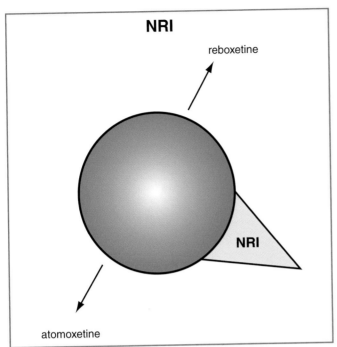

FIGURE 2-48 Icon of a selective norepinephrine reuptake inhibitor. Reboxetine and atomoxetine are two antidepressants that have selective actions at the norepinephrine reuptake inhibitor (NRI).

Selective norepinephrine reuptake inhibitors (NRIs)

Although some tricyclic antidepressants (e.g., desipramine, maprotilene) block norepinephrine reuptake more potently than serotonin reuptake, even these tricyclics are not really selective, since they still block many other receptors such as alpha 1, histamine 1, and muscarinic cholinergic receptors, as all tricyclics do. Tricyclic antidepressants are discussed later in this chapter.

The first truly selective noradrenergic reuptake inhibitor marketed in Europe and other countries is reboxetine; the first in the United States is atomoxetine (Figure 2-48 and Table 2-2). Both of these compounds are selective NRIs (Figure 2-49) and lack the additional undesirable binding properties of tricyclic antidepressants. Reboxetine is approved as an antidepressant in Europe but not in the United States. Extensive testing in the United States suggested inconsistent efficacy in major depression with the possibility of less effectiveness than the SSRIs, so reboxetine was dropped from further development as an antidepressant. Atomoxetine was never developed as an antidepressant but is marketed for the treatment of attention deficit hyperactivity disorder in the United States and other countries.

Many of the important concepts about NET inhibition have already been covered in the section on SNRIs above. This includes the observations that NET inhibition raises not only NE diffusely throughout all NE neuronal projections but also DA levels in the prefrontal cortex (Figure 2-36). It also includes both the therapeutic and side effect profile of NET inhibition. There is some question about whether NET inhibition by itself has any different clinical profile than when NET inhibition occurs simultaneously with SERT inhibition, as when administering an SNRI or giving a selective NRI with an SSRI. One thing that may be different is that NET inhibitors that are selective tend to be dosed so that there is a greater proportion of NET occupancy, close to saturation, compared to NET

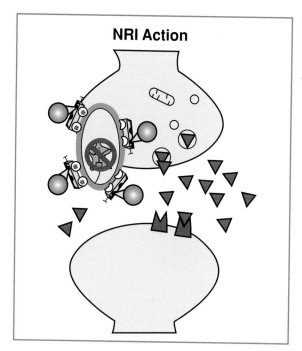

NRI Action

FIGURE 2-49 NRI actions. In this figure, the norepinephrine reuptake inhibitor (NRI) is inserted into the norepinephrine reuptake pump, thus blocking it and mediating the drug's effects.

occupancy when dosed as an SNRI or as an NDRI, which, as mentioned above, may occupy substantially fewer NETs at clinically effective antidepressant doses. This higher degree of NET occupancy of selective NET inhibitors may be necessary for optimal efficacy for either depression or ADHD if there is no simultaneous SERT or DAT inhibition with which to add or synergize. One of the interesting observations is that high degrees of selective NET inhibition, although often activating, can also be sedating in some patients. Perhaps this is due to "over-tuning" noradrenergic input to cortical pyramidal neurons.

There is less documentation that NET inhibition is as helpful for anxiety disorders as SERT inhibition, and neither of the selective NRIs shown here (Figure 2-48) is approved for anxiety disorders, although atomoxetine is approved for adult ADHD, which is frequently comorbid with anxiety disorders.

Alpha 2 antagonists as serotonin norepinephrine disinhibitors (SNDIs)

Blocking the reuptake pumps for monoamines is not the only way to increase their levels or their release. Another way to raise both serotonin and norepinephrine levels is to block alpha 2 receptors (Figure 2-50 and Table 2-2). This results in disinhibition of both serotonin and norepinephrine release by a mechanism to be explained below and is why this mechanism is sometimes also called SNDI action (Table 2-2).

Recall that norepinephrine turns off its own release by interacting with presynaptic alpha 2 autoreceptors on noradrenergic neurons (Figures 1-33 and 1-34); norepinephrine also turns off serotonin release by interacting with presynaptic alpha 2 heteroreceptors on serotonergic neurons (Figure 1-36). If an alpha 2 antagonist is administered, norepinephrine can no longer turn off its own release and noradrenergic neurons are thus

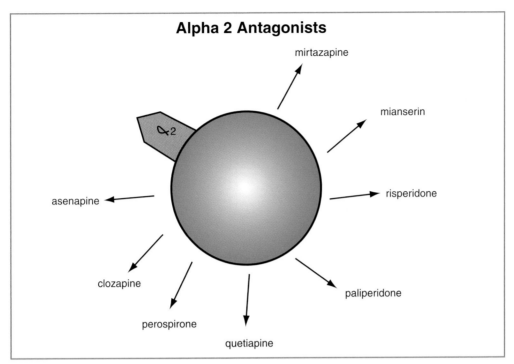

FIGURE 2-50 Alpha 2 antagonists. Blockade of alpha 2 receptors by alpha 2 antagonists can increase both serotonergic and noradrenergic neurotransmission, since alpha 2 antagonism causes serotonin and norepinephrine disinhibition. Dual enhancement of both serotonin and norepinephrine release by alpha 2 antagonism thus generates an antidepressant effect. Alpha 2 antagonists include mirtazapine, mianserin, risperidone, paliperidone, quetiapine, perospirone, clozapine, and asenapine.

disinhibited (Figure 2-51). That is, the alpha 2 antagonist "cuts the brake cable" of the noradrenergic neuron and norepinephrine release is therefore increased.

Similarly, alpha 2 antagonists do not allow norepinephrine to turn off serotonin release. Therefore serotonergic neurons become disinhibited (Figure 2-52). Like their actions at noradrenergic neurons, alpha 2 antagonists act at serotonergic neurons to "cut the brake cable" of noradrenergic inhibition (NE brake on 5HT shown in Figures 1-36 and 1-38). Serotonin release is therefore increased (Figure 2-52).

A second mechanism to increase serotonin release after an alpha 2 antagonist is administered may be even more important. Recall that norepinephrine neurons from the locus coeruleus innervate the cell bodies of serotonergic neurons in the midbrain raphe (Figures 1-35 and 1-38). This noradrenergic input enhances serotonin release via a postsynaptic alpha 1 receptor. Thus, when norepinephrine is disinhibited in the noradrenergic pathway to the raphe, it will increase norepinephrine release there, stimulating alpha 1 receptors and thereby provoking more serotonin release (Figure 2-53). This is like stepping on the serotonin accelerator. Thus alpha 2 antagonists both "cut the brake cable" and "step on the accelerator" for serotonin release (Figure 2-54). The bottom line is that an alpha 2 antagonist is a serotonin and norepinephrine disinhibitor (SNDI) (Table 2-2).

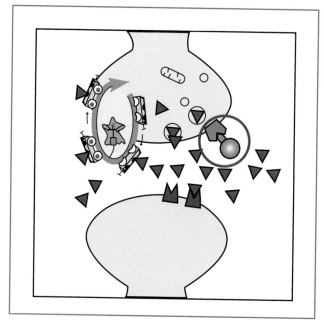

FIGURE 2-51 Alpha 2 antagonists and norepinephrine. Alpha 2 antagonists can increase noradrenergic neurotransmission by "cutting the brake cable" for noradrenergic neurons. That is, alpha 2 antagonists block presynaptic alpha 2 autoreceptors (red circle), which are the "brakes" on noradrenergic neurons. This causes noradrenergic neurons to become disinhibited, since norepinephrine can no longer block its own release. Thus noradrenergic neurotransmission is enhanced.

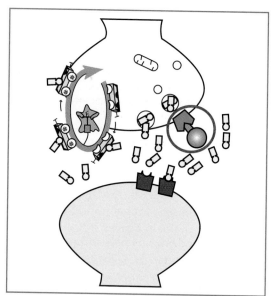

FIGURE 2-52 Alpha 2 antagonists and serotonin. Alpha 2 antagonists can also increase serotonergic neurotransmission by "cutting the brake cable" for serotonergic neurons (compare with Figure 2-51). That is, alpha 2 antagonists block presynaptic alpha 2 heteroreceptors (red circle), the "brakes" on serotonergic neurons. This causes serotonergic neurons to become disinhibited, since norepinephrine can no longer block serotonin release. Thus serotonergic neurotransmission is enhanced.

    Alpha 2 antagonist actions therefore yield dual enhancement of both 5HT and NE release (see Figures 2-51 through 2-54) but, unlike SNRIs, they have this effect by a mechanism independent of blockade of monoamine transporters. These two mechanisms, monoamine transport blockade and alpha 2 antagonism, are synergistic, so that blocking them simultaneously gives a much more powerful disinhibitory signal to these two neurotransmitters than if only one mechanism were blocked. For this reason, the alpha 2 antagonist mirtazapine is often combined with an SNRI to treat patients who do not

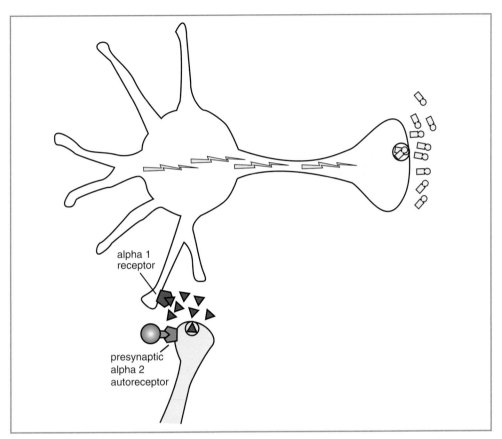

FIGURE 2-53 Alpha 2 antagonists and serotonin. Alpha 2 antagonists can also increase serotonergic neurotransmission by "stepping on the serotonin accelerator." First, antagonism of alpha 2 autoreceptors increases norepinephrine output from noradrenergic neurons in the locus coeruleus (bottom). Norepinephrine then stimulates postsynaptic excitatory alpha 1 receptors on the cell bodies of serotonergic neurons in the midbrain raphe. This increases serotonergic neuronal firing and serotonin release from the serotonin nerve terminal (right).

respond to an SNRI alone. This is discussed further in the section on antidepressants in clinical practice later in this chapter (i.e., "California rocket fuel").

Although no selective alpha 2 antagonist is available for use as an antidepressant, there are several drugs with prominent alpha 2 properties (Figure 2-50), including some atypical antipsychotics, and at least one antidepressant, mirtazapine (Figure 2-55). Although mirtazapine does not block any monoamine transporter, it has additional potent antagonist actions upon 5HT2A receptors, 5HT2C receptors, 5HT3 receptors, and histamine 1 receptors (Figure 2-55).

A summary of the serotonergic actions of mirtazapine is shown in Figure 2-56. When mirtazapine disinhibits serotonin release by the alpha 2 antagonist mechanism, it causes serotonin to be released onto all serotonin receptors; however, mirtazapine simultaneously blocks the actions of serotonin at 5HT2A, 5HT2C, and 5HT3 receptors, leaving net stimulation of only 5HT1A receptors (Figure 2-56).

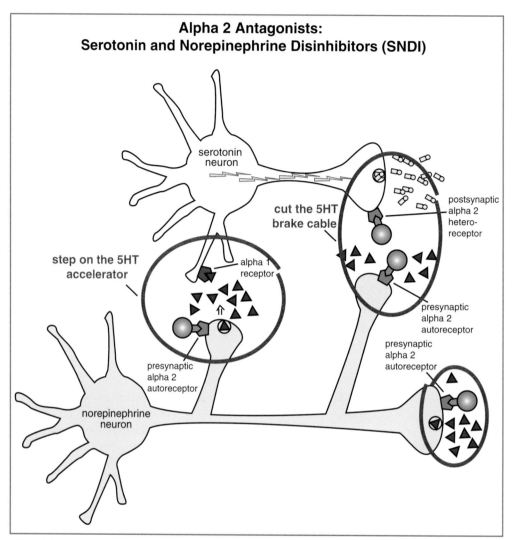

FIGURE 2-54 Alpha 2 antagonists: serotonin and norepinephrine disinhibitors (SNDI). This figure shows how both noradrenergic and serotonergic neurotransmission are enhanced by alpha 2 antagonists. The noradrenergic neuron at the bottom is interacting with the serotonergic neuron at the top. The noradrenergic neuron is disinhibited at all of its axon terminals because an alpha 2 antagonist is blocking all of its presynaptic alpha 2 autoreceptors. This has the effect of "cutting the brake cables" for norepinephrine (NE) release at all of its noradrenergic nerve terminals (NE released in all three red circles). Serotonin (5HT) release is enhanced by NE via two distinct mechanisms. First, alpha 2 antagonists "step on the 5HT accelerator" when NE stimulates alpha 1 receptors on the 5HT cell body and dendrites (left red circle). Second, alpha 2 antagonists "cut the 5HT brake cable" when alpha 2 presynaptic heteroreceptors are blocked on the 5HT axon terminal (middle red circle).

Net 5HT1A agonist action of mirtazapine due to serotonin itself stimulating 5HT1A receptors results in release of dopamine. This would theoretically be helpful for depression and cognition (Figure 2-56). Mirtazapine is anecdotally useful in many anxiety disorders but is not approved for this use.

5HT2A/5HT2C antagonist actions of mirtazapine should theoretically contribute to anxiolytic, sleep-restoring, and antidepressant effects while not causing sexual dysfunction

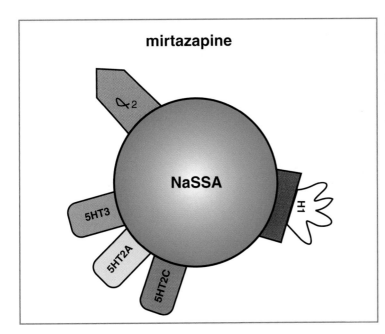

mirtazapine

α2

NaSSA

5HT3

5HT2A

5HT2C

H1

(Figure 2-56). In fact, mirtazapine is one of the few antidepressants that can increase serotonin release and not cause significant sexual dysfunction. In terms of antidepressant effects, 5HT2A antagonist action can be difficult to separate from 5HT2C antagonist actions. Both may contribute to increasing dopamine and norepinephrine release, as discussed in Chapter 1 for antidepressants and illustrated in Figure 1-40.

5HT2C antagonist action as a mechanism for increasing both NE and DA release in prefrontal cortex may be more important than 5HT2A antagonist actions for a drug such as mirtazapine, which lacks the D2 antagonism of an atypical antipsychotic. It turns out that 5HT2A regulation of dopamine release is quite complex and depends on the specific circuit, the area of the brain where 5HT2A receptors are located, and the baseline amount of dopamine and serotonin release as well as the presence of other simultaneous pharmacological mechanisms, such as D2 antagonism. However, 5HT2C antagonism may be more consistently linked to norepinephrine and dopamine disinhibition in the prefrontal cortex regardless of these various factors. The bottom line is that in addition to being an SNDI (serotonin norepinephrine disinhibitor; Table 2-2) due to alpha 2 antagonist properties, mirtazapine is also an NDDI (norepinephrine and dopamine disinhibitor; Table 2-2) due to 5HT2C (and possibly 5HT2A) antagonist properties. Both of these concepts of SNDI and NDDI are novel explanations for the pharmacological actions of this established antidepressant (Table 2-2). These novel concepts may also help to explain the antidepressant actions not only of some atypical antipsychotics but also of several new drugs in development (discussed in the section on future antidepressants, below).

Although it is not clear that 5HT2C antagonist properties alone can cause weight gain, when combined with mirtazapine's simultaneous H1 antihistamine properties (Figure 2-55), weight gain appears more likely.

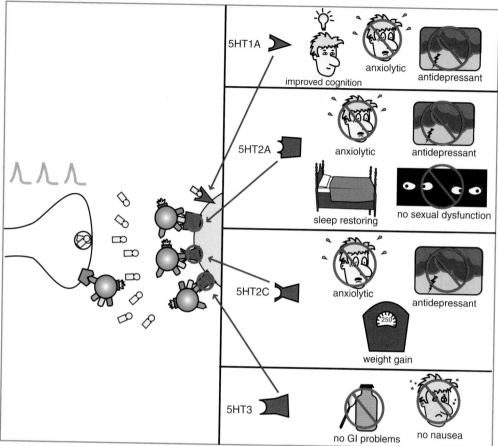

FIGURE 2-56 Mirtazapine actions at serotonin (5HT) synapses. When presynaptic alpha 2 heteroreceptors are blocked by mirtazapine, 5HT is released with the potential to activate any 5HT receptors. However, because mirtazapine blocks 5HT2C, 5HT2A, and 5HT3 receptors, the increased serotonin release is directed largely to the 5HT1A receptor. The result is that antidepressant and anxiolytic actions are preserved but the side effects associated with stimulating 5HT2A, 5HT2C, and 5HT3 are blocked. Mirtazapine's antagonism of 5HT2C receptors could contribute to weight gain.

5HT3 antagonist action should theoretically reduce any nausea or gastrointestinal problems caused by mirtazapine's ability to increase serotonin release (Figure 2-56).

H1 antihistamine actions of mirtazapine (Figure 2-57) should theoretically relieve insomnia at night and improve anxiety during the day, but they could also cause drowsiness during the day. Combined with the 5HT2C antagonist properties described above, the H1 antihistamine actions of mirtazapine could also cause weight gain (Figure 2-57). Interestingly, the histamine 1 antagonist properties of mirtazapine are so potent that both mirtazapine and its active enantiomer esmirtazapine can be given in such low doses that they are essentially selective histamine 1 antagonists. The active enantiomer at very low doses is under investigation as a novel hypnotic.

So, there you have it. Mirtazapine is a molecule with very complex pharmacology that does not block any monoamine transporter yet is a very effective antidepressant. In summary, the therapeutic actions of mirtazapine are thought to be mainly mediated through its alpha 2 antagonist and 5HT2C antagonist properties. The other properties add to

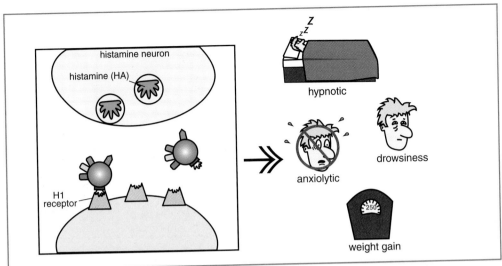

FIGURE 2-57 Mirtazapine at histamine 1 receptors. When mirtazapine blocks histamine 1 receptors, it can cause anxiolytic actions and possibly reduce nighttime insomnia, but it may also contribute to weight gain and daytime drowsiness.

therapeutic actions, cause some side effects, but probably allow patients to tolerate the powerful alpha 2 and 5HT2C antagonist actions that boost serotonin, norepinephrine, and possibly dopamine. An integrated view of mirtazapine's pharmacological actions is shown in Figure 2-58. Because of these unique pharmacological properties, it is worthwhile to understand this molecule and add it to the therapeutic armamentarium for depression, especially as an augmenting agent for difficult cases.

Two other alpha 2 antagonists are marketed as antidepressants in some countries (but not the United States), namely mianserin (worldwide except in the United States) and setiptilene (Japan). Unlike mirtazapine, mianserin has potent alpha 1 antagonist properties that tend to mitigate its ability to enhance serotonergic neurotransmission, so that this drug enhances predominantly noradrenergic neurotransmission yet with associated 5HT2A, 5HT2C, 5HT3, and histamine 1 antagonist properties. Yohimbine is also an alpha 2 antagonist, but its alpha 1 antagonist properties similarly mitigate its pro-serotonergic actions. Several selective alpha 2 antagonists, including idazoxan and fluparoxan, have been tested, but they have not demonstrated sufficiently robust antidepressant efficacy with sufficient tolerability, as they may provoke panic, anxiety, and prolonged erections in men, side effects that are not generally observed with alpha 2 antagonists such as mirtazapine, which have additional pharmacological properties that tend to block these side effects.

Serotonin antagonist/reuptake inhibitors (SARIs)

Several antidepressants share the ability to block serotonin 2A and 2C receptors as well as serotonin reuptake. The prototype drug with this antidepressant mechanism is trazodone (Figure 2-59), which is classified as a serotonin antagonist/reuptake inhibitor (SARI) (Table 2-2) or, more fully, as a serotonin 2A/2C antagonist and serotonin reuptake inhibitor (Figure 2-60). However, moderate to high doses of trazodone are required to inhibit SERT and 5HT2C receptors as well as 5HT2A receptors sufficiently for trazodone to be an effective antidepressant.

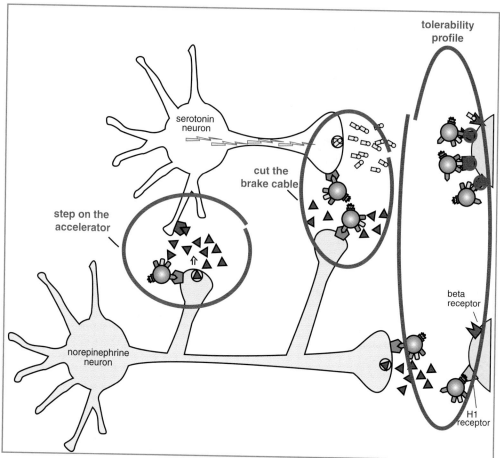

FIGURE 2-58 Overview of mirtazapine's actions. Mirtazapine's actions include those of alpha 2 antagonism, already shown in Figure 2-54: therapeutic actions of cutting the norepinephrine (NE) brake cable while stepping on the serotonin (5HT) accelerator (left circle) as well as cutting the 5HT brake cable (middle circle). This increases both 5HT and NE neurotransmission. On the right are the additional actions of mirtazapine beyond alpha 2 antagonism. These postsynaptic actions mainly account for the tolerability profile of mirtazapine.

    Doses of trazodone lower than those effective for antidepressant action are frequently used for the effective treatment of insomnia. Low doses exploit trazodone's potent actions as a 5HT2A antagonist and also its properties as an antagonist of histamine 1 and alpha 1 adrenergic receptors, but they do not adequately exploit its SERT or 5HT2C inhibition properties, which are weaker (Figure 2-59). As discussed in Blocking the brain's arousal system with histamine 1 and alpha 1 antagonism can cause sedation or sleep; along with 5HT2A antagonist properties, this may explain the mechanism of how a low dose of trazodone works as a hypnotic. Since insomnia is one of the most frequent residual symptoms of depression after treatment with an SSRI (discussed earlier in this chapter and illustrated in Figure 2-9), a hypnotic is often necessary for patients with a major depressive episode. A hypnotic can not only potentially relieve the insomnia itself but – as recent data suggest – treating insomnia in patients with major depression also increases remission rates due to improvement of other symptoms, such as loss of energy and depressed mood. This ability of low doses of trazodone to improve sleep

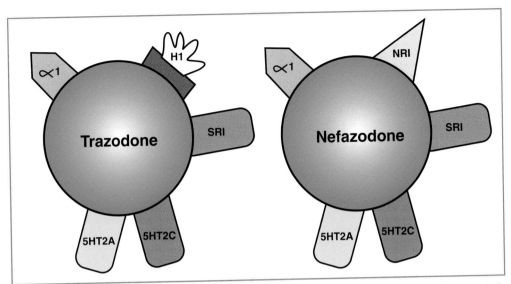

FIGURE 2-59 Serotonin antagonist/reuptake inhibitors. Shown here are icons for two serotonin 2A antagonist/reuptake inhibitors (SARIs): trazodone and nefazodone. These agents have a dual action, but the two mechanisms are different from the dual action of the serotonin norepinephrine reuptake inhibitors (SNRIs). The SARIs act by potent blockade of serotonin 2A (5HT2A) receptors as well as dose-dependent blockade of serotonin 2C (5HT2C) receptors and the serotonin transporter (SRI). SARIs also block alpha 1 adrenergic receptors. In addition, trazodone has the unique property of histamine 1 receptor antagonism and nefazodone has the unique property of norepinephrine reuptake inhibition (NRI).

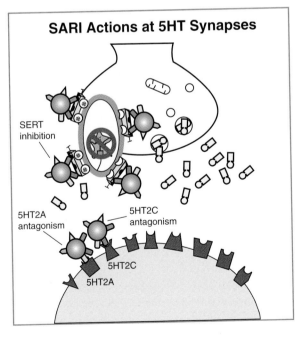

SARI Actions at 5HT Synapses

SERT inhibition

5HT2A antagonism

5HT2C antagonism

5HT2C

5HT2A

FIGURE 2-60 SARI actions at serotonin (5HT) synapses. This figure shows the dual actions of a serotonin 2A antagonist/reuptake inhibitor (SARI). This agent acts both presynaptically and postsynaptically. Presynaptic actions are indicated by the serotonin reuptake inhibitor (SRI) portion of the icon, which is inserted into the serotonin reuptake pump, blocking it. Postsynaptic actions are indicated by the serotonin 2A receptor antagonist portion of the icon (5HT2A) inserted into the 5HT2A receptor and by the serotonin 2C antagonist portion of the icon (5HT2C) inserted into the 5HT2C receptor. It is believed that all three blocking actions contribute to the antidepressant effects of SARIs. The 5HT2A antagonist actions are more potent than the serotonin reuptake properties or 5HT2C antagonism.

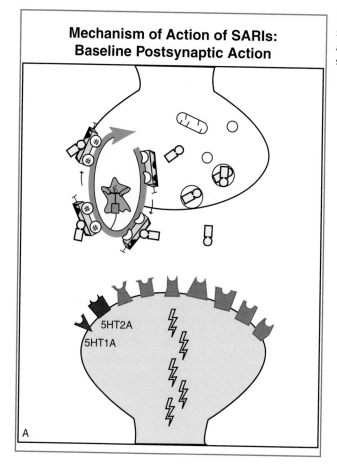

**Mechanism of Action of SARIs:
Baseline Postsynaptic Action**

5HT2A
5HT1A

FIGURE 2-61A Mechanism of action of SARIs, part 1: baseline postsynaptic actions. Shown here is a postsynaptic serotonin neuron with baseline firing.

A

in depressed patients may thus be an important mechanism whereby trazodone can augment the efficacy of other antidepressants.

Beyond the treatment of insomnia associated with depression, recruiting SERT inhibition with trazodone by increasing the dose is an important pharmacological mechanism that can be potentially synergistic with 5HT2A/5HT2C antagonism for broader antidepressant actions (Figures 2-61 through 2-64). However, in order to get this synergy of multiple mechanisms with trazodone monotherapy, a moderate to high dose must be used, which can often be attained without unacceptable daytime sedation by slow dose titration, allowing tolerance to develop, or giving the dose mostly at night to avoid unacceptable daytime sedation. Controlled-release formulations of trazodone are also in testing to reduce peak-dose sedation. Alternatively, low to moderate doses of trazodone can be added to a full dose of a known SERT inhibitor such as an SSRI or an SNRI to exploit 5HT2A/SERT synergy, as shown in Figures 2-60 through 12-63. An interesting aspect of trazodone's actions is the relative lack of sexual side effects at any dose, something it shares with mirtazapine, another 5HT2A/5HT2C antagonist.

How does 5HT2A/2C antagonism synergize with SERT inhibition to enhance the treatment of depressive symptoms other than insomnia? There are four possible ways in which this happens; these are illustrated in Figures 2-61 though 2-64.

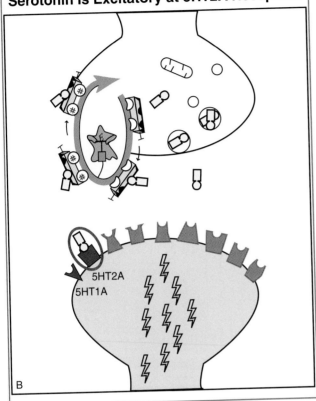

**Mechanism of Action of SARIs:
Serotonin Is Excitatory at 5HT2A Receptors**

5HT2A
5HT1A

B

FIGURE 2-61B Mechanism of action of SARIs, part 2: serotonin (5HT) is excitatory at 5HT2A receptors. Stimulation of 5HT2A receptors by 5HT (red circle) increases firing of the postsynaptic 5HT neuron compared to baseline.

Serotonin 2A antagonism potentiates the inhibitory action of serotonin at 5HT1A receptors (Figure 2-61A)

Recall that Serotonin 1A receptors in general can have the opposite actions of serotonin 2A receptors. Thus, serotonin itself is excitatory at 5HT2A receptors (compare Figures 2-61A and 2-61B) and inhibitory at 5HT1A receptors (compare Figures 2-61A and 2-61C). Whether serotonin excites or inhibits the neuron depends on the density of each receptor at a given synapse and the amount of serotonin released. If the excitatory action of serotonin at 5HT2A receptors is blocked, this potentiates the inhibitory action of 5HT1A receptors (compare Figure 2-61D with Figures 2-61C and 2-61A).

Trazodone will cause 5HT2A inhibition at essentially any clinical dose, but to get the potentiation of serotonin's inhibition at 5HT1A receptors, there must be SERT inhibition that raises serotonin in the synapse and therefore increases serotonin levels so serotonin itself can interact at 5HT1A receptors at the same time that trazodone is blocking 5HT2A receptors (Figure 2-61D). This can be accomplished either by raising the trazodone dose or by adding a SERT inhibitor. The potentiation of 5HT1A inhibition of serotonin neurons may also be useful in relieving anxiety and in reducing overactivity in neuronal circuits in some brain regions associated with the various symptoms of depression (see reduction in

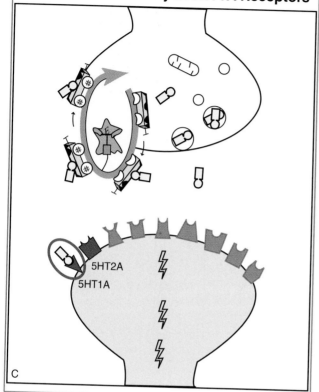

**Mechanism of Action of SARIs:
Serotonin Is Inhibitory at 5HT1A Receptors**

5HT2A
5HT1A

C

FIGURE 2-61C Mechanism of action of SARIs, part 3: serotonin (5HT) is inhibitory at 5HT1A receptors. Stimulation of 5HT1A receptors by 5HT (red circle) decreases firing of the postsynaptic 5HT neuron compared to baseline.

nerve impulse flow shown in Figure 2-61D and hypothetical areas of neuronal hyperactivity in depression in Figure 1-64).

Serotonin 2A antagonism potentiates gene expression stimulated by 5HT1A receptors (Figure 2-62)

Another action of serotonin at 5HT1A receptors that is opposed by serotonin actions at 5HT2A receptors is the stimulation of gene expression. That is, 5HT1A receptors stimulate gene expression by signal transduction through a second messenger system that utilizes cAMP (Figure 2-62A). Serotonin blocks this signal cascade system through actions downstream from 5HT2A receptors (Figure 2-62B). When this action of serotonin at 5HT2A receptors is blocked, the stimulation of gene expression by serotonin actions at 5HT1A receptors is potentiated (Figure 2-62C). Again, any clinical dose of trazodone will block 5HT2A receptors, but a higher dose of trazodone or a concomitantly administered SERT inhibitor is necessary to increase serotonin levels so that there is stimulation of 5HT1A receptors and thus 5HT2A/SERT synergy (Figure 2-62C). Potentiation of gene expression may be helpful in facilitating the regulation of neurotransmitter receptors or neurotrophic factors associated with improvement in the symptoms of depression.

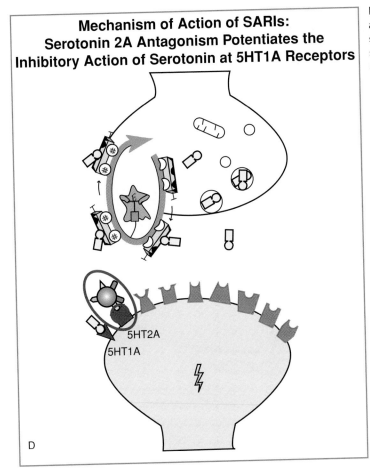

Mechanism of Action of SARIs: Serotonin 2A Antagonism Potentiates the Inhibitory Action of Serotonin at 5HT1A Receptors

5HT2A

5HT1A

D

FIGURE 2-61D Mechanism of action of SARIs, part 4: synergy between 5HT1A stimulation and 5HT2A antagonism. When 5HT2A receptors are pharmacologically blocked rather than stimulated, the inhibitory actions of 5HT at 5HT1A receptors are potentiated.

Serotonin 2A antagonism potentiates the inhibitory action of serotonin 1A on glutamate release from cortical pyramidal neurons (Figure 2-63)

Serotonin stimulates glutamate release from pyramidal neurons in prefrontal cortex by its actions at 5HT2A receptors (Figure 2-63A) but inhibits glutamate release from these same neurons by its actions at 5HT1A receptors (Figure 2-63B). When 5HT2A receptors are blocked, it potentiates the inhibitory actions of serotonin at 5HT1A receptors (Figure 2-63C), but this can occur only if trazodone's potent 5HT2A antagonist properties are coupled with simultaneous SERT inhibition. Preventing the release of too much glutamate from dysfunctional pyramidal neurons that have inefficient information processing may improve information processing and reduce symptoms of depression in patients who have abnormal pyramidal cell functioning in various prefrontal cortex areas that mediate specific symptoms of depression (Figure 2-63C and Figure 1-64).

Serotonin 2A/2C potentiation of NE and DA disinhibition at serotonin 1A receptors (Figure 2-64)

Finally, as already discussed above in the sections on fluoxetine (Figure 2-25) and mirtazapine, serotonin's actions at 5HT2C receptors inhibit both DA and NE release (Figure 2-64). This same inhibition may also occur under certain circumstances at 5HT2A

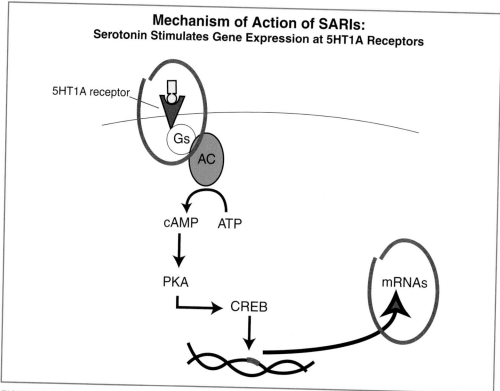

Mechanism of Action of SARIs:
Serotonin Stimulates Gene Expression at 5HT1A Receptors

FIGURE 2-62A Serotonin (5HT) stimulates gene expression through 5HT1A receptors. The molecular consequences of 5HT1A stimulation alone, shown here, result in a certain amount of gene expression corresponding to the pharmacological actions shown in Figure 2-61C. 5HT occupancy of its 5HT1A receptor (top red circle) causes a certain amount of gene transcription (see bottom red circle on the right). The 5HT1A receptor is coupled to a stimulatory G protein (Gs) and adenylate cyclase (AC), which produces the second messenger cyclic AMP from ATP. This, in turn, activates protein kinase A (PKA), so that transcription factors such as cyclic AMP response element binding protein (CREB) can activate gene expression (mRNAs).

receptors. Also already discussed is how stimulation of serotonin 1A receptors acutely reduces the serotonergic inhibition of DA and NE release at 5HT2C receptors and possibly at 5HT2A receptors, thus disinhibiting DA and NE release (Figure 2-64). Because this 5HT1A mechanism tends to desensitize, it may be important to potentiate this action of serotonin at 5HT1A receptors by simultaneously blocking 5HT2C and/or 5HT2A receptors, leading to release of both DA and NE in prefrontal cortex (Figure 2-64). The bottom line is that producing disinhibition of NE and DA in prefrontal cortex by whatever mechanism could theoretically help to enhance the efficiency of information processing there and lead to a reduction in the symptoms of depression mediated in this brain region.

Nefazodone is another SARI with robust 5HT2A antagonist actions and weaker 5HT2C antagonism and SERT inhibition, but it is no longer commonly used because of rare liver toxicity (Figure 2-59). Several tricyclic antidepressants – such as amitriptyline, nortriptyline, doxepin, and amoxapine – also have a combination of serotonin 2A and 2C antagonism with serotonin reuptake inhibition along with several other pharmacological actions; these are discussed later in this chapter in the section on tricyclic antidepressants. Since the potency of blockade of serotonin 2A and 2C receptors varies considerably among

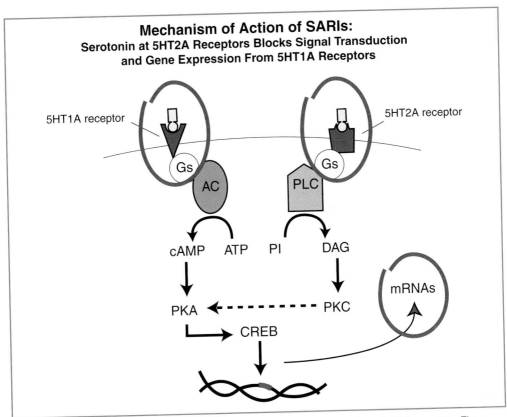

Mechanism of Action of SARIs:
Serotonin at 5HT2A Receptors Blocks Signal Transduction
and Gene Expression From 5HT1A Receptors

FIGURE 2-62B Serotonin (5HT) at 5HT2A receptors blocks gene expression from 5HT1A receptors. The molecular consequence of 5HT2A receptor stimulation concomitant with 5HT1A receptor stimulation is to reduce the gene expression of 5HT1A stimulation alone (i.e., that shown in Figure 2-62A). These molecular consequences correlate with the pharmacological actions of simultaneous 5HT1A and 5HT2A stimulation. Simultaneous activation of the 5HT2A receptor by 5HT (top right red circle) will alter the consequences of activating 5HT1A receptors (top left red circle) in a negative way and reduce the gene expression of 5HT1A receptors acting alone (Figure 2-62A). Thus, occupancy of 5HT2A receptor (top circle) causes coupling of a stimulatory G protein (Gs) with the enzyme phospholipase C (PLC). This, in turn, activates calcium flux and converts phosphatidylinositol (PI) into diacylglycerol (DAG). This activates the enzyme phosphokinase C (PKC), which has an inhibitory action on phosphokinase A (PKA). This reduces the activation of transcription factors such as cyclic AMP response element binding protein (CREB) and leads to a decrease in gene expression (bottom red circle).

the tricyclics, it is not clear how important this action is to the therapeutic actions of tricyclic antidepressants in general.

Many other drugs are 5HT2A/2C antagonists, including mirtazapine, just discussed in the previous section, and the atypical antipsychotics, all of which are potent 5HT2A antagonists and some of which are also potent 5HT2C antagonists. The use of atypical antipsychotics as augmenting agents for treatment-resistant depression is discussed later in this chapter in the section on antidepressants in clinical practice; their use for treatment of bipolar depression is discussed in Chapter 3, on mood stabilizers.

YM992 is another SARI (serotonin 2A/2C antagonist with moderately potent serotonin reuptake inhibition properties) that is in testing as an antidepressant. Selective 5HT2A antagonists, however, do not appear to be effective antidepressants. On the other hand, drugs

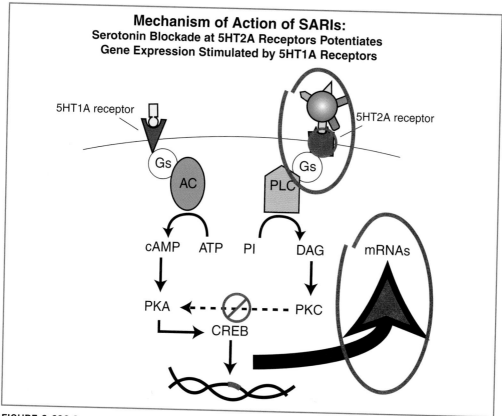

Mechanism of Action of SARIs:
Serotonin Blockade at 5HT2A Receptors Potentiates
Gene Expression Stimulated by 5HT1A Receptors

FIGURE 2-62C Serotonin (5HT) blockade at 5HT2A receptors potentiates gene expression from 5HT1A receptors. The molecular consequence of 5HT1A receptor disinhibition by 5HT2A receptor blockade is shown here – namely, enhanced gene expression. These molecular events are the consequence of the pharmacological actions shown in Figure 2-61D. Simultaneous inhibition of the 5HT2A receptor (top right circle) can stop the negative consequences that 5HT2A receptor stimulation by 5HT can have on gene expression, as shown in Figure 2-62B. Thus gene expression of the 5HT1A receptor is enhanced when 5HT2A receptors are blocked (bottom red circle) rather than diminished when they are stimulated (Figure 2-62B).

with 5HT2A/2C antagonist properties plus direct-acting 5HT1A agonist properties are in testing as potential novel antidepressants and disinhibitors of DA release for improving sexual dysfunction, including the agents flibanserin, adatanserin, BMS181,101, and others. One particularly novel agent with 5HT2C antagonist properties in testing as an antidepressant is agomelatine, discussed in the section on future antidepressants below.

Classic antidepressants: monoamine oxidase inhibitors

The first clinically effective antidepressants to be discovered were inhibitors of the enzyme monoamine oxidase (MAO). They were discovered by accident when an antituberculosis drug, iproniazid, was observed to help depression that coexisted in some of the patients who had tuberculosis. This antituberculosis drug was eventually found to work in depression by inhibiting the enzyme MAO. However, inhibition of MAO was unrelated to its antituberculosis actions.

This discovery soon led to the synthesis of more drugs in the 1950s and 1960s that inhibited MAO but lacked unwanted additional properties (such as antituberculosis properties and liver toxicity). Although best known as powerful antidepressants, the MAOIs are

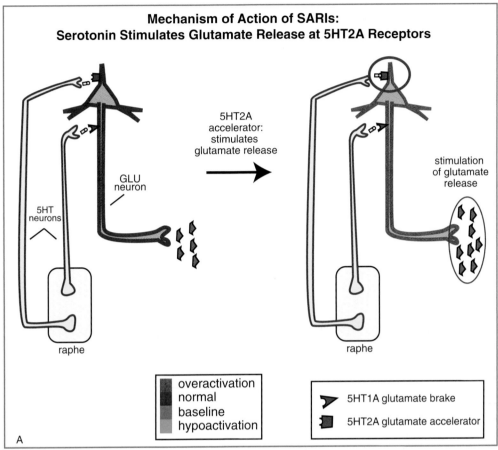

Mechanism of Action of SARIs:
Serotonin Stimulates Glutamate Release at 5HT2A Receptors

5HT2A accelerator: stimulates glutamate release

stimulation of glutamate release

GLU neuron

5HT neurons

raphe

raphe

overactivation
normal
baseline
hypoactivation

5HT1A glutamate brake

5HT2A glutamate accelerator

A

FIGURE 2-63A Serotonin (5HT) stimulates glutamate release at 5HT2A receptors. 5HT projections from the midbrain raphe synapse with pyramidal glutamate neurons in the prefrontal cortex (right). Binding of 5HT to 5HT2A receptors stimulates glutamate release from pyramidal neurons (left).

also highly effective therapeutic agents for certain anxiety disorders, such as panic disorder and social phobia. MAO inhibitors, however, tend to be underutilized in clinical practice. There are many reasons for this, including the fact that there are many other options for treatment today, preventing modern-day clinicians from becoming familiar with them. Since these are old drugs, and there is essentially no marketing for them, there is a good deal of misinformation and mythology about their dietary and drug interaction dangers. For these reasons, these agents are discussed in this chapter, which in this respect is uncharacteristic of modern psychopharmacology texts. Readers with no interest in MAO inhibitors can, of course, skip this section as well as the following section on tricyclic antidepressants and go on to antidepressant pharmacokinetics, but in so doing they may miss information on a few secret weapons in the therapeutic armamentarium for patients who fail to respond to the better-known agents.

Three of the original MAO inhibitors that are still available for clinical use today are phenelzine, tranylcypromine, and isocarboxazid (Table 2-4). These are all irreversible enzyme inhibitors and thus bind to MAO covalently and irreversibly and destroy its function forever. Enzyme activity returns only after new enzyme is synthesized. Sometimes such

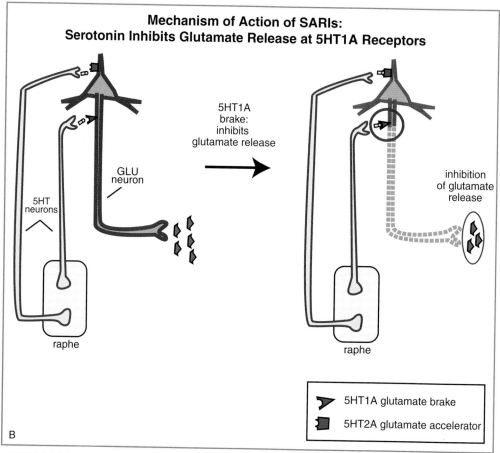

Mechanism of Action of SARIs:
Serotonin Inhibits Glutamate Release at 5HT1A Receptors

5HT1A
brake:
inhibits
glutamate release

GLU
neuron

5HT
neurons

inhibition
of glutamate
release

raphe

raphe

> 5HT1A glutamate brake

▶ 5HT2A glutamate accelerator

B

FIGURE 2-63B Serotonin (5HT) inhibits glutamate release at 5HT1A receptors. Binding of 5HT to 5HT1A receptors inhibits glutamate release from pyramidal neurons (left).

enzyme inhibitors are called "suicide inhibitors," because once this kind of inhibitor binds to the enzyme, the enzyme essentially commits suicide in that it can never function again until a new enzyme protein is synthesized by the neuron's DNA in the cell nucleus. This is an unfortunate terminology for a very effective class of antidepressants and perhaps is a concept better utilized by enzymologists, not by clinicians.

Amphetamine is itself a weak MAO inhibitor (Table 2-5). Some MAO inhibitors, such as tranylcypromine, have chemical structures modeled on amphetamine; thus, in addition to MAO inhibitor properties, they also have amphetamine-like dopamine-releasing properties (Tables 2-4 and 2-5). Amphetamine acts on the dopamine transporter (DAT) to trigger dopamine release. Tranylcypromine has these same actions on DAT as well. Selegiline itself does not have amphetamine-like properties but is metabolized to both l-amphetamine and l-methamphetamine, which do have inhibitory actions on DAT and dopamine-releasing properties (Tables 2-4 and 2-5). Thus there is a close mechanistic link between some MAO inhibitors and DAT inhibition as well as between the MAO-inhibiting properties and DAT-inhibiting properties of amphetamine itself (Tables 2-4 and 2-5). It is therefore not surprising that one of the augmenting agents utilized to boost MAO inhibitors in

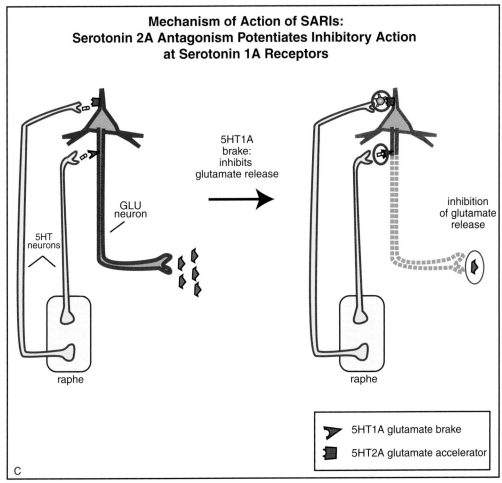

Mechanism of Action of SARIs: Serotonin 2A Antagonism Potentiates Inhibitory Action at Serotonin 1A Receptors

5HT1A brake: inhibits glutamate release

GLU neuron

5HT neurons

inhibition of glutamate release

raphe

raphe

▶ 5HT1A glutamate brake

◀ 5HT2A glutamate accelerator

C

FIGURE 2-63C Serotonin (5HT) 2A antagonism potentiates inhibitory action at 5HT1A receptors. Blockade of 5HT2A receptors can potentiate the inhibitory actions of serotonin at 5HT1A receptors on glutamate release (left).

treatment-resistant patients is amphetamine, administered by experts with great caution while monitoring blood pressure.

MAO subtypes

MAO exists in two subtypes, A and B (Table 2-6). Both forms are inhibited by the original MAO inhibitors, which are therefore nonselective (Table 2-4). The A form preferentially metabolizes the monoamines most closely linked to depression (i.e., serotonin and norepinephrine), whereas the B form preferentially metabolizes trace amines such as phenethylamine (Table 2-6). Both MAO-A and MAO-B metabolize dopamine and tyramine (Table 2-6). Both MAO-A and MAO-B are in the brain (Table 2-6). Noradrenergic neurons (Figure 1-31) and dopaminergic neurons are thought to contain both MAO-A and MAO-B, with perhaps MAO-A activity predominant, whereas serotonergic neurons are thought to contain only MAO-B. With the exception of platelets and lymphocytes, which have MAO-B, MAO-A is the major form of this enzyme outside of the brain (Table 2-6).

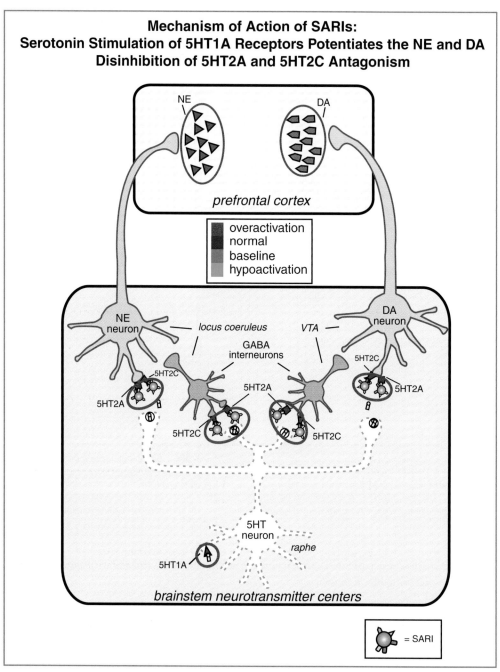

Mechanism of Action of SARIs: Serotonin Stimulation of 5HT1A Receptors Potentiates the NE and DA Disinhibition of 5HT2A and 5HT2C Antagonism

FIGURE 2-64 Stimulation of 5HT1A receptors: disinhibition of norepinephrine and dopamine. Serotonin (5HT) actions at 5HT2C and 5HT2A receptors inhibit both norepinephrine (NE) and dopamine (DA) release. Indirect stimulation of presynaptic 5HT1A receptors via SERT inhibition by high doses of trazodone can reduce this inhibition of NE and DA by 5HT via reducing the concentrations of 5HT at postsynaptic sites on NE and DA neurons. Furthermore, if 5HT2C and 5HT2A receptors are blocked, this may potentiate the disinhibiting effects of 5HT1A stimulation on NE and DA.

TABLE 2-4 Currently approved MAO inhibitors

Name (trade name)	Inhibition of MAO-A	Inhibition of MAO-B	Amphetamine properties
phenelzine (Nardil)	+	+	
tranylcypromine (Parnate)	+	+	+
isocarboxazid (Marplan)	+	+	
amphetamines (at high doses)	+	+	+
selegiline transdermal system (Emsam)			
brain	+	+	+
gut	+/−	+	+
selegiline low dose oral (Deprenyl, Eldepryl)	−	+	+
rasaligine (Agilect/Azilect)	−	+	−
moclobemide (Aurorix, Manerix)	+	−	−

TABLE 2-5 MAO inhibitors with amphetamine actions or amphetamines with MAO inhibition?

Drug	Comment
amphetamine	MAOI at high doses
tranylcypromine (Parnate)	also called phenylcyclopropylamine
selegiline	metabolized to L-methamphetamine
	metabolized to L-amphetamine
	less amphetamine formed transdermally

TABLE 2-6 MAO enzymes

	MAO-A	MAO-B
Substrates	5-HT	Phenylethylamine
	NE	DA
	DA	Tyramine
	Tyramine	
Tissue distribution	Brain, gut, liver, placenta, skin	Brain, platelets, lymphocytes

Brain MAO-A must be inhibited for antidepressant efficacy to occur (Figure 2-65). This is not surprising, since this is the form of MAO that preferentially metabolizes serotonin and norepinephrine, two of the three components of the trimonoaminergic neurotransmitter system linked to depression and to antidepressant actions, both of which demonstrate increased brain levels after MAO-A inhibition (Figure 2-65). MAO-A, along with MAO-B, also metabolizes dopamine, but inhibition of MAO-A alone does not appear to lead to robust increases in brain dopamine levels, since MAO-B can still metabolize dopamine (Figure 2-65).

Inhibition of MAO-B is not effective as an antidepressant, as there is no direct effect on either serotonin or norepinephrine metabolism and little or no dopamine accumulates owing to the continued action of MAO-A (Figure 2-66). What, therefore, is the therapeutic value of MAO-B inhibition? When this enzyme is selectively inhibited, it can boost the action of concomitantly administered levodopa in Parkinson's disease. Evidently, in the presence

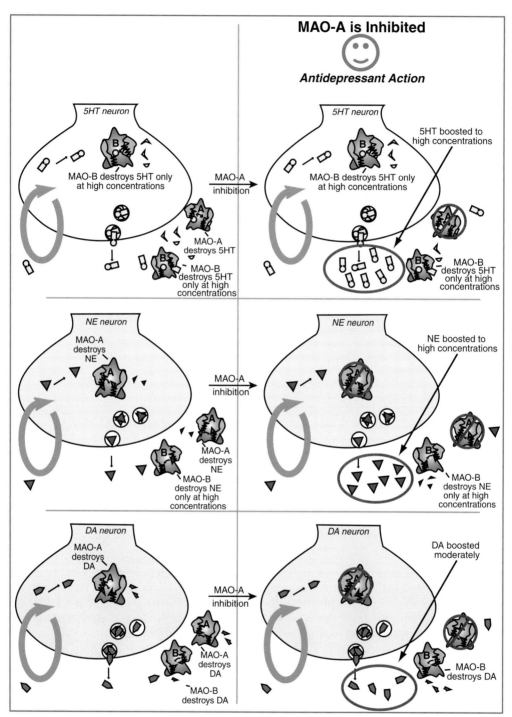

FIGURE 2-65 Monoamine oxidase A (MAO-A) inhibition. The enzyme MAO-A metabolizes serotonin (5HT) and norepinephrine (NE) as well as dopamine (DA) (left panels). Monoamine oxidase B (MAO-B) also metabolizes DA, but it metabolizes 5HT and NE only at high concentrations (left panels). This means that MAO-A inhibition increases 5HT, NE, and DA (right panels) but that the increase in DA is not as great as that of 5HT and NE because MAO-B can continue to destroy DA (bottom right panel). Inhibition of MAO-A is an efficacious antidepressant strategy.

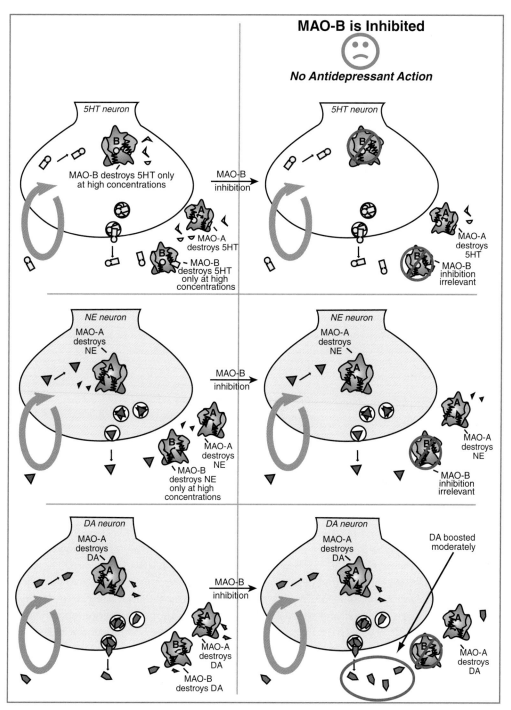

FIGURE 2-66 Monoamine oxidase B (MAO-B) inhibition. Selective inhibitors of MAO-B do not have antidepressant efficacy. This is because MAO-B metabolizes serotonin (5HT) and norepinephrine (NE) only at high concentrations (top two left panels). Since MAO-B's role in destroying 5HT and NE is small, its inhibition is not likely to be relevant to the concentrations of these neurotransmitters (top two right panels). Selective inhibition of MAO-B also has somewhat limited effects on dopamine (DA) concentrations, because MAO-A continues to destroy DA. However, inhibition of MAO-B does increase DA to some extent, which can be therapeutic in other disease states, such as Parkinson's disease.

of a large load of dopamine derived from administration of a large dose of its precursor levodopa, selective MAO-B inhibition is sufficient to boost dopamine action in the brain. MAO-B is also thought to convert some environmentally derived amine substrates, called protoxins, into toxins that may cause damage to neurons and possibly contribute to the cause or decline of function in Parkinson's disease. Inhibition of MAO-B may thus halt this process, and there is speculation that this might slow the degenerative course of various neurodegenerative disorders, including Parkinson's disease. Thus, two MAO inhibitors in Table 2-4, selegiline and rasaligine, when administered orally in doses selective for inhibition of MAO-B, are approved for use in patients with Parkinson's disease but are not effective at these selective MAO-B doses as antidepressants.

Perhaps the most important role of MAO-B in psychopharmacology is when it is inhibited simultaneously with MAO-A (Figure 2-67). In that case, there is a triple and very robust monoaminergic boost of dopamine as well as serotonin and norepinephrine (Figure 2-67). This would theoretically provide the most powerful antidepressant efficacy across the range of depressive symptoms, from diminished positive affect to increased negative affect (see Figure 1-55). Thus MAO-A plus B inhibition is one of the few therapeutic strategies available to increase dopamine in depression and therefore to treat refractory symptoms of diminished positive affect. This is a good reason for specialists in psychopharmacology to become adept at administering MAO inhibitors, so that they can have an additional strategy within their armamentarium for patients with treatment-resistant symptoms of diminished positive affect, which is a very common problem in a referral practice.

Tyramine reactions and dietary restrictions

One of the biggest barriers to utilizing MAO inhibitors has traditionally been the risk that a patient taking one of these drugs might develop a hypertensive reaction after ingesting tyramine in the diet. How does the combination of tyramine in the diet plus MAO-A inhibition in the gut lead to a dangerous elevation in blood pressure? Tyramine works to elevate blood pressure because it is a potent releaser of norepinephrine. Normally, NE is not allowed to accumulate to dangerous levels, owing in part to efficient destruction of NE by MAO-A once NE is released during neurotransmission (Figure 2-68). Thus there is no vasoconstriction and no elevated blood pressure because there is no excessive stimulation of postsynaptic alpha 1 or other adrenergic receptors (Figure 2-68). When foods high in tyramine content – such as tap beers, smoked meat or fish, fava beans, aged cheeses, sauerkraut, or soy – are ingested (Table 2-7), MAO-A in the intestinal wall goes to work, safely destroying tyramine before it is absorbed; MAO-A in the liver safely destroys any tyramine that gets absorbed; and even if any tyramine reaches the noradrenergic sympathetic neuron (Figure 2-69), the MAO-A there destroys any synaptic norepinephrine that this tyramine would release. The body thus has a huge capacity for processing tyramine, and the average person is able to handle around 400 mg of ingested tyramine before blood pressure is elevated. A high-tyramine meal, by contrast, represents only around 40 mg of tyramine.

However, when MAO-A is inhibited, this capacity to handle dietary tyramine is much reduced, and a high-tyramine meal is sufficient to raise blood pressure when a substantial amount of MAO-A is irreversibly inhibited (Figure 2-70). In fact, it may take as little as 10 mg of dietary tyramine to increase blood pressure when MAO-A is essentially knocked out by high doses of an MAO inhibitor. Some blood pressure elevations can be very large, sudden, and dramatic, causing a condition known as a hypertensive crisis (Table 2-8), which can rarely cause intracerebral hemorrhage or even death. This risk is normally controlled

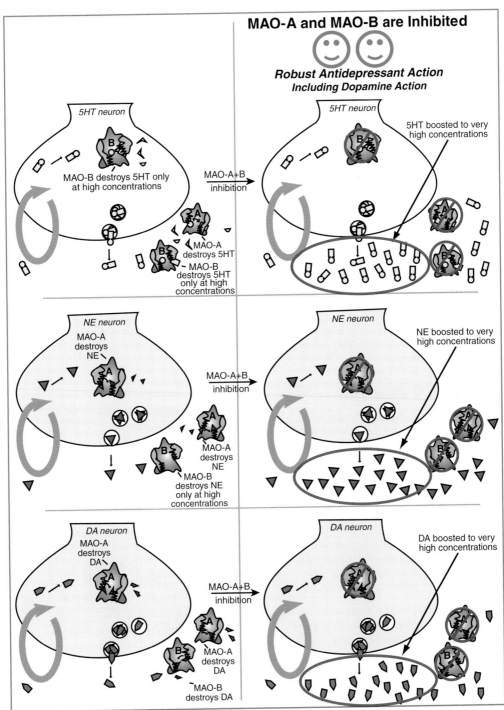

FIGURE 2-67 Combined inhibition of monoamine oxidase A (MAO-A) and monoamine oxidase B (MAO-B).
Combined inhibition of MAO-A and MAO-B may have robust antidepressant actions owing to increases not only in serotonin (5HT) and norepinephrine (NE) but also dopamine (DA). Inhibition of both MAO-A, which metabolizes 5HT, NE, and DA, and MAO-B, which metabolizes primarily DA (left panels), leads to greater increases in each of these neurotransmitters than inhibition of either enzyme alone.

TABLE 2-7 Suggested tyramine dietary modifications for MAO inhibitors*

Food to avoid	Food allowed
Dried, aged, smoked, fermented, spoiled, or improperly stored meat, poultry, and fish	Fresh or processed meat, poultry, and fish
Broad bean pods	All other vegetables
Aged cheeses	Processed and cottage cheese, ricotta cheese, yogurt
Tap and nonpasteurized beers	Canned or bottled beers and alcohol (have little tyramine)
Marmite, sauerkraut	Brewer's and baker's yeast
Soy products/tofu	

*No dietary modifications needed for low doses of transdermal selegiline or for low oral doses of selective MAO-B inhibitors.

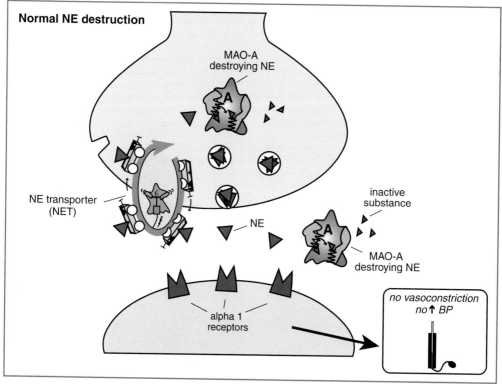

FIGURE 2-68 Normal destruction of norepinephrine. Monoamine oxidase A (MAO-A) is the enzyme that normally acts to destroy norepinephrine (NE) to keep it in balance. Since accumulated NE can cause vasoconstriction and elevated blood pressure via increased binding at alpha 1 and other adrenergic receptors, its normal destruction by MAO-A helps prevent these negative effects.

by restricting the diet so that foods dangerously high in tyramine content are eliminated (Table 2-7). Until recently, the risk of hypertensive crisis and the hassle of restricting diet have generally been the price that a patient has had to pay in order to get the therapeutic benefits of the MAO inhibitors in treating depression.

Because of the potential danger of a hypertensive crisis from a tyramine reaction in patients taking irreversible MAO inhibitors, a certain mythology has grown up around

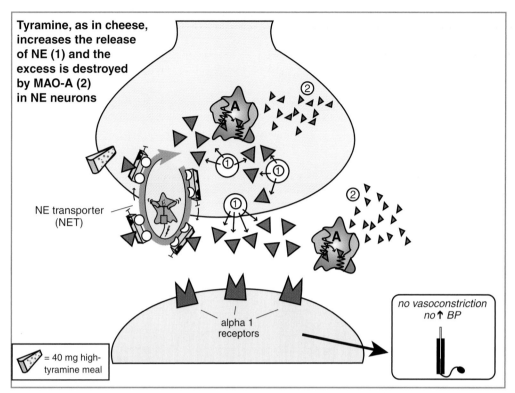

Tyramine, as in cheese, increases the release of NE (1) and the excess is destroyed by MAO-A (2) in NE neurons

NE transporter (NET)

② ①

alpha 1 receptors

no vasoconstriction no ↑ BP

= 40 mg high-tyramine meal

FIGURE 2-69 Tyramine increases norepinephrine release. Tyramine is an amine present in various foods, including cheese. Indicated in this figure is how a high-tyramine meal (40 mg, depicted here as cheese) acts to increase the release of norepinephrine (NE) (1). However, in normal circumstances the enzyme monoamine oxidase A (MAO-A) readily destroys the excess NE released by tyramine (2), and no harm is done (i.e., no vasoconstriction or elevation in blood pressure).

how much tyramine is in various foods and therefore what dietary restrictions are necessary. Since the tyramine reaction is sometimes called a "cheese reaction," there is a myth that all cheese must be restricted. However, that is true only for aged cheeses such as English Stilton, but not for most processed cheese (Figure 2-71) or for most cheeses utilized in most commercial chain pizzas (Figure 2-72). Thus, it is not true that a patient on an MAO inhibitor must avoid all ingestion of any cheese. Also, it is not true that such patients must avoid all wine and beer. Canned and bottled beer are low in tyramine; generally only tap and nonpasteurized beers must be avoided (Table 2-8), and many wines, including Chianti, are actually quite low in tyramine (Figure 2-73). Thus, unless someone taking an irreversible inhibitor of MAO-A is going to eat 25 to 100 pieces of pizza or drink 25 to 100 glasses of wine or beer at a party, it is likely that he or she can still have a moderate amount of fun. Of course, every prescriber should counsel patients taking the classic MAO inhibitors about diet and keep up to date with the tyramine content of foods their patients wish to eat.

New developments for MAO inhibitors

Two developments have occurred with MAO inhibitors in recent years that appear to mitigate the risk of tyramine reactions. One is the production of inhibitors that are not only selective for MAO-A but also reversible. The other is the production of an MAO

TABLE 2-8 Hypertensive crisis

Defined by diastolic blood pressure >120 mm Hg

Potentially fatal reaction characterized by:

    Occipital headache which may radiate frontally

    Palpitation

    Neck stiffness or soreness

    Nausea

    Vomiting

    Sweating (sometimes with fever)

    Dilated pupils, photophobia

    Tachycardia or bradycardia, which can be associated with constricting chest pain

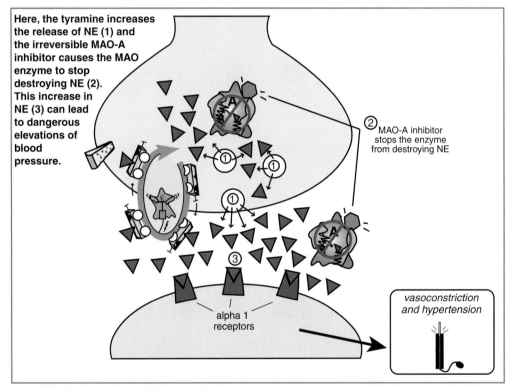

FIGURE 2-70 Inhibition of monoamine oxidase A (MAO-A) and tyramine. Here tyramine is releasing norepinephrine (NE) (1) just as shown in Figure 2-69. However, this time MAO-A is also being inhibited by an irreversible MAO-A inhibitor (2). This results in MAO-A stopping its destruction of NE (2). As indicated in Figure 2-65, such MAO-A inhibition in itself causes accumulation of NE. When MAO-A inhibition is taking place in the presence of tyramine, the combination can lead to a very large accumulation of NE (3). Such a great NE accumulation can lead to excessive stimulation of postsynaptic adrenergic receptors (3) and therefore dangerous vasoconstriction and elevation of blood pressure.

inhibitor that can be delivered through a skin patch such that both MAO-A and MAO-B are inhibited in the brain but much less MAO-A is inhibited in the gut. Neither of these innovations enhances the efficacy of MAO inhibition in depression, but both reduce the risk of hypertensive crisis, which can occur when tyramine is ingested in the diet after MAO-A is inhibited in the gut. One of these innovations is listed in Table 2-4 as moclobemide, a

Tyramine Content of Cheese

Cheese		mg per 15 g serving
English STILTON	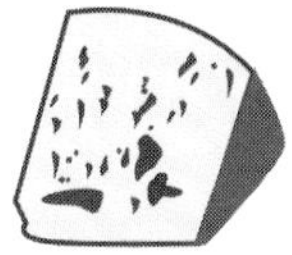	17.3
Kraft ® grated PARMESAN	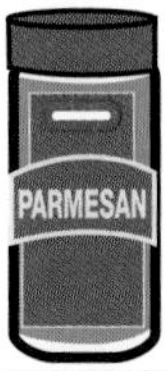	0.2
Philadelphia ® CREAM CHEESE	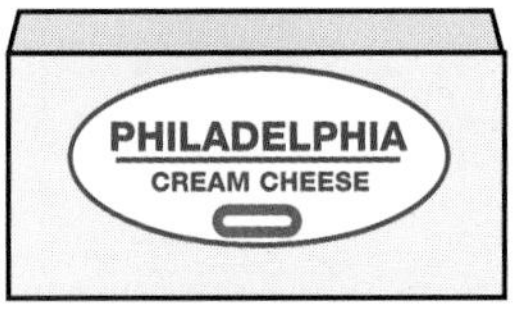	0

FIGURE 2-71 Tyramine content of cheese, part 1. The tyramine content of different types of cheeses varies. Aged cheeses such as English Stilton are high in tyramine; however, most processed cheeses are quite low in tyramine.

selective and reversible inhibitor of MAO-A, sometimes also called a RIMA (or reversible inhibitor of MAO-A). This agent is approved in Canada, Mexico, and many European and other countries but not in the United States.

The other innovation listed in Table 2-4 is the transdermal delivery system for selegiline, cleverly dosed high when delivered to the brain to inhibit both MAO-A and MAO-B there for antidepressant actions yet simultaneously dosed low when delivered to the gut to inhibit, preferentially, MAO-B so as to reduce hypertensive reactions to tyramine. Transdermal selegiline is currently available only in the United States. How it attains this clever differential inhibition of brain versus gut MAO-A is explained below.

RIMAs

The RIMAs are a nifty development in new drug therapeutics for depression because they have the potential of providing MAO-A inhibition yet with decreased risk of a tyramine reaction (Figure 2-74). How can one inhibit MAO-A to have antidepressant actions yet not inhibit MAO-A to avoid tyramine reactions? Enter the reversible inhibitors of MAO-A. If someone taking a RIMA eats aged cheese with high tyramine content in a meal, as the tyramine is absorbed it will release norepinephrine, but this will chase the reversible inhibitor off the MAO-A enzyme, reactivating MAO-A in the intestine, liver, and sympathomimetic neurons and therefore allowing the dangerous amines to be destroyed

Tyramine Content of Commercial-Chain Pizzas

Serving		mg per serving
1/2 medium double cheese, double pepperoni	Domino's Pizza™	0.378
1/2 medium double cheese, double pepperoni	Pizza Hut	0.063
1/2 medium double cheese, double pepperoni	pizza pizza	0

FIGURE 2-72 Tyramine content of cheese, part 2. The tyramine content of several commercial chain pizzas is shown here. As can be seen, these types of cheese are actually quite low in tyramine content.

(Figures 2-74 and 2-75). This is sort of like having your cake – or cheese – and eating it too. The RIMAs may thus have the same therapeutic profile as the irreversible inhibitors of MAO, particularly when they are adequately dosed, but without the same likelihood of a cheese reaction if a patient inadvertently eats otherwise dangerous dietary tyramine. However, many regulators in different countries still post a warning about tyramine reactions associated with moclobemide; thus some degree of dietary caution or restriction of tyramine intake is generally still recommended with this drug.

Transdermal delivery of selective MAO-B inhibitor

In the case of selective MAO-B inhibitors administered at low doses, no significant amount of MAO-A is inhibited and there is very little risk of hypertension from dietary amines. Patients taking MAO-B inhibitors to prevent the progression of Parkinson's disease, for example, do not require any special diet. On the other hand, MAO-B inhibitors are not effective antidepressants at doses that are selective for MAO-B. Only when the MAO-B inhibitor selegiline is given orally in doses that make it lose its selectivity and inhibit MAO-A as well is this agent effective orally as an antidepressant. However, these oral doses also cause tyramine reactions.

How can selegiline be administered so that it irreversibly inhibits MAO-A and MAO-B in the brain to provide robust antidepressant actions yet inhibits MAO-B only in the gut to avoid tyramine reactions? The answer is to deliver selegiline by a transdermal patch

FIGURE 2-73 Tyramine content of wine. Although patients taking a monoamine oxidase inhibitor (MAOI) have historically been told to avoid all wine and beer because of the risk of a tyramine reaction, canned and bottled beers as well as many wines are actually low in tyramine.

(Figure 2-76). That is, transdermal administration through a skin patch is like an intravenous infusion without the needle, delivering drug directly into the systemic circulation, hitting the brain in high doses, and avoiding a first pass through the liver (Figure 2-76). By the time drug recirculates to the intestine and liver, it has much decreased levels and significantly inhibits only MAO-B in these tissues. This action is sufficiently robust that, at least for low doses of transdermal selegiline, no dietary restrictions are necessary (Figure 2-77).

To show the profound reduction in risk of tyramine reactions with transdermal selegiline, it is useful to compare how much tyramine it takes to make blood pressure rise when patients take various MAO inhibitors, remembering that a high-tyramine diet is 40 mg of tyramine and that normals can handle around 400 mg of tyramine before blood pressure is increased (Figure 2-77). As stated earlier, perhaps as little as 10 mg of dietary tyramine is all that it takes for a traditional nonselective and irreversible oral MAO inhibitor to cause a tyramine reaction (Figure 2-77, first column). In that case, MAO-A and MAO-B are both inhibited in the brain for antidepressant actions, and they are also both inhibited in the gut, which increases the risk of tyramine reactions.

Contrast this with the patient taking an oral selective MAO-B inhibitor, who has only MAO-B inhibited in the brain and in the gut and can ingest as much tyramine as someone not taking any MAO inhibitor (Figure 2-77, the two far right columns). No tyramine reaction, but also no antidepressant action.

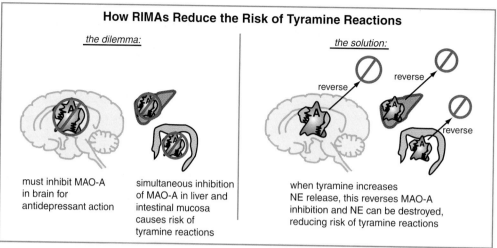

How RIMAs Reduce the Risk of Tyramine Reactions

the dilemma:

must inhibit MAO-A in brain for antidepressant action

simultaneous inhibition of MAO-A in liver and intestinal mucosa causes risk of tyramine reactions

the solution:

reverse

reverse

reverse

when tyramine increases NE release, this reverses MAO-A inhibition and NE can be destroyed, reducing risk of tyramine reactions

FIGURE 2-74 Reversible inhibitors of monoamine oxidase A (RIMAs). Inhibition of monoamine oxidase A (MAO-A) in the brain is necessary for an antidepressant effect. However, MAO-A is present not only in the brain but also in the gut. Inhibition of MAO-A in the liver and intestinal mucosa poses the risk of a tyramine reaction. How can the effects in the brain be preserved while those in the gut are avoided? Reversible inhibitors of monoamine oxidase A (RIMAs) can be removed from the enzyme by competitors. Thus when tyramine increases norepinephrine (NE) release, it is increasing the competition for MAO-A, which leads to the reversal of MAO-A inhibition; thus NE can be destroyed, reducing risk of a tyramine reaction.

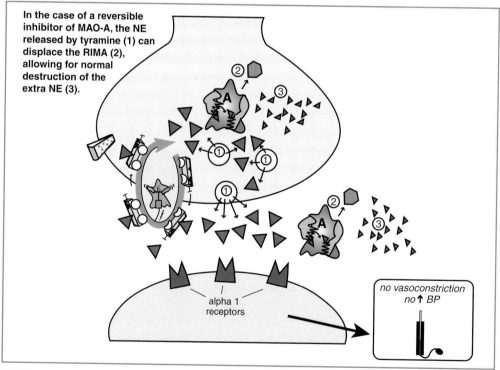

In the case of a reversible inhibitor of MAO-A, the NE released by tyramine (1) can displace the RIMA (2), allowing for normal destruction of the extra NE (3).

alpha 1 receptors

no vasoconstriction no↑ BP

FIGURE 2-75 Reversible inhibition of monoamine oxidase A (MAO-A). Shown in this figure is the combination of an MAO-A inhibitor and tyramine. However, in this case the MAO-A inhibitor is of the reversible type (reversible inhibitor of MAO-A, or RIMA). The accumulation of norepinephrine (NE) released by tyramine (1) can displace the RIMA (2), allowing for normal destruction of the extra NE (3).

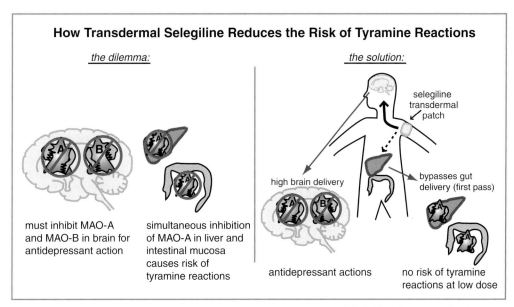

How Transdermal Selegiline Reduces the Risk of Tyramine Reactions

the dilemma:

must inhibit MAO-A and MAO-B in brain for antidepressant action

simultaneous inhibition of MAO-A in liver and intestinal mucosa causes risk of tyramine reactions

the solution:

selegiline transdermal patch

high brain delivery

bypasses gut delivery (first pass)

antidepressant actions

no risk of tyramine reactions at low dose

FIGURE 2-76 **Transdermal selegiline.** The selective monoamine oxidase B (MAO-B) inhibitor selegiline has antidepressant efficacy only when given at doses high enough also to inhibit monoamine oxidase A (MAO-A); yet when it is administered orally at these doses, it can also cause a tyramine reaction. How can selegiline inhibit both MAO-A and MAO-B in the brain to have antidepressant effects while inhibiting MAO-B only in the gut, so as to avoid a tyramine reaction? Transdermal administration of selegiline delivers the drug directly into the systemic circulation, hitting the brain in high doses and thus having antidepressant effects but avoiding a first pass through the liver and thus reducing risk of a tyramine reaction.

What is interesting are the two columns in Figure 2-77 for transdermal selegiline, showing that the average patient can take in much more than 40 mg of tyramine in a meal before showing a hypertensive reaction. At low doses of transdermal selegiline, there is substantial inhibition of both MAO-A and MAO-B in the brain but sufficiently selective inhibition of MAO-B in the gut such that no dietary restrictions are currently warranted. At high doses of transdermal selegiline, there is probably some MAO-A inhibition in the gut, with less tyramine therefore needed to raise blood pressure but still about twice as much as in a high-tyramine meal. Thus, at high doses of transdermally administered selegiline, some dietary caution against very high dietary intake of tyramine may be prudent.

Dangerous drug interactions: decongestants and drugs that boost sympathomimetic amines

Although the MAO inhibitors are famous in any pharmacology textbook for their notorious tyramine reactions, the truth is that drug–drug interactions are potentially more important clinically than dietary interactions because drug interactions are potentially more common, and some drug interactions can be much more dangerous and even lethal. Thus, when drugs that boost adrenergic stimulation by other mechanisms are added to MAO inhibitors that boost adrenergic stimulation by MAO inhibition, dangerous hypertensive reactions can ensue (Table 2-8). These interactions are generally well recognized; but, as for tyramine reactions, a certain mythology has grown up around what drugs can be given safely with MAO inhibitors.

It is true, for example, that many decongestants can adversely interact with MAO inhibitors to elevate blood pressure (Table 2-9 and Figure 2-78). However, that does

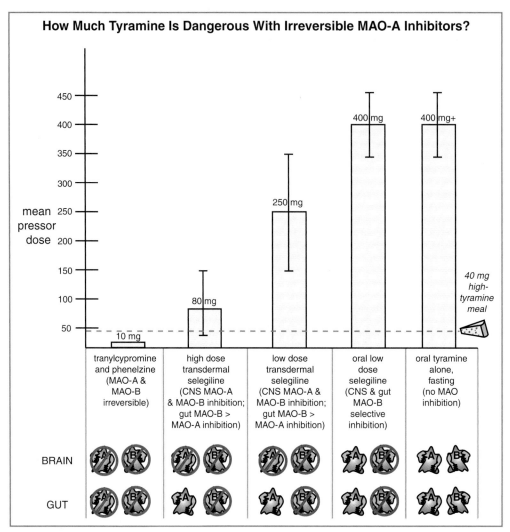

FIGURE 2-77 Dangerous tyramine levels with irreversible monoamine oxidase A (MAO-A) inhibitors. When it contains 40 mg of tyramine, a meal is considered high in this substance; however, in normal individuals (i.e., those not taking an MAO-A inhibitor) it takes as much as 400 mg of tyramine to elevate blood pressure (far right column). Patients taking low dose oral selegiline, which inhibits monoamine oxidase B (MAO-B) only, may ingest as much tyramine as someone not taking any MAO inhibitor; however, they also will not experience antidepressant effects (fourth column). In contrast, patients who take nonselective irreversible MAO inhibitors such as tranylcypromine or phenelzine may be able to ingest as little as 10 mg of tyramine before experiencing a tyramine reaction (first column). These patients experience antidepressant effects but are highly at risk for a tyramine reaction. Transdermal selegiline, on the other hand, inhibits MAO-A and MAO-B in the brain but only MAO-B in the gut; this means that it achieves antidepressant efficacy but is less likely to cause tyramine reactions. Patients taking transdermal selegiline may be able to ingest a high-tyramine meal of 40 mg or more with safety.

not mean that a patient can never take any cold preparation with an MAO inhibitor. What must be avoided are agents that add to the pro-noradrenergic actions of MAO inhibition to stimulate alpha 1 postsynaptic vascular receptors excessively (Figure 2-78). Currently, this applies mostly to phenylephrine, a relatively selective alpha 1 agonist, since three other related agents have been withdrawn from the U.S. and some other

TABLE 2-9 Potentially dangerous hypertensive combos: agents when combined with MAOIs that can cause hypertension (theoretically via adrenergic stimulation)

Decongestants
phenylephrine (alpha 1 selective agonist)
ephedrine* (ma huang, ephedra) (alpha and beta agonist; central NE and DA releaser)
pseudoephedrine* (active stereoisomer of ephedrine – same mechanism as ephedrine)
phenylpropanolamine* (alpha 1 agonist; less effective central NE/DA releaser than ephedrine)

Stimulants
amphetamines
methylphenidate

Antidepressants with NRI
TCAs
NRIs
SNRIs
NDRIs

Appetite suppressants with NRI
sibutramine
phentermine

*withdrawn from markets in the United States and some other countries.

markets – namely ephedrine, pseudoephedrine, and phenylpropanolamine (Table 2-9). Another ingredient in cold preparations that should be avoided is the cough suppressant and opiate derivate dextromethorphan, discussed in more detail in the following section.

Stimulants such as methylphenidate, which potentiate NE at adrenergic synapses by blocking NE reuptake, and amphetamines, which do not only this but also release NE and DA, can elevate blood pressure; in combination with MAO inhibitors, they should either be avoided or used with the utmost caution and monitoring in heroic cases (Table 2-10). Any drugs that block norepinephrine reuptake, from antidepressants to ADHD drugs to appetite suppressants, should also be avoided or utilized only by experts when the risks and benefits are justified in an individual patient who is given adequate monitoring.

The mechanism of excessive noradrenergic stimulation when MAO inhibitors are combined with these various agents mentioned in Table 2-9 is illustrated in Figure 2-78. Specifically, decongestants work by vasoconstricting nasal blood vessels. When topically applied or given in reasonable oral doses, however, they generally do not have sufficient systemic actions to elevate blood pressure by themselves (Figure 2-78A). Nevertheless, in some vulnerable patients, these agents can elevate blood pressure even by themselves. MAO inhibitors given by themselves do potentiate norepinephrine, but this generally is not sufficient to cause hypertension, as shown in Figure 2-78B and as already discussed above. In fact, if anything, MAO inhibitors administered by themselves may be more likely to cause hypotension, especially orthostatic hypotension. The problem comes when the two mechanisms of decongestants and MAO inhibitors are combined, especially in vulnerable patients, in whom the pro-noradrenergic actions of MAO inhibition in concert with the direct stimulation of alpha 1 receptors by an agent such as phenylephrine can result in elevated blood pressure or even a hypertensive crisis (Figure 2-78C).

Interaction of Decongestants and MAO Inhibitors

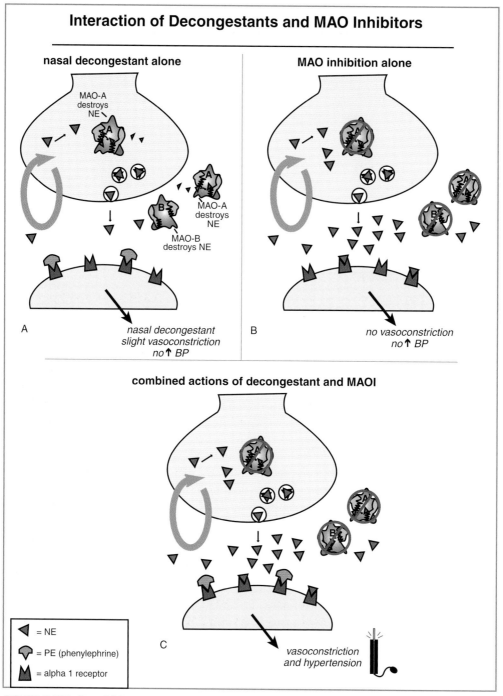

FIGURE 2-78A, B, and C Interaction of decongestants and monoamine oxidase (MAO) inhibitors.
Decongestants that stimulate postsynaptic alpha 1 receptors, such as phenylephrine, may interact with MAO inhibitors to increase risk of a tyramine reaction. Decongestants work by constricting nasal blood vessels, but they do not typically elevate blood pressure at the doses used (**A**). An MAO inhibitor given alone (and without the ingestion of tyramine) increases norepinephrine but does not usually cause vasoconstriction or hypertension (**B**). However, the noradrenergic actions of an MAO inhibitor combined with the direct alpha 1 stimulation of a decongestant may be sufficient to cause hypertension or even hypertensive crisis (**C**).

TABLE 2-10 Potentially lethal combos: agents when combined with MAOIs that can cause hyperthermia/serotonin syndrome (theoretically via SERT inhibition)

Antidepressants

SSRIs

SNRIs

TCAs (especially clomipramine)

Other TCA structures

cyclobenzaprine

carbamazepine

Appetite suppressants with SRI

sibutramine

Opioids

dextromethorphan

meperidine

tramadol

methadone

propoxyphene

Dangerous drug interactions: combining MAO inhibition with serotonin reuptake blockade

More dangerous than the combination of adrenergic stimulants with MAO inhibitors may be the combination of agents that inhibit serotonin reuptake with MAO inhibitors. Although experts can sometimes cautiously administer some of the agents listed in Table 2-9 concomitantly with MAO inhibitors under heroic circumstances, one can essentially never combine agents that have potent serotonin reuptake inhibition (listed in Table 2-10) with agents given in doses that cause substantial MAO inhibition. This includes certainly any SSRI (serotonin selective reuptake inhibitor), any SNRI (serotonin norepinephrine reuptake inhibitor, including the appetite suppressant sibutramine), and the tricyclic antidepressant clomipramine (Table 2-10). Occasionally, tricyclics with weak serotonin reuptake inhibition can be combined with MAO inhibitors for heroic cases by experts, but this is rarely done any more because of the presence of many powerful and less dangerous therapeutic options. Opioids that block serotonin reuptake, especially meperidine but also methadone and even propoxyphene, dextromethorphan, and tramadol, especially at high doses, must be avoided when an MAO inhibitor is being given. Coadministration of an MAO inhibitor with an injection of mepiridine may be the drug combination from the lists in Tables 2-9 and 2-10 that most frequently causes serious complications and even death. In fact, any agent with serotonin reuptake blockade has the potential to cause a fatal "serotonin syndrome," noted by hyperthermia, coma, seizures, brain damage, and death. Theoretically, agents with a tricyclic structure such as carbamazepine and cyclobenzaprine are put on this list as a precautionary measure, but they are not known for potent serotonin reuptake blockade (Table 2-10).

The mechanism whereby serotonin reuptake inhibition combined with MAO-A inhibition causes the serotonin syndrome and its complications is illustrated in Figure 2-79. Already discussed is the serotonin reuptake pump, or serotonin transporter, also known as SERT, and the consequences of SERT inhibition (see Figure 2-79A and Figure 2-17). We have also discussed the actions of irreversible MAO-A and B inhibitors in increasing

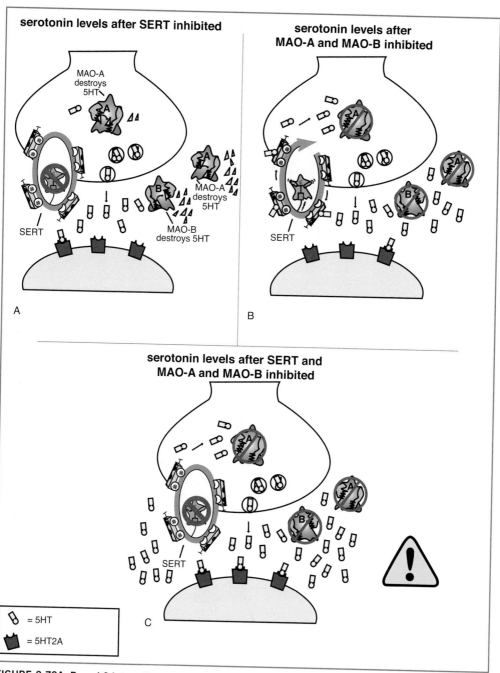

FIGURE 2-79A, B, and C Interaction of serotonin reuptake inhibitors (SRIs) and monoamine oxidase (MAO) inhibitors. Inhibition of the serotonin transporter (SERT) leads to increased synaptic availability of serotonin (**A**). Similarly, inhibition of MAO leads to increased serotonin levels (**B**). These two mechanisms in combination can cause excessive stimulation of postsynaptic serotonin receptors, which may lead to hyperthermia, seizures, coma, cardiovascular collapse, or even death.

TABLE 2-11 Some tricyclic antidepressants still in use

Generic name	Trade name
clomipramine	Anafranil
imipramine	Tofranil
amitriptyline	Elavil, Endep, Tryptizol, Loroxyl
nortriptyline	Pamelor, Endep, Aventyl
protriptyline	Vivactil
maprotiline	Ludiomil
amoxapine	Asendin
doxepin	Sinequan, Adapin
desipramine	Norpramin, Pertofran
trimipramine	Surmontil
dothiepin	Prothiaden
lofrepramine	Deprimyl, Gamanil
tianeptine	Coaxil, Stablon

synaptic concentrations of serotonin by the mechanism of MAO inhibition (see Figure 2-79B as well as Figures 2-65 to 2-67). When these two mechanisms are combined, dangerous consequences can ensue (Figure 2-79C).

Theoretically, excessive stimulation of postsynaptic serotonin receptors, possibly the most important of which is the 5HT2A receptor in the hypothalamus, causes, among other things, a disruption in thermoregulation, resulting in dangerous hyperthermia and temperatures $\geq 106°$ F or over $40°$ C. Perhaps because the serotonin neuron has MAO-B (the "wrong" form of MAO for a substrate that is metabolized preferentially by MAO-A), preventing excessive concentrations of serotonin from accumulating may be quite dependent on the serotonin reuptake pump. In contrast, norepinephrine and dopamine neurons are equipped with the "right" form of MAO (namely, MAO-A). Thus, blocking SERT alone elevates 5HT robustly at 5HT neurons, and when the extrasynaptic removal of 5HT by MAO-A is also inhibited, a potentially disastrous accumulation of 5HT can occur. The consequences can range from migraines, myoclonus, diarrhea, agitation, and even psychosis on the milder end of the spectrum of potential symptomatology to hyperthermia, seizures, coma, cardiovascular collapse, permanent hyperthermic brain damage, and even death at the severe end of the spectrum of symptoms. For this reason, it is important to monitor closely all concomitant medication for patients on MAO inhibitors, even in patients taking the new RIMAs or the selegiline patch, where these drug interactions also apply.

Classic antidepressants: tricyclic antidepressants

The tricyclic antidepressants (Table 2-11) were so named because their chemical structure contains three rings (Figure 2-80). The tricyclic antidepressants were synthesized about the same time as other three-ringed molecules that were shown to be effective tranquilizers for schizophrenia (i.e., the early antipsychotic neuroleptic drugs such as chlorpromazine) (Figure 2-80). The tricyclic antidepressants were a disappointment when tested as antipsychotics. Even though they had a three-ringed structure, they were not effective in the treatment of schizophrenia and were almost discarded. However, during testing for schizophrenia, they were discovered to be antidepressants. That is, careful clinicians detected

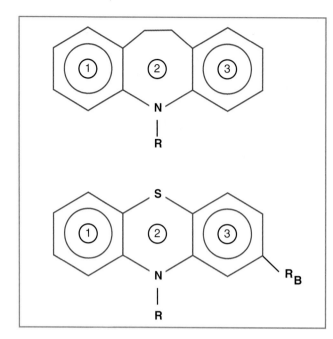

FIGURE 2-80 Tricyclic structure. At top is the chemical structure of a tricyclic antidepressant (TCA). The three rings show how this group of drugs got its name. At bottom is the general chemical formula for the phenothiazine antipsychotic drugs. These drugs also have three rings, and the first antidepressants – the TCAs – were modeled after such drugs.

antidepressant properties in schizophrenic patients, although not antipsychotic properties in these patients. Thus, the antidepressant properties of the tricyclic antidepressants were serendipitously observed in the 1950s and 1960s and eventually the TCAs were marketed for the treatment of depression.

Long after their antidepressant properties were observed, the tricyclic antidepressants were discovered to block the reuptake pumps for norepinephrine or for both norepinephrine and serotonin. Some tricyclics have much more potency for inhibition of the serotonin reuptake pump (e.g., clomipramine) (Figures 2-81A and 2-82); others are more selective for norepinephrine over serotonin (e.g., desipramine, maprotiline, nortriptyline, protriptyline) (Figures 2-81B and 2-83). Most, however, block both serotonin and norepinephrine reuptake to some extent.

In addition, some tricyclic antidepressants have antagonist actions at 5HT2A and 5HT2C receptors. Although these properties have not been emphasized in classic explanations of the mechanism of action of these drugs, recent developments showing the importance of blocking 5HT2A and 5HT2C receptors in mediating the mechanism of therapeutic action of other drugs strongly suggest that these properties could contribute to the therapeutic profile of those tricyclics that have such pharmacologic actions (Figures 2-84 and 2-85). Specifically, blocking 5HT2A receptors is associated with improvement of sleep and has a potential antidepressant action in its own right (Figure 2-84), possibly linked to the ability of 5HT2A/5HT2C receptor blockade to disinhibit both DA and NE release. This was discussed extensively above in relation to SARI action and trazodone and illustrated in Figure 2-64.

The major limitation to the tricyclic antidepressants has never been their efficacy: these are quite efficacious agents. The problem with drugs in this class is the fact that all of them share at least four other unwanted pharmacological actions shown in Figure 2-81, namely,

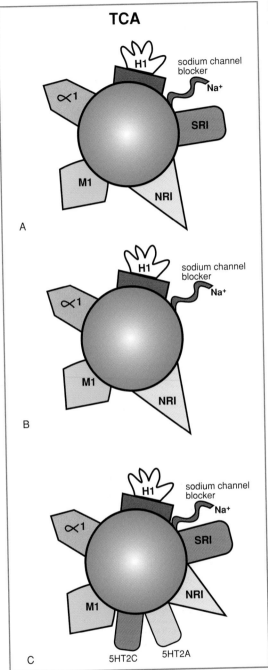

A

B

C

FIGURE 2-81 Icons of tricyclic antidepressants.
All tricyclic antidepressants block reuptake of
norepinephrine and are antagonists at histamine 1,
alpha 1 adrenergic, and muscarinic cholinergic
receptors; they also block voltage-sensitive sodium
channels (**A, B, and C**). Some tricyclic
antidepressants are also potent inhibitors of the
serotonin reuptake pump (**A**), and some may
additionally be antagonists at serotonin 2A and 2C
receptors (**C**).

blockade of muscarinic cholinergic receptors, histamine 1 receptors, alpha 1 adrenergic
receptors, and voltage-sensitive sodium channels (see Figures 2-86 through 2-88).

Blockade of histamine 1 receptors, also called antihistaminic action, causes sedation
and may cause weight gain (Figure 2-86). Blockade of M1 muscarinic cholinergic receptors,
also known as anticholinergic actions, causes dry mouth, blurred vision, urinary retention,

SRI Inserted

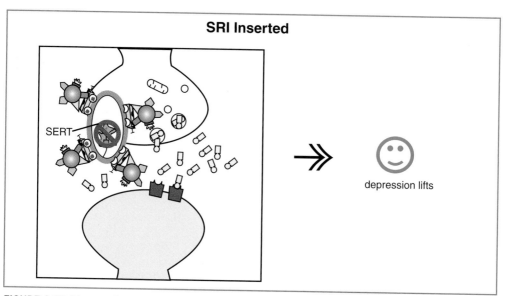

depression lifts

FIGURE 2-82 Therapeutic actions of tricyclic antidepressants (TCAs), part 1. In this figure, the icon of the TCA is shown with its serotonin reuptake inhibitor (SRI) portion inserted into the serotonin transporter (SERT), blocking it and causing an antidepressant effect.

NRI Inserted

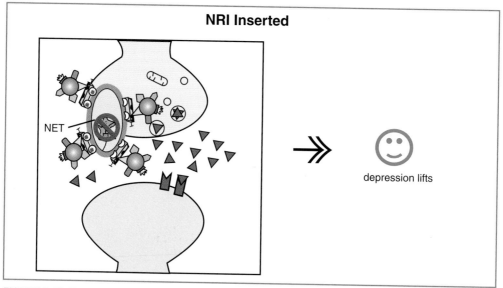

depression lifts

FIGURE 2-83 Therapeutic actions of tricyclic antidepressants (TCAs), part 2. In this figure, the icon of the TCA is shown with its norepinephrine reuptake inhibitor (NRI) portion inserted into the norepinephrine transporter (NET), blocking it and causing an antidepressant effect. Thus both the serotonin reuptake portion (see Figure 2-82) and the norepinephrine reuptake portion of the TCA act pharmacologically to cause an antidepressant effect.

and constipation (Figure 2-87). To the extent that these agents can block M3 cholinergic receptors, they may interfere with insulin action. Blockade of alpha 1 adrenergic receptors causes orthostatic hypotension and dizziness (Figure 2-88). Tricyclic antidepressants also weakly block voltage-sensitive sodium channels in the heart and brain; in overdose, this action is thought to be the cause of coma and seizures due to central

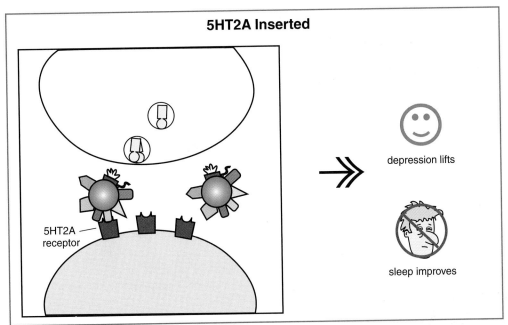

FIGURE 2-84 Therapeutic actions of tricyclic antidepressants (TCAs), part 3. In this figure, the icon of the TCA is shown with its 5HT2A portion inserted into the 5HT2A receptor, blocking it and causing an antidepressant effect as well as potentially improving sleep.

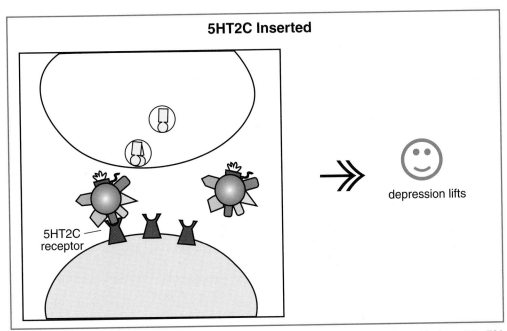

FIGURE 2-85 Therapeutic actions of tricyclic antidepressants (TCAs), part 4. In this figure, the icon of the TCA is shown with its 5HT2C portion inserted into the 5HT2C receptor, blocking it and causing an antidepressant effect.

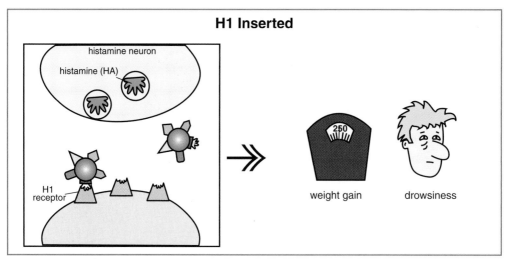

FIGURE 2-86 Side effects of tricyclic antidepressants (TCAs), part 1. In this figure, the icon of the TCA is shown with its antihistamine (H1) portion inserted into histamine receptors, causing the side effects of weight gain and drowsiness.

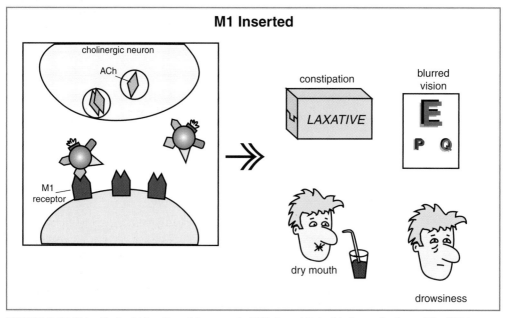

FIGURE 2-87 Side effects of tricyclic antidepressants (TCAs), part 2. In this figure, the icon of the TCA is shown with its anticholinergic/antimuscarinic (M1) portion inserted into acetylcholine receptors, causing the side effects of constipation, blurred vision, dry mouth, and drowsiness.

nervous system (CNS) actions as well as cardiac arrhythmias and cardiac arrest and death due to peripheral cardiac actions (Figure 2-89).

The term "tricyclic antidepressant" is archaic in today's pharmacology. First, the antidepressants that block monoamine transporters are not all tricyclic anymore: the new agents can have one, two, three, or four rings in their structures. Second, the tricyclic antidepressants are not merely antidepressants, since some of them have anti–obsessive compulsive

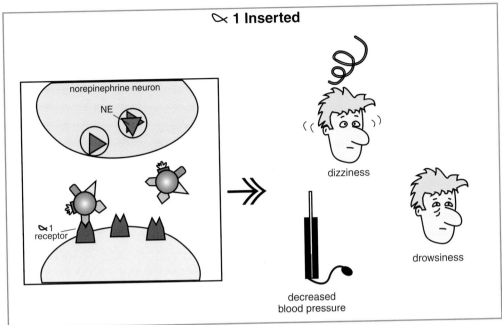

FIGURE 2-88 Side effects of tricyclic antidepressants (TCAs), part 3. In this figure, the icon of the TCA is shown with its alpha-adrenergic antagonist (alpha) portion inserted into alpha 1 adrenergic receptors, causing the side effects of dizziness, drowsiness, and decreased blood pressure.

disorder effects and others have anti-panic effects. Because of their side effects and potential for death in overdose, tricyclic antidepressants have fallen into second-line use for depression. However, there remains considerable use of these agents for difficult-to-treat patients, and the cost of these agents is quite low.

Antidepressant pharmacokinetics

The CYP450 enzymes and the **pharmacokinetic** actions they represent must be contrasted with the **pharmacodynamic** actions of antidepressants discussed in the previous sections of this chapter, focusing on the various mechanisms of action of antidepressants. Although most of this book deals with the **pharmacodynamics** of psychopharmacological agents, especially how drugs act on the brain, the following section provides a quick overview of the **pharmacokinetics** of antidepressants.

CYP450 1A2

One CYP450 enzyme of specific relevance to antidepressants is 1A2 (Figures 2-90, 2-91, and 2-92). Certain tricyclic antidepressants (TCAs) are **substrates** for this enzyme, especially the secondary amines like clomipramine and imipramine (Figure 2-90). CYP450 1A2 demethylates such TCAs but does not thereby inactivate them. In this case, the desmethyl metabolite of the TCA is still an active drug (e.g., desmethylclomipramine, desipramine, and nortriptyline; see Figure 2-90).

CYP450 1A2 is **inhibited** by the serotonin selective reuptake inhibitor (SSRI) fluvoxamine (Figure 2-91). Thus, when fluvoxamine is given concomitantly with other drugs that

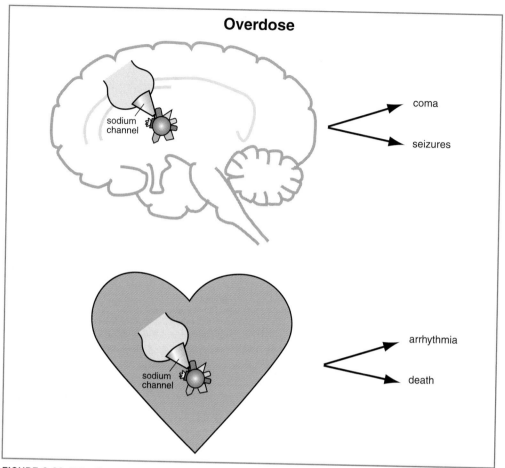

FIGURE 2-89 Side effects of tricyclic antidepressants (TCAs), part 4. In this figure, the icon of the TCA is shown with its sodium channel blocker portion blocking voltage-sensitive sodium channels in the brain (top) and heart (bottom). In overdose, this action can lead to coma, seizures, arrhythmia, and even death.

use 1A2 for their metabolism, those drugs can no longer be metabolized as efficiently. Two instances of potentially important drug interactions are seen when fluvoxamine is given along with either duloxetine or theophyllin (Figure 2-92). In those cases, the duloxetine (or theophyllin) dose must often be lowered or else the blood levels of drug will rise and possibly cause side effects or even be toxic. The same may occur with caffeine.

CYP450 2D6

Another important CYP450 enzyme for antidepressants is 2D6. Tricyclic antidepressants are **substrates** of 2D6, which hydroxylates and thereby inactivates the TCAs. Several other antidepressants from the SSRI class are substrates of CYP2D6, and some are both substrates and inhibitors. We have already discussed venlafaxine as an important substrate of CYP2D6, as this antidepressant is converted into its active metabolite desvenlafaxine by CYP2D6, as shown in Figure 2-37. Most antidepressants that are substrates for CYP2D6, however, are converted into inactive metabolites, (e.g., the metabolites of duloxetine, paroxetine, atomoxetine, and tricyclic antidepressants are inactive) (Figure 2-93). There is a wide range of potency for 2D6 inhibition by many antidepressants, with paroxetine, fluoxetine,

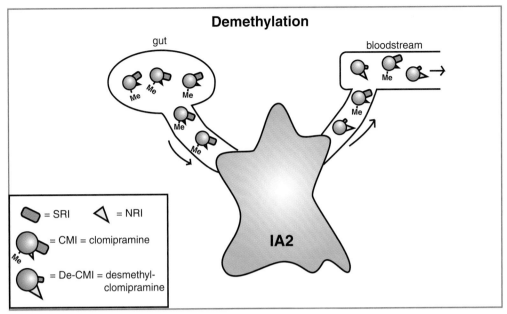

FIGURE 2-90 Substrates for CYP450 1A2. Certain tricyclic antidepressants, especially secondary amines such as clomipramine and imipramine, are substrates for CYP450 1A2. By demethylation, this enzyme converts the tricyclics into active metabolites to form desmethylclomipramine and desipramine, respectively.

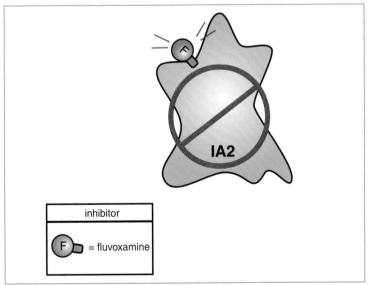

FIGURE 2-91 Inhibitors of CYP450 1A2. The serotonin selective reuptake inhibitor (SSRI) fluvoxamine is a potent inhibitor of the enzyme CYP450 1A2.

and duloxetine among the more potent inhibitors and reboxetine, bupropion, fluvoxamine, sertraline, and citalopram among those that are less potent (Figure 2-94).

One of the most important drug interactions that antidepressants can cause through inhibition of 2D6 is to raise plasma drug levels of tricyclic antidepressants (TCAs) when TCAs are given concomitantly with SSRIs or when there is switching between TCAs and SSRIs. Since TCAs are substrates for 2D6 and various antidepressants are inhibitors of

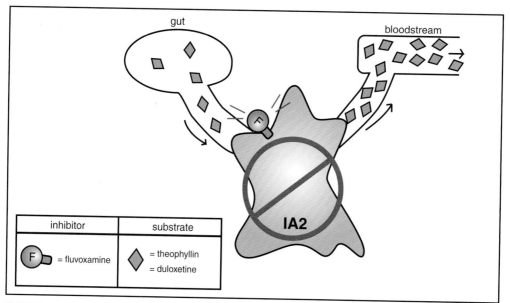

FIGURE 2-92 Consequences of CYP450 1A2 inhibition. Theophylline and duloxetine are substrates for CYP450 1A2. Thus, in the presence of the CYP450 1A2 inhibitor fluvoxamine, their levels will rise; therefore their dose must often be lowered in order to avoid side effects.

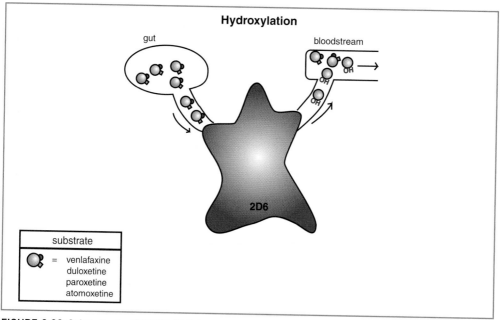

FIGURE 2-93 Substrates for CYP450 2D6. Venlafaxine, duloxetine, paroxetine, and atomoxetine are substrates for CYP450 2D6, which converts these antidepressants to active (desvenlafaxine) or inactive metabolites.

2D6 (Figure 2-94), concomitant administration will raise TCA levels, perhaps to toxic levels (Figure 2-95). Concomitant administration of an SSRI and a TCA thus requires monitoring of the plasma drug concentrations of the TCA and probably requires a dose reduction of the TCA.

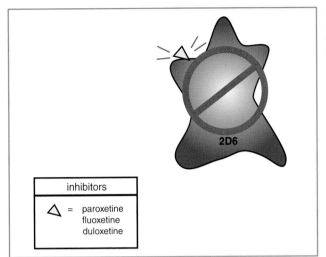

FIGURE 2-94 Inhibitors of CYP450 2D6. Some antidepressants (paroxetine, fluoxetine, duloxetine) are inhibitors of CYP450 2D6.

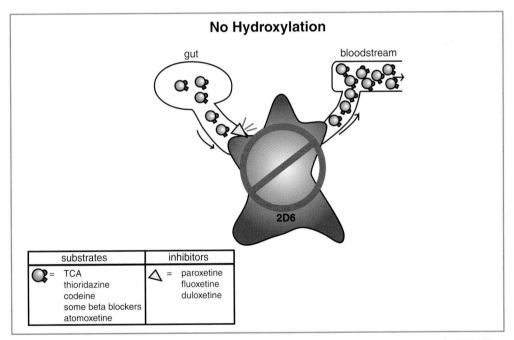

FIGURE 2-95 Consequences of CYP450 2D6 inhibition. If a tricyclic antidepressant (a substrate for CYP450 2D6) is given concomitantly with a serotonin selective reuptake inhibitor or a serotonin norepinephrine reuptake inhibitor that is an inhibitor of CYP450 2D6, this will cause the levels of the tricyclic antidepressant to increase, which can be toxic. Therefore either monitoring of tricyclic plasma concentration with dose reduction or avoidance of this combination is required.

Other substrates of 2D6 whose plasma drug levels can be raised by antidepressants that are 2D6 inhibitors include venlafaxine, duloxetine, paroxetine, and atomoxetine; however, clinical experience suggests that only atomoxetine commonly requires dosage reduction when administered with a 2D6 inhibitor. These interactions among antidepressants are important to bear in mind for prescribers who commonly use one antidepressant to augment

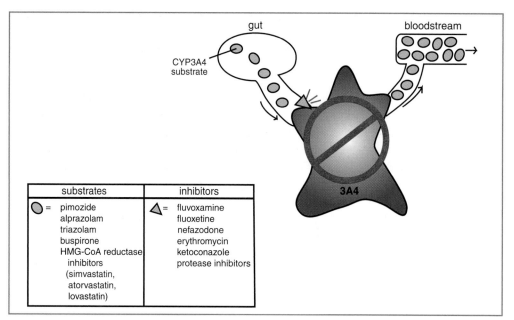

substrates	inhibitors
◐ = pimozide alprazolam triazolam buspirone HMG-CoA reductase inhibitors (simvastatin, atorvastatin, lovastatin)	△ = fluvoxamine fluoxetine nefazodone erythromycin ketoconazole protease inhibitors

FIGURE 2-96 Substrates and inhibitors for CYP450 3A4. The antipsychotic pimozide, the benzodiazepines alprazolam and triazolam, the anxiolytic buspirone, and HMG-CoA reductase inhibitors are all substrates for CYP450 3A4. Fluvoxamine, fluoxetine, and nefazodone are moderate CYP450 3A4 inhibitors, as are some nonpsychotropic agents.

another or who switch patients from one antidepressant to another without a full washout of the first antidepressant. Concomitant administration of an antidepressant that is a 2D6 inhibitor could theoretically interfere with the analgesic actions of codeine (which must be converted to an active metabolite by 2D6 in order to work) and could theoretically raise the plasma drug levels of some beta blockers, as well as thioridazine, and cause dangerous arrhythmias.

CYP450 3A4

A third important CYP450 enzyme for antidepressants is 3A4 (Figure 2-96). Some antidepressants are substrates for 3A4 and others are inhibitors of this enzyme. Many drugs, including some antidepressants that are substrates for 3A4, are also substrates for several other metabolic pathways; in these cases, inhibition of 3A4 does not necessarily raise the plasma drug levels of such agents. Generally, the most important thing for a clinician to know is which drugs can have clinically important increases in their plasma drug levels when 3A4 is inhibited. It is thus important to know which of these drugs are substrates and which are inhibitors of 3A4.

Among psychotropic drugs, the antipsychotic pimozide, the anticonvulsant and mood stabilizer carbamazepine, the benzodiazepines alprazolam and triazolam, and the anxiolytic buspirone are all **substrates** of 3A4 (Figure 2-96). Among nonpsychotropic drugs, certain cholesterol-lowering HMG-CoA reductase inhibitors (e.g., simvastatin, atorvastatin, and lovastatin but not pravastatin or fluvastatin) are also **substrates** for 3A4 (Figure 2-96).

Among the antidepressants, fluvoxamine, fluoxetine, and nefazodone are moderately potent 3A4 **inhibitors**, with reboxetine and sertraline weaker 3A4 **inhibitors**

(Figure 2-96). Among nonpsychotropic drugs, certain protease inhibitors for the treatment of human immunodeficiency virus (HIV) infection, certain azole antifungals (e.g., ketoconazole), and macrolide antibiotics (e.g., erythromycin) are all potent 3A4 **inhibitors** (Figure 2-96).

Clinically important consequences of combining 3A4 substrates with 3A4 inhibitors

Combining a 3A4 inhibitor with the 3A4 substrate pimozide can result in elevated plasma pimozide levels, with consequent QTc prolongation and dangerous cardiac arrhythmias. Combining a 3A4 inhibitor with carbamazepine, alprazolam, or triazolam can cause significant sedation due to elevated plasma drug levels of the latter agents. Combining a 3A4 inhibitor with certain cholesterol-lowering drugs that are 3A4 substrates (e.g., simvastatin, atorvastatin, and lovastatin but not pravastatin or fluvastatin) can increase the risk of muscle damage and rhabdomyolysis from elevated plasma levels of these statins.

Drug interactions mediated by CYP450 enzymes are constantly being discovered; the active clinician who combines drugs must be alert to these and thus remain continually up to speed on what drug interactions are important. Here we present only the general concepts of drug interactions at CYP450 enzyme systems, but the specifics should be found in a comprehensive and up-to-date reference source before prescribing.

CYP450 inducers

Finally, drugs can not only be substrates or inhibitors for CYP450 enzymes; they can also be **inducers**. An inducer increases the activity of the enzyme over time because it induces the synthesis of more copies of the enzyme. One example of this is the effects of the anticonvulsant and mood stabilizer carbamazepine, which induces 3A4 over time. Another example of CYP450 enzyme induction is cigarette smoking, which induces 1A2 over time. The consequence of such enzyme induction is that substrates for the induced enzyme will be more efficiently metabolized over time, and thus their levels in the plasma will fall. Doses of such substrate drugs may therefore need to be increased over time to compensate for this.

For example, carbamazepine is both a substrate and an inducer of 3A4. Thus, as treatment becomes chronic, 3A4 is induced and carbamazepine blood levels fall. Failure to recognize this and to increase carbamazepine dosage to compensate may lead to a failure of anticonvulsant or mood stabilizing efficacy, with breakthrough symptoms occurring as a result.

Another important thing to remember about a CYP450 inducer is what happens if the inducer is stopped. Thus, if one stops smoking, levels of drugs that are 1A2 substrates will rise. If one stops carbamazepine, levels of drugs that are 3A4 substrates will rise.

In summary, many antidepressant drug interactions require dosage adjustment of one of the drugs. A few combinations must be strictly avoided. Many drug interactions are statistically but not clinically significant. By following the principles outlined here, the skilled practitioner will learn whether any given drug interaction is clinically relevant.

Trimonoaminergic modulators (triple monoamine modulators, or TMMs)

An increasing number of agents now appear to modulate the trimonoaminergic neurotransmitter system of 5HT, NE, and DA by mechanisms other than inhibition of monoamine transporters and in a manner that may be more effective when given with a monoamine

TABLE 2-12 Trimonoamine modulators (TMMs)

- folate
- L-MTHF (L-methyl-tetrahydrofolate)
- estrogen
- estrogen replacement therapy
- thyroid hormones (T3/T4)
- lithium
- brain stimulation
- psychotherapy

transport inhibitor rather than as a monotherapy (Tables 2-2 and 2-12). These therapeutic interventions range from hormones to vitamins, medical foods, ions, electrical and magnetic brain stimulation, and even psychotherapy (Table 2-12). A few of these key therapeutics are reviewed here very briefly to provide a quick overview of this evolving concept. All are categorized as "trimonoaminergic modulators," or TMMs (Tables 2-2 and 2-12), because their various mechanisms of action are all postulated to share in common the modulation of one or more of the monoamines. Thus, TMMs theoretically boost the action of antidepressants in the treatment of depressive episodes, particularly when given as augmenting agents for the treatment of depressive episodes that fail to remit with traditional antidepressant treatment.

Estrogen as a trimonoaminergic, GABA, and glutamate modulator

The hormone estrogen has a profound impact on mood and on the trimonoamine neurotransmitter system and thus can be considered a trimonoaminergic modulator (TMM). Estrogen also modulates the activity of other neurotransmitters, including GABA (gamma-aminobutyric acid) and glutamate, as will be discussed below. Many of estrogen's effects upon various neurotransmitter systems appear to be the result of estrogen binding to nuclear hormone receptors, known as estrogen receptors (Figure 2-97). Receptors for estrogen may also exist in neuronal cell membranes, but these are not yet well characterized. However, it is well established that nuclear ligand receptors specifically for estrogen are transformed into nuclear ligand–activated transcription factors when estrogen binds to them.

Estrogen and nuclear hormone receptors

Estrogen modulates gene expression by binding to nuclear hormone receptors for estrogen – i.e., "estrogen receptors" (Figure 2-97A). Receptors for estrogen differ from tissue to tissue and may differ from brain region to brain region. In addition to various subtypes of estrogen receptors, there are also nuclear hormone receptors for progesterone and androgens as well as for other steroids such as glucocorticoids and mineralocorticoids. Unlike neurotransmitter receptors located on neuronal membranes, nuclear ligand–activated receptors for estrogen are located in the neuronal cell nucleus, so estrogen must penetrate the neuronal membrane and the nuclear membrane to find its receptors, which are located near the genes that estrogen influences (Figure 2-97). These genes are called estrogen response elements (Figure 2-97B). Activation of estrogen response elements by estrogen requires receptor

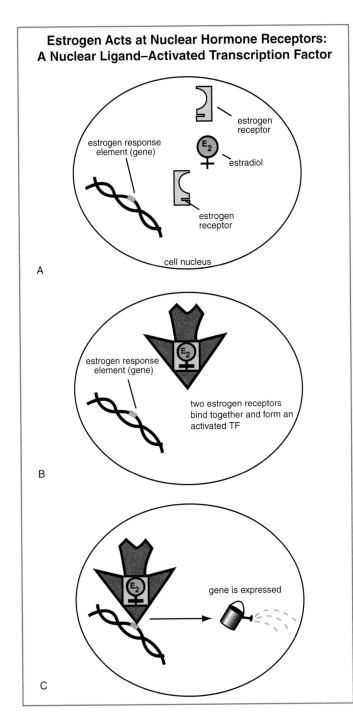

Estrogen Acts at Nuclear Hormone Receptors: A Nuclear Ligand–Activated Transcription Factor

A

- estrogen receptor
- E₂ / estradiol
- estrogen receptor
- estrogen response element (gene)
- cell nucleus

B

- estrogen response element (gene)
- two estrogen receptors bind together and form an activated TF

C

- gene is expressed

FIGURE 2-97A, B, and C

Estrogen and nuclear hormone receptors. Estrogen modulates gene expression by binding to estrogen receptors. Estrogen receptors differ from tissue to tissue and may differ from brain region to brain region. (**A**) Unlike neurotransmitter receptors located on neuronal membranes, receptors for estradiol are located in the neuronal cell nucleus, so estradiol must penetrate the neuronal membrane and the nuclear membrane to find its receptors, which are therefore located near the genes to be influenced. These genes are called estrogen response elements. (**B**) The expression of estrogen response elements within the DNA of the neuron must be initiated by estrogen and its receptor. Activation of these genes by estradiol requires "dimerization" (i.e., coupling of two copies of the estrogen receptor) when estrogen binds to the receptor to form an active transcription factor (TF) capable of "turning on" the estrogen response element. (**C**) Once the estrogen receptors are activated by estradiol into transcription factors, they activate gene expression by the estrogen response elements in the neuron's DNA. The gene products expressed include direct trophic factors such as nerve growth factor (NGF) and brain-derived neurotrophic factor (BDNF), which can facilitate synaptogenesis and prevent apoptosis and neurodegeneration.

"dimerization" (i.e., the coupling of two copies of the estrogen receptor) when estrogen binds to them; this forms an active transcription factor capable of "turning on" estrogen response elements (Figure 2-97B). Once estrogen receptors are activated as transcription factors, they activate gene expression in the neuron by binding to estrogen response elements in the neuron's DNA (Figure 2-97C).

Estrogen and trophic actions on dendritic spine formation

Gene products that are regulated by estrogen include trophic factors such as brain-derived neurotrophic factor (BDNF) as well as neurotransmitter synthesizing and metabolizing enzymes and various neurotransmitter receptors. Dramatic evidence of estrogen's trophic properties can be observed in hypothalamic and hippocampal neurons in adult female experimental animals within days and across a single menstrual (estrus) cycle (Figures 2-98 and 2-99). During the early phase of the cycle, estradiol levels rise, causing dendritic spines to form specifically in the ventromedial hypothalamus and on pyramidal neurons in the hippocampus of female rats. Progesterone administration rapidly potentiates this, so spine formation is at its greatest when both estrogen and progesterone peak just after the first half of the cycle (Figure 2-98). However, once estrogen levels fall significantly and progesterone continues to rise, the presence of progesterone without estrogen triggers downregulation of these spines by the end of the estrus cycle (Figure 2-98).

Estrogen as a GABA (gamma-aminobutyric acid) inhibitor

One hypothesis to explain the mechanism of this cyclical formation and then loss of dendritic spines is that estrogen regulates a type of spine formation that occurs when neurons are active and that reverses when neurons are inactive, known as "activity-dependent" dendritic spine formation (Figure 2-99). As estrogen levels rise and fall during the menstrual cycle, estrogen can cause a corresponding cyclical rather than continuous activation of neurons in certain brain areas. The cyclical activation of these neurons is explained by the fact that estrogen exerts a cyclical inhibitory influence on GABA interneurons (Figure 2-99). Estrogen inhibits this inhibition. This is not psychopharmacological double talk but a well-known phenomenon called disinhibition, just a fancy way of saying "activated."

By inhibiting GABAergic inhibition, estrogen thus activates pyramidal neurons (Figure 2-99B). Estrogen does this by downregulating and thus reducing the synthesis of glutamic acid decarboxylase (GAD), the enzyme that synthesizes GABA. This, in turn, reduces the synthesis of GABA itself, which diminishes the release of GABA from GABAergic interneurons. No GABA, no inhibition; no inhibition, pyramidal neurons are activated.

Estrogen as a glutamate activator

When estrogen activates pyramidal neurons, these neurons release glutamate (Figures 2-99B and 2-99C). As estrogen levels rise during the first half of the menstrual cycle, so does pyramidal neuron activation by glutamate from other pyramidal neurons (Figure 2-99B); as estrogen levels fall during the last half of the menstrual cycle, pyramidal cells lose their activation (Figure 2-99C).

The cyclical formation of dendritic spines that is the consequence of these cyclical changes in estrogen levels is shown for a single menstrual (estrus) cycle in Figure 2-99A, B, and C. Thus, at the beginning of the cycle, estrogen levels are low, so GABA interneurons are active. When GABA interneurons are active, they inhibit pyramidal neurons (Figure 2-99A). However, as estrogen levels rise during the first half of the cycle, GABA interneurons are progressively inhibited, causing progressive disinhibition of pyramidal neurons (Figure 2-99B).

Disinhibited pyramidal neurons release glutamate (Figure 2-99B). Glutamate then interacts at a number of glutamate receptors, including postsynaptic NMDA receptors on other pyramidal neurons (Figure 2-99B). Sustained activation of NMDA receptors can

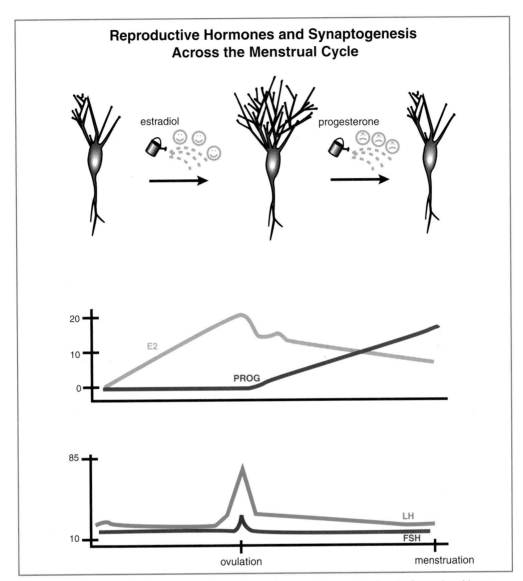

FIGURE 2-98 Reproductive hormones and synaptogenesis across the menstrual cycle. Dramatic evidence of estrogen's trophic properties can be observed in hypothalamic and hippocampal neurons in adult female experimental animals within days and across a single menstrual (estrus) cycle. During the early phase of the cycle, estradiol levels rise, and this trophic influence induces dendritic spine formation and synaptogenesis. Progesterone administration rapidly potentiates this, so spine formation is at its greatest when both estrogen and progesterone peak just after the first half of the cycle. However, once estrogen levels fall significantly and progesterone continues to rise, the presence of progesterone without estrogen triggers downregulation of these spines and removal of the synapses by the end of the estrus cycle.

trigger long-term potentiation and trophic changes in postsynaptic neurons, including the formation of dendritic spines by the middle of the cycle (Figure 2-99C). Once estrogen levels fall by the end of the cycle, glutamate neurons again become inactive, and activity-dependent dendritic spine formation is not maintained (back to Figure 2-99A).

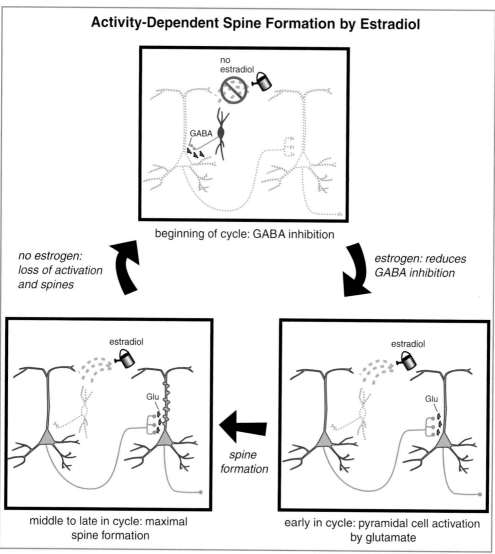

FIGURE 2-99 Activity-dependent spine formation by estradiol. Estrogen exerts a cyclical inhibitory influence on gamma-aminobutyric acid (GABA) interneurons, which in turn regulate pyramidal neurons. When estrogen levels are low, GABA interneurons are active; thus pyramidal neurons are inhibited (**A**). As estrogen levels rise early in the menstrual cycle, GABA inhibition is reduced, thus disinhibiting pyramidal neurons and leading to glutamate release (**B**). Sustained activation of N-methyl-d-aspartate (NMDA) receptors by glutamate, achieved by the middle or late cycle, can trigger long-term potentiation and trophic changes that include the formation of dendritic spines (**C**). As estrogen levels fall by the end of the menstrual cycle, GABA interneurons become active again and resume inhibition of pyramidal neurons, preventing the maintenance of dendritic spine formation (**A**).

Estrogen regulation and major depression over a woman's life cycle

Estrogen levels shift rather dramatically across the female life cycle in relation to various types of reproductive events (Figure 2-100). Such shifts are also linked to the onset or recurrence of major depressive episodes (Figures 2-100 and 2-101). In men, the incidence of depression rises in puberty and then is essentially constant throughout life, despite a slowly declining testosterone level from age twenty-five onward (Figure 2-102). By contrast, in

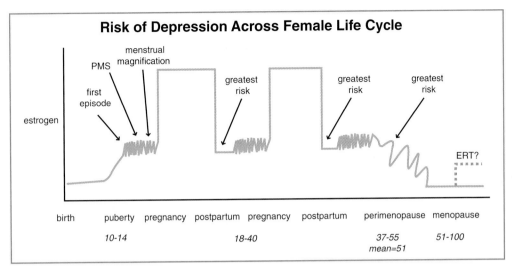

FIGURE 2-100 Risk of depression across female life cycle. Several issues of importance in assessing women's vulnerability to the onset and recurrence of depression are illustrated here. These include first onset in puberty and young adulthood, premenstrual syndrome (PMS), and menstrual magnification as harbingers of future episodes or incomplete recovery states from prior episodes of depression. There are two periods of especially high vulnerability for first episodes of depression or for recurrence if a woman has already experienced an episode, namely, the postpartum period and the perimenopausal period. ERT, estrogen replacement therapy.

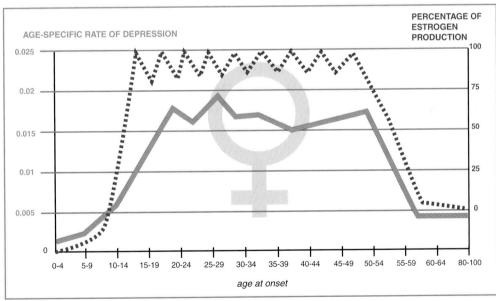

FIGURE 2-101 Incidence of depression across female life cycle. The incidence of depression in women mirrors their changes in estrogen across the life cycle. As estrogen levels rise during puberty, the incidence of depression also rises; it falls again during menopause, when estrogen levels fall. Thus before puberty and after menopause, women have the same frequency of depression as men (see Figure 2-102). During their childbearing years, however, when estrogen is high and cycling, the incidence of depression in women is two to three times as high as it is in men (see Figure 2-102).

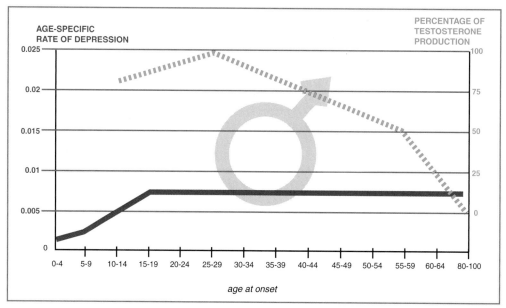

FIGURE 2-102 Incidence of depression across the male life cycle. In men, the incidence of depression rises in puberty and then is essentially constant throughout life, despite a slowly declining testosterone level from age twenty-five onward.

women, the incidence of depression in many ways mirrors their changes in estrogen across the life cycle (Figure 2-101). That is, as estrogen levels rise during puberty, the incidence of depression skyrockets in women; then, after menopause, it falls again (Figure 2-101). Thus, women have the same frequency of depression as men before puberty and after menopause. However, during their childbearing years, when estrogen is high and cycling, the incidence of depression in women is two to three times higher than it is in men (compare Figures 2-101 and 2-102).

Depression and its treatment during childbearing years and pregnancy

As estrogen levels first begin to rise and then cycle during puberty, first episodes of depression often begin (Figure 2-100). Unfortunately these episodes are frequently unrecognized and untreated. Although antidepressant efficacy is not well documented under the age of eighteen for most antidepressants and suicidality is thought to be increased in patients under the age of twenty-five for all antidepressants, treatment of first episodes of depression at any age should be seriously considered, including evaluation and initiation of treatment with antidepressants for unipolar depression or with mood stabilizers for bipolar disorder (Figure 2-103).

Throughout the childbearing years, most women experience some irritability during the late luteal phase just prior to menstrual flow of menstrual cycles; however, if this is actually incapacitating, it may be a form of mood disorder known as premenstrual dysphoric disorder (PMDD) or as premenstrual syndrome (PMS) (Figure 2-100). PMDD can be treated cyclically with oral contraceptive hormones or alternatively with antidepressants, sometimes just during the late luteal phase (Figure 2-103). In some patients, this end-of-cycle worsening is really the unmasking of a mood disorder that is actually present during the whole cycle but is sufficiently worse at the end of the cycle that it becomes obvious as a phenomenon called "menstrual magnification" (Figure 2-100). This may be a harbinger of

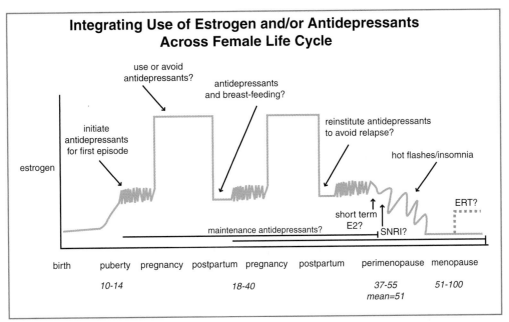

FIGURE 2-103 Use of estrogen and/or antidepressants across the female life cycle. This figure illustrates some of the issues involved in integrating endocrine shifts and events related to a woman's life cycle with treatment of a mood disorder with antidepressants and/or estrogen. These include use of antidepressants prior to age eighteen if necessary, calculating risks versus benefits of antidepressant maintenance during pregnancy and breast-feeding, and deciding whether to include estrogens or antidepressants in the treatment of perimenopausal symptoms or after menopause. E2, estradiol; SNRI, serotonin norepinephrine reuptake inhibitor; ERT, estrogen replacement therapy.

further worsening or may also represent a state of incomplete recovery of a previous episode of depression. Nevertheless, both PMS and menstrual magnification are important not only for the symptoms they cause in the short run but also for the risk they represent for a full recurrence in the future, signaling the potential need both for symptomatic and preventive treatment (Figure 2-103).

Regular cycling of estrogen persists during the childbearing years except during pregnancy, when a woman's estrogen levels skyrocket (Figure 2-100). Estrogen levels then plummet precipitously immediately postpartum, and regular menstrual cycles begin again once the woman stops nursing (Figure 2-100). Rapid changes in estrogen levels in the postpartum period are considered a major risk factor for the onset or recurrence of a major depressive episode, psychotic depressive episode, or bipolar manic episode (Figure 2-100).

One of the most controversial and unsettled areas of modern psychopharmacology is the selection of therapeutic interventions for the treatment of major depressive disorder and prevention of recurrence of depression in women during their childbearing years, when they may be pregnant or become pregnant (Figure 2-103).

What about risks of treatment to the girl, adolescent, or woman of childbearing potential? Antidepressants are not generally approved for the treatment of major depression and may even cause increased suicidality in girls before age eighteen, with one of the lowest benefits and highest risks for antidepressants over the female life cycle (Figure 2-11). Antidepressants, although proven effective in women between the ages of eighteen and twenty-five, may also cause increased suicidality up to the age of twenty-five, with a less than ideal benefit-to-risk ratio for antidepressant treatment (Figure 2-11).

TABLE 2-13 Risks of antidepressant use or avoidance during pregnancy

Risks: Damned if you do

Congenital cardiac malformations (especially first trimester; paroxetine)
Newborn persistent pulmonary hypertension (third trimester; SSRIs)
Neonatal withdrawal syndrome (third trimester; SSRIs)
Prematurity, low birth weight
Long-term neurodevelopmental abnormalities
Increased suicidality due to antidepressant use (up to age 25)
Medical–legal risks of using antidepressants

Risks: Damned if you don't

Relapse of major depression
Increased suicidality due to antidepressant non-use
Poor self-care
Poor motivation for prenatal care
Disruption of mother–infant bonding
Low birth weight, developmental delay in children of women with untreated depression
Self-harm
Harm to infant
Medical–legal risks of not using antidepressants

What about risks of treatment to the patient's fetus? Some antidepressants may pose risks to the fetus, including increased risk for serious congenital malformations if administered during the first trimester; increased risk for other fetal abnormalities and for fetal withdrawal symptoms after birth if administered during the third trimester; and increased risks of prematurity, low birth weight, and possibly long-term neurodevelopmental abnormalities if given any time during pregnancy (Table 2-13).

At the same time, lack of treatment during pregnancy is not without risks to mother and fetus (Table 2-13). For the mother with untreated depression, the risks include relapse or worsening of depression, poor self-care, and possible self-harm (Table 2-13). Not only is there risk of increased suicidality when young mothers are treated with antidepressants, there is also the risk of suicide when seriously depressed mothers of any age are not treated with antidepressants (Table 2-13). There are also numerous risks to the baby if the mother is not treated with antidepressants, including risk of poor prenatal care due to low motivation in the mother, risk of low birth weight and early developmental delay, disruption of maternal–infant bonding in the children of women with untreated depression, and even risk of harm to the infant by seriously depressed mothers in the postpartum period (Table 2-13).

Thus it seems that the psychopharmacologist is "damned if you do" treat pregnant patients with antidepressants, and "also damned if you don't" (Table 2-13, Figure 2-103). Without clear guidelines, clinicians are best advised to assess risks and benefits for both child and mother on a case-by-case basis. For mild cases of depression, psychotherapy and psychosocial support may be sufficient. However, in many cases, the benefits of continuing antidepressant treatment during pregnancy outweigh the risks. Since patients with unipolar or bipolar depression (especially children and adolescents) may be prone to impulsive behavior, it is a good idea for girls and women of childbearing potential who take antidepressants to receive counseling and possibly contraceptives to reduce the risk of unplanned pregnancies and first-trimester exposure of fetuses to antidepressants.

Depression and its treatment during the postpartum period and while breast-feeding

What about taking antidepressants during the postpartum period, when the mother is lactating and may be nursing (Figure 2-103)? This is a very high risk period for the onset or recurrence of a major depressive episode in women (Figure 2-100). Should a mother with depression avoid antidepressants in order to avoid risk of exposing the baby to antidepressants in the mother's breast milk (Figure 2-103)? How about a mother with past depression now in remission who is weighing the risk of her own relapse against the risk of exposing the baby to antidepressants in breast milk (Figure 2-103)? In these circumstances there are no firm guidelines that fit all cases and a risk–benefit ratio must be calculated for each situation, taking into consideration the risk of recurrence to the mother if she does not take antidepressants (given her own personal and family history of mood disorder), and the risk to her bonding to her baby if she does not breast-feed or to her baby if there is exposure to trace amounts of antidepressants in her breast milk. Although estrogen replacement therapy (ERT) has been reported to be effective in some patients with postpartum depression or postpartum psychosis, this is still considered experimental and should be reserved for use, if at all, only in patients resistant to antidepressants.

Whereas the risk to the infant of exposure to small amounts of antidepressants in breast milk is only now being clarified, it is quite clear that the mother with a prior postpartum depression who neglects to take antidepressants after a subsequent pregnancy has a 67% risk of recurrence if she does not take antidepressants, and only one-tenth of that risk of recurrence if she does take antidepressants postpartum. Also, up to 90% of all postpartum psychosis and bipolar episodes occur within the first four weeks after delivery. Such high risk patients will require appropriate treatment of their mood disorder, so the decision here is about whether to breast feed, not whether the mother should be treated.

Depression and its treatment during perimenopause

Another very high risk period for the onset or recurrence of major depression is perimenopause (Figure 2-100). Regular cycling of estrogen stops during the perimenopausal transition to menopause, when menstrual cycles are on-again, off-again, and intermittently anovulatory prior to their complete cessation (Figure 2-100). Irregular estrogen cycles may provide a trigger to new onset or recurrence of major depressive episodes in women during perimenopause. This is a long-lasting period of risk, since perimenopause can last for five to seven years until menopause begins (i.e., the complete cessation of menstruation). Hormone levels can thus be chaotic and unpredictable for many years, and these fluctuations are often experienced as both physiological and psychological stressors. Vasomotor symptoms (i.e., hot flushes or hot flashes), often accompanied by sweating and insomnia, are well-known stressors that accompany perimenopause and are a clinical signal for the presence of irregularly fluctuating estrogen levels. Vasomotor symptoms may also be a harbinger of onset or relapse of major depression, since fluctuating estrogen levels may be the physiological trigger for major depressive episodes during perimenopause.

The links between vasomotor symptoms and depression are both clinical and neurobiological. The clinical link is demonstrated by the high degree of overlap between the symptoms of depression and the symptoms of perimenopause and menopause (Figure 2-104). The neurobiological link between vasomotor symptoms and depression is that both are regulated by the trimonoamine neurotransmitter system. The specific circuits hypothesized to mediate the various symptoms of major depressive disorder have already been discussed in Chapter 1 and illustrated in Figures 1-45 to 1-55. Also mentioned in the present chapter has been the fact that estrogen affects the trimonoamine neurotransmitter system by

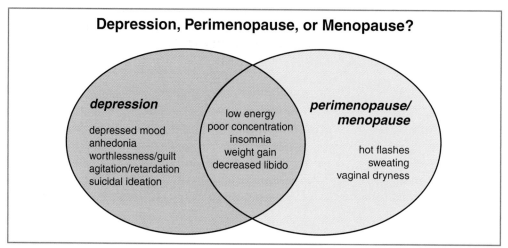

FIGURE 2-104 Depression, perimenopause, or menopause? There is a high degree of overlap between symptoms of depression and those of perimenopause and menopause. Overlapping symptoms may include low energy, poor concentration, insomnia, weight gain, and decreased libido.

regulating the expression of genes for numerous neurotransmitter receptors, synthesizing enzymes, and metabolizing enzymes (shown conceptually in Figure 2-97).

Thus, dysregulation of trimonoaminergic neurotransmitter systems within circuits that mediate the various symptoms of depression caused by irregular fluctuation of estrogen levels could lead to neurotransmitter deficiencies that trigger a major depressive episode (Figure 2-105A), consistent with the monoamine hypothesis of depression (Figure 1-42). Similarly, dysregulation of neurotransmitter systems within hypothalamic thermoregulatory centers by irregular fluctuation of estrogen levels could lead to neurotransmitter deficiencies that trigger vasomotor symptoms (Figure 2-106A). It is thus not surprising that other symptoms related to dysregulation of neurotransmitters within the hypothalamus can occur in both perimenopause and in depression (Figure 2-104), namely insomnia, weight gain, and decreased libido (Figures 1-47, 1-48, and 1-52).

How are vasomotor symptoms mediated? It appears that hypothalamic thermoregulatory centers are the homeostatic control sites for integrating internal core body temperature and peripheral temperature signals with vascular and neurochemical signals. Noradrenergic and serotonergic input to the hypothalamus are two of the key neurochemical signals. If estrogen causes dysregulation of noradrenergic and serotonergic circuits throughout the brain, it is not surprising that this could lead not only to the various symptoms of depression (Figure 2-105A and Figures 1-45 to 1-55) but also to vasomotor symptoms and other symptoms of perimenopause and menopause (Figure 2-106A), with considerable overlap between them (Figure 2-104).

The clinical and neurobiological links between vasomotor symptoms and depression predict links between the treatments for these two conditions as well. Classically, estrogen replacement therapy (ERT) has been the approved treatment for vasomotor symptoms, presumably smoothing out the chaotic fluctuations or deficient levels of estrogen that cause these symptoms in perimenopausal or postmenopausal women. Numerous studies suggest that ERT may also be effective in treating depression or may be useful in augmenting antidepressants in some women during perimenopause, although ERT has never been approved for this use (Figure 2-103). Moreover, in recent years, significant concerns have

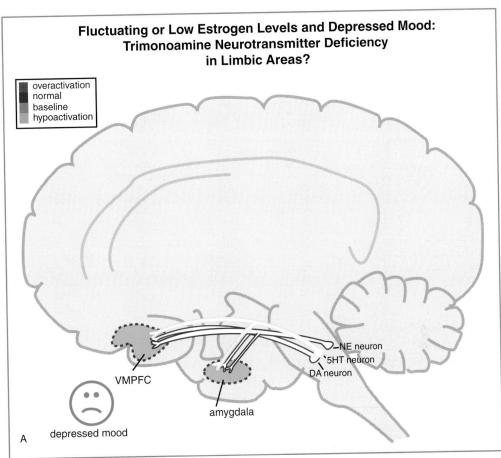

FIGURE 2-105A Estrogen interaction with monoamines may lead to depressed mood. Irregular fluctuation of estrogen levels can cause dysregulation of trimonoaminergic neurotransmitter systems within circuits mediating symptoms of depression, such as depressed mood, and thus contribute to the development of a major depressive episode.

arisen over the long-term safety of ERT, and many women and their physicians now opt out of ERT treatment.

This has created the need for a novel treatment for vasomotor symptoms, and given the clinical and neurobiological link between vasomotor symptoms and the symptoms of depression, it was logical to look at antidepressants that target the trimonoaminergic neurotransmitter system to find a treatment for vasomotor symptoms. Early studies have shown promising if inconsistent results with some SSRIs (Figure 2-106B) as well as with the alpha 2 agonist clonidine and even the anticonvulsant and chronic pain treatment gabapentin. However, the most promising results to date seem to be with SNRIs, especially the SNRI desvenlafaxine. Perhaps it is necessary to target both the profound hypothalamic regulation of temperature by norepinephrine as well as serotonin to achieve optimal efficacy in the treatment of vasomotor symptoms (Figure 2-106C) rather than targeting just serotonin regulation of temperature with an SSRI (Figure 2-106B). Studies of desvenlafaxine treatment of women with vasomotor symptoms (but not major depression) show that they achieve a

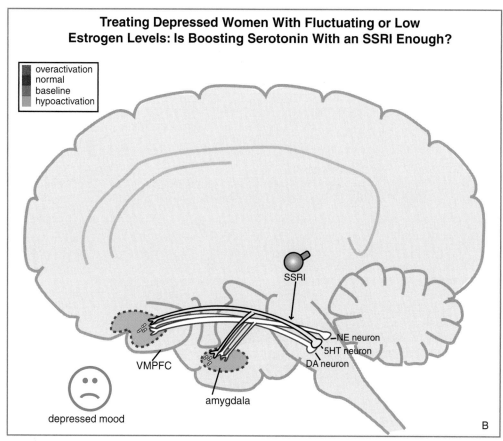

FIGURE 2-105B Treating depressed women with fluctuating estrogen: SSRI. Early studies provide inconsistent results as to the efficaciousness of serotonin selective reuptake inhibitors (SSRIs) for depressed mood in postmenopausal women who are not taking estrogen replacement therapy. This suggests that the presence of estrogen may boost the efficacy of SSRIs and the absence of estrogen may reduce the efficacy of SSRIs in some depressed women.

50% reduction of hot flushes in about a week, with approximately half of women eventually attaining a 75% reduction in hot flushes.

The question now is whether psychopharmacologists should identify and treat vasomotor symptoms as well as the traditional symptoms of depression in perimenopausal women (Figure 2-104). Since the treatments for these two conditions overlap, this may not be difficult. Vasomotor symptoms are not only stressful to experience but their persistence can stand in the way of a perimenopausal woman reaching full remission of a major depressive episode or of sustaining that remission over the long run. Remission of the classic symptoms of depression while vasomotor symptoms persist is likely a signal that fluctuating estrogen levels are still affecting the brain, at least in hypothalamic regulatory centers. Further research is necessary to determine whether targeting vasomotor symptoms in women with depression (Figures 2-105A and 2-106A) will lead to a better chance of achieving and sustaining remission from depression and also whether targeting vasomotor symptoms in women who do not have depression but are at risk for the onset or recurrence of depression will prevent new episodes of depression. In the meantime, it makes sense for psychopharmacologists to consider taking this approach of targeting not just the classic mood symptoms

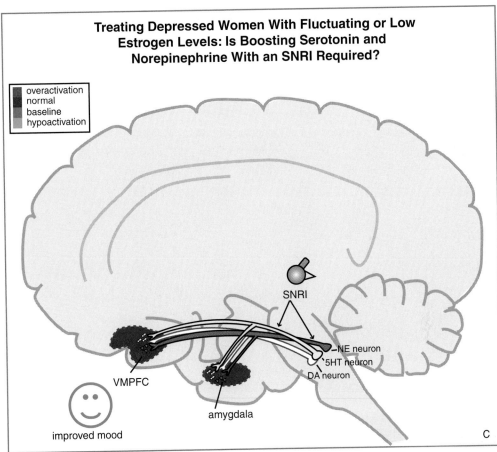

Treating Depressed Women With Fluctuating or Low Estrogen Levels: Is Boosting Serotonin and Norepinephrine With an SNRI Required?

overactivation
normal
baseline
hypoactivation

SNRI

NE neuron
5HT neuron
DA neuron

VMPFC

amygdala

improved mood

C

FIGURE 2-105C Treating depressed women with fluctuating estrogen: SNRI. Recent data suggest that serotonin norepinephrine reuptake inhibitors (SNRIs) may have efficacy for depressed mood in postmenopausal women whether or not they are taking estrogen. It may be that actions on both the serotonergic and noradrenergic systems are required to treat depression in some women when estrogen levels are low.

of depression (Figure 2-105A) but also vasomotor symptoms in perimenopausal women (Figure 2-106A).

Depression and its treatment during menopause

Menopause is the final stage of transition of estrogen in the female life cycle and is either a state of relative estrogen deficiency or, in a dwindling number of women, a state associated with estrogen replacement therapy (ERT). Despite the lack of chaotic estrogen fluctuations, many women continue to experience vasomotor symptoms after the onset of menopause. This may be due to the loss of expression of sufficient numbers of brain glucose transporters due to low concentrations of estrogen. Theoretically, this would cause inefficient CNS transport of glucose, which would be detected in hypothalamic centers that would react by triggering a noradrenergic alarm, with vasomotor response, increased blood flow to the brain, and compensatory increases in brain glucose transport. The situation would be potentially exacerbated in the large number of menopausal women with diabetes and prediabetes. Presumably, SNRI treatment could reduce an overreactive hypothalamus and thus minimize consequent vasomotor symptoms.

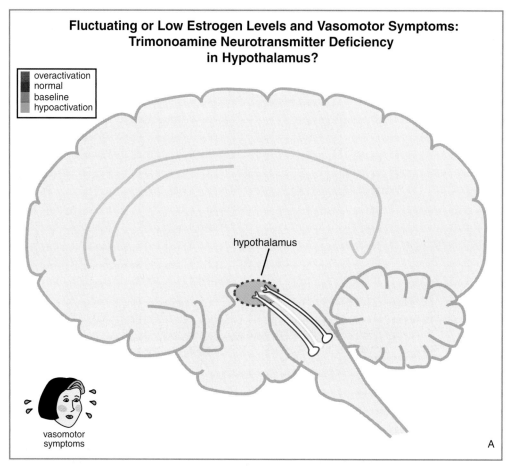

FIGURE 2-106A Estrogen interaction with monoamines may lead to vasomotor symptoms. Irregular fluctuation of estrogen levels can cause dysregulation of trimonoaminergic neurotransmitter projections to the hypothalamus and thus lead to vasomotor symptoms.

What about the treatment of depression in postmenopausal women (Figures 2-103, 2-104, 2-105B, and 2-105C)? Although depression is less of a risk after menopause than during perimenopause and all antidepressants are potentially useful, there are some special considerations for treating women with depression after menopause. One issue of note relates to the observation that SSRIs seem to work better in women in the presence of estrogen than in the absence of estrogen (Figure 2-105B). Thus, SSRIs may have more reliable efficacy in premenopausal women (who have normal cycling estrogen levels) and in postmenopausal women who are taking ERT than in postmenopausal women who are not taking ERT. By contrast, SNRIs seem to have consistent efficacy in both pre- and postmenopausal women whether they are taking ERT or not (Figure 2-105C). Furthermore, there appears to be a relative advantage of SNRIs over SSRIs for treating depression in women over the age of fifty, especially those women who are not taking ERT. Thus, the treatment of depression in postmenopausal women should take into consideration whether they have vasomotor symptoms and whether they are taking ERT before deciding whether to prescribe an SSRI (Figure 2-105B) or an SNRI (Figure 2-105C).

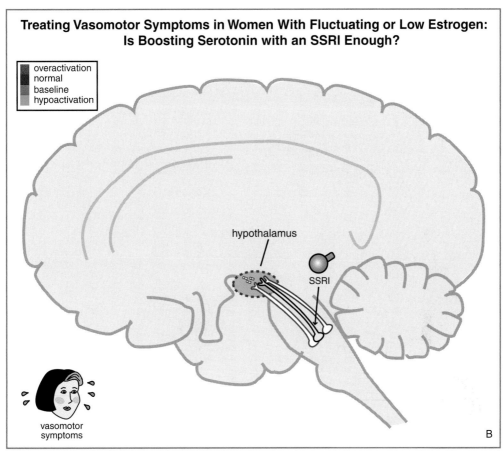

Treating Vasomotor Symptoms in Women With Fluctuating or Low Estrogen: Is Boosting Serotonin with an SSRI Enough?

overactivation
normal
baseline
hypoactivation

hypothalamus

SSRI

vasomotor
symptoms

B

FIGURE 2-106B Treating vasomotor symptoms: SSRI. Early studies provide inconsistent results as to the ability of serotonin selective reuptake inhibitors (SSRIs) to improve vasomotor symptoms.

L-methylpholate (6-(S)-5-methyl-tetrahydrofolate, or MTHF) as a trimonoamine modulator (TMM)

MTHF, derived from folate (Figure 2-107), is an important regulator of a critical cofactor for trimonoamine neurotransmitter synthesis, namely tetrahydrobiopterin or BH4 (Figure 2-108A). Because BH4 is a critical enzyme cofactor, there are several mechanisms that lead to its formation, two of which are intimately entwined with MTHF metabolism (Figure 2-108).

The trimonoamine synthetic enzymes that require BH4 as a cofactor are both tryptophan hydroxylase, the rate-limiting enzyme for serotonin synthesis, and tyrosine hydroxylase, the rate-limiting enzyme for dopamine and norepinephrine synthesis (Figure 2-109). MTHF is thus considered to be a TMM (trimonoamine modulator) because of its role as an indirect regulator of trimonoamine neurotransmitter synthesis and concentrations.

Numerous studies now suggest that low plasma, red blood cell, and/or cerebrospinal fluid (CSF) levels of folate or MTHF (Figure 2-107) may be associated with depression in some patients (Figure 2-110). Since MTHF indirectly regulates monoamine levels (Figures 2-108 and 2-109), low CNS levels of MTHF could lead to reduced activity of trimonoaminergic neurotransmitter synthesizing enzymes, causing monoamine deficiency (Figure 2-110A), consistent with the monoamine hypothesis of depression (Figure 1-42).

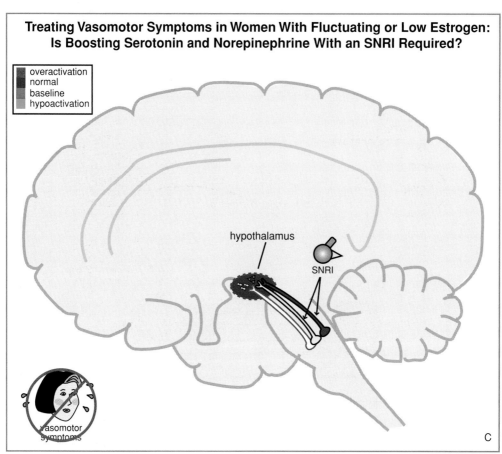

Treating Vasomotor Symptoms in Women With Fluctuating or Low Estrogen: Is Boosting Serotonin and Norepinephrine With an SNRI Required?

overactivation
normal
baseline
hypoactivation

hypothalamus

SNRI

vasomotor symptoms

C

FIGURE 2-106C Treating vasomotor symptoms: SNRI. Recent data suggest that serotonin norepinephrine reuptake inhibitors (SNRIs), especially desvenlafaxine, may have efficacy for vasomotor symptoms. It may be that actions on both the serotonergic and noradrenergic systems are required to improve these symptoms.

Those at greatest risk for low CNS MTHF levels may be those with a common genetic variant of an enzyme that reduces their ability to convert folate to MTHF (specifically, the C677T variant of the enzyme methylene THF-R, or methylene tetrahydrofolate reductase, which converts folic acid to MTHF) (see Figures 2-107 and 2-108). This genetic variant may be present more frequently in depressed patients than in individuals who are not depressed.

Several studies have shown that administration of folate, MTHF, or another folate derivative known as folinic acid (Leucovorin) may all boost the therapeutic efficacy of antidepressants in patients with major depressive disorder who fail to respond adequately to their antidepressant and who may or may not have measurable folate deficiency. Current research specifically suggests that MTHF may be indicated for depressed patients with low plasma, red blood cell, and/or CSF folate levels and who have not responded adequately to antidepressants (Figure 2-110B). Theoretically, patients with inadequate responses to a monoamine-enhancing antidepressant might benefit from MTHF treatment, which elevates their BH4 levels (Figure 2-108), leading to enhancement of their trimonoamine neurotransmitter synthesis (Figures 2-109 and 2-110B).

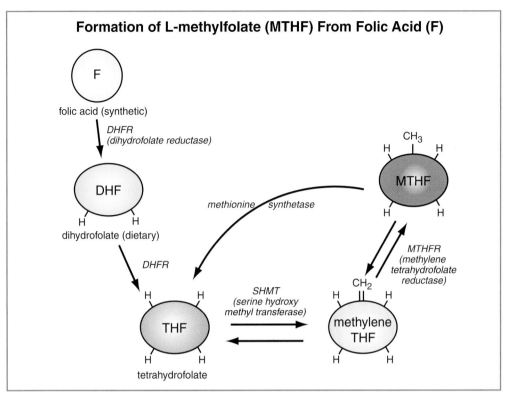

Formation of L-methylfolate (MTHF) From Folic Acid (F)

FIGURE 2-107 L-5-methyl-tetrahydrofolate (MTHF). MTHF is a trimonoamine modulator naturally synthesized from the vitamin folate for use within the central nervous system. Folic acid (synthetic) is converted to dihydrofolate (DHF) by the enzyme dihydrofolate reductase (DHFR), and DHF, in turn, is converted to tetrahydrofolate (THF), again by DHFR. Serine hydroxyl methyl transferase (SHMT) then converts THF to methylene THF. Finally, methylene THF is converted by methylene tetrahydrofolate reductase (MTHFR) to MTHF.

Why MTHF rather than folic acid for depression?

Folate is one of the thirteen essential vitamins. Dihydrofolate, a mixture of polyglutamates (i.e., a number of glutamatic acid entities) is the form of folate obtained from dietary intake of green vegetables, yeast, liver, kidney, and egg yolk. Folic acid is the synthetic form of folate contained in over-the-counter vitamin supplements (usually mixed with several other vitamins and nutrients and present in low doses). Folic acid is also the synthetic form of folate contained in prescriptions written by a licensed practitioner in higher doses for medical use.

Dihydrofolate and folic acid are converted to monoglutamate entities by the enzyme alpha-L-glutamyl transferase in the intestinal wall as they are absorbed. Once absorbed, monoglutamate entities are converted to MTHF, the only form of folate that passes into the brain and is utilized by trimonoamine neurons to facilitate neurotransmitter synthesis (Figure 2-107). Normally, ingesting folate either from dihydrofolate in the diet or from folic acid in synthetic supplements will result in adequate delivery of MTHF levels to the brain, especially in those individuals with the more efficient variant of the enzyme methylene THF reductase and who do not have depression.

However, robust levels of MTHF in the brain which may be necessary to maximize the chances of boosting trimonoamine neurotransmitter synthesis (Figures 2-108, 2-109, and 2-110B) are more likely attained after administration of MTHF rather than

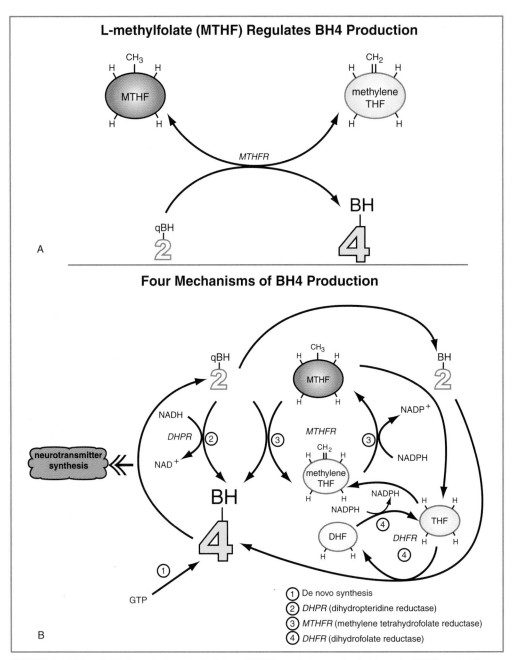

FIGURE 2-108A and B L-5-methyl-tetrahydrofolate (MTHF) regulates tetrahydrobiopterin (BH4) production.
BH4 is a critical enzyme cofactor for trimonoamine neurotransmitter synthesis. There are several mechanisms that lead to its production (**B**), the most important of which may be the actions of MTHF to create BH4 (**A**).

folic acid. Thus MTHF may have significant advantages over folic acid as a TMM for depressed patients who do not respond adequately to antidepressant treatment, who may or may not be folate-deficient, who may or may not have the inefficient form of the MTHF synthesizing enzyme methylene THF reductase, and who may or may not be taking various anticonvulsant mood stabilizers that interfere with folic acid absorption.

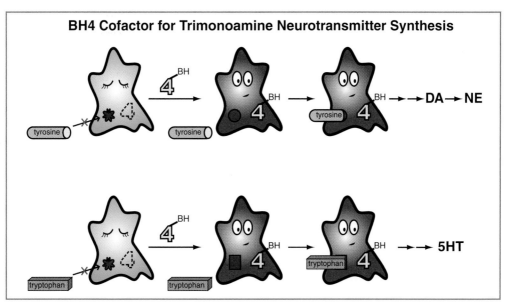

FIGURE 2-109 Tetrahydrobiopterin (BH4) cofactor for trimonoamine neurotransmitter synthesis. BH4 is a critical enzyme cofactor for tyrosine hydroxylase, the rate-limiting enzyme for dopamine and norepinephrine synthesis, and tryptophan hydroxylase, the rate-limiting enzyme for serotonin. Because L-5-methyl-tetrahydrofolate (MTHF) regulates BH4 production, it therefore plays an indirect role in regulating trimonoamine synthesis and concentrations. Thus MTHF is considered to be a trimonoaminergic modulator.

Specifically, it may take as much as 7 mg of oral folic acid to generate the same plasma levels of MTHF as giving 1 mg of oral MTHF itself. How much folic acid is this? The recommended daily allowance of folic acid from food or dietary supplements is 0.4 mg (0.8 mg for pregnant women); over-the-counter multivitamin supplements typically provide between 0.25 and 1 mg of folic acid; normal "prescription strength" folic acid is 1 mg of pure folic acid; high-dose prescription folic acid for treating pregnant women to reduce the risk of neural tube defects is between 4 and 5 mg of folic acid. By comparison, the lowest dose of MTHF studied in depression to augment antidepressant treatment is 7.5 mg, roughly equivalent to 52 mg of folic acid. Although high doses of folic acid can be administered orally, the precursors of MTHF may compete with MTHF for entry into the brain by binding to folate transport receptors and thus limit the amount of MTHF that can get into the brain (Figure 2-110B). Thus high doses of MTHF itself are likely to provide substantially more active MTHF moiety to the brain than high doses of folic acid. The exact dose of MTHF to treat depression is not fully determined, but since MTHF works indirectly to boost monoamine synthesis, high doses are likely to be necessary to optimize this action.

MTHF itself is available by prescription in the United States as a "medical food" also called L-methylfolate (Deplin) and not as an over-the-counter dietary supplement or vitamin. According to the FDA, a medical food is different both from a drug and a food and is defined as a food that is formulated to be consumed orally "under the supervision of a physician and which is intended for the specific dietary management of a disease or condition for which distinctive nutritional requirements, based on recognized scientific principles, are established by medical evaluation." Medical foods are required when dietary management cannot achieve the specific nutrient requirements. Treatment with MTHF seems to be safe,

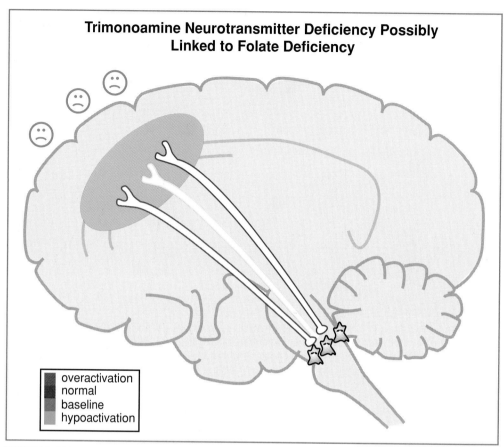

Trimonoamine Neurotransmitter Deficiency Possibly Linked to Folate Deficiency

- overactivation
- normal
- baseline
- hypoactivation

FIGURE 2-110A Folate deficiency and monoamines. Because L-5-methyl-tetrahydrofolate (MTHF) indirectly regulates trimonoamine neurotransmitter synthesis, deficiency of folate, from which it is derived, can lead to reduced monoamine levels and thus to symptoms of depression. In fact, studies show that low levels of folate or MTHF may be linked to depression in some patients.

apparently has few if any side effects, and is generally less expensive than augmenting with a second antidepressant. Further research is necessary to determine the exact priority that should be given to this approach in treatment algorithms for major depression.

S-adenosyl-methionine (SAMe), MTHF, and methylation

MTHF may have additional actions on monoamine neurotransmitter metabolism through another mechanism – namely, its well–known ability to regulate methylation reactions (Figure 2-111). Another agent possibly useful for augmenting antidepressants in patients with inadequate responses is S-adenosyl-methionine (SAMe), which shares with MTHF the ability to regulate methylation (Figure 2-111). Both MTHF and SAMe may thus affect the regulation of various critical components of monoamine neurotransmitter activity not only by indirect modulation of neurotransmitter synthesis by promoting the synthesis of BH4 enzymatic cofactor but also by modulating catabolic enzymes, monoamine transporters, and neurotransmitter receptors via methylation and its downstream effects (Figure 2-111). These complex mechanisms are under active investigation to determine how the natural products and putative TMMs MTHF and SAMe may contribute to the treatment of depression.

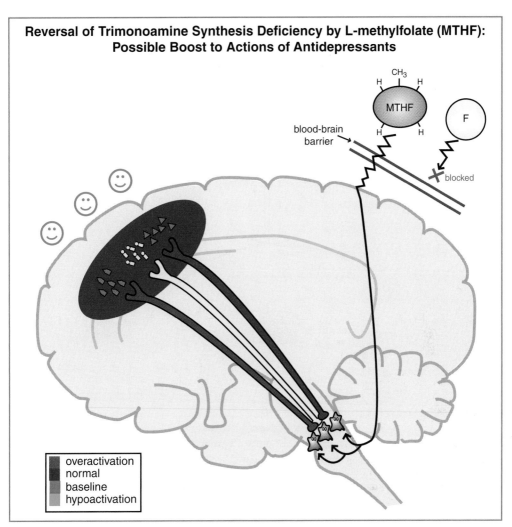

FIGURE 2-110B L-5-methyl-tetrahydrofolate (MTHF) and antidepressants. Administration of MTHF, folate, or folinic acid in conjunction with an antidepressant may boost the therapeutic effects of antidepressant monotherapy. High doses of oral MTHF may be the most efficient of these for boosting BH4 production in the central nervous system and thus enhancing brain trimonoamine neurotransmitter levels.

Thyroid

Thyroid hormones are other examples of hormones that bind to nuclear ligand receptors to form a nuclear ligand–activated transcription factor. Abnormalities in thyroid hormone levels have long been associated with depression (Figure 2-112A), and various forms and doses of thyroid hormones have long been utilized as augmenting agents to antidepressants either to boost their efficacy in patients with inadequate response or to speed up their onset of action (Figure 2-112B). Thyroid hormones have many complex cellular actions, including actions that may boost trimonoaminergic neurotransmitters as downstream consequences of thyroid's known abilities to regulate neuronal organization, arborization, and synapse formation (Figure 2-112B). Thus it may be appropriate to classify thyroid hormones as another form of trimonoaminergic modulator in order to explain their ability to enhance antidepressant action in some patients.

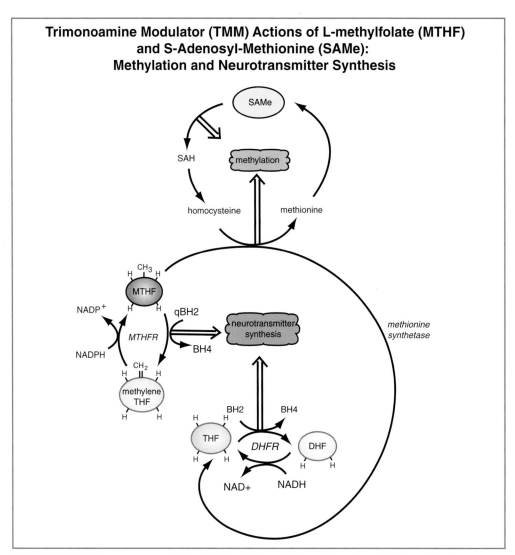

FIGURE 2-111 Trimonoamine modulation (TMM) of L-5-methyl-tetrahydrofolate (MTHF) and S-adenosyl-methionine (SAMe). MTHF regulates methylation reactions, as does SAMe, another agent that has been used to augment antidepressants. Regulation of methylation can affect modulation of catabolic enzymes, monoamine transporters, and receptors and thus is another means to regulate monoamine activity.

Lithium

The mechanism of action of lithium is still debated and not yet firmly established. Actions of lithium at other sites of the signal transduction cascade for neurotransmitters are discussed in Chapter 3, on mood stabilizers. In addition to these actions, lithium can boost the actions of monoamines, perhaps by one of these actions or by other mechanisms yet poorly understood (Figure 2-113). It is clear that, in addition to mood stabilizing actions, lithium can be effective as an augmenting agent to many antidepressants in patients with major depressive episodes who have inadequate responses to antidepressants, although perhaps not as a monotherapy for such patients. Lithium as a mood stabilizing monotherapy, especially for

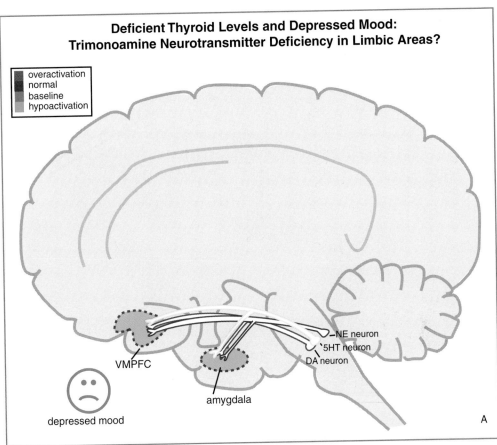

Deficient Thyroid Levels and Depressed Mood: Trimonoamine Neurotransmitter Deficiency in Limbic Areas?

overactivation
normal
baseline
hypoactivation

NE neuron
5HT neuron
DA neuron

VMPFC

amygdala

depressed mood

A

FIGURE 2-112A Thyroid levels and depressed mood. Abnormal thyroid levels have been linked to depression. This may be because thyroid hormones are involved in neuronal organization, arborization, and synapse formation, which in turn can affect levels of trimonoaminergic neurotransmitters. Deficient thyroid levels may be associated with monoamine deficiency in limbic regions and thus cause depressed mood.

mania, is discussed in Chapter 3, on mood stabilizers. Actions of lithium on antidepressants can be considered to be a form of trimonoaminergic modulation, and lithium should be part of the therapeutic armamentarium for unipolar depression in patients with inadequate responses to prior treatment with antidepressants (Figure 2-113).

Brain stimulation: creating a "perfect storm" in brain circuits of depressed patients

Electroconvulsive therapy (ECT) is the classic therapeutic form of brain stimulation for depression. ECT is a highly effective treatment for depression whose mechanism of action remains a mystery. Failure to respond to a variety of antidepressants, singly or in combination, is a key factor for considering ECT, although it may also be utilized in urgent and severely disabling high-risk circumstances such as psychotic, suicidal, or postpartum depressions. ECT is the only therapeutic agent for the treatment of depression that is rapid in onset; its therapeutic actions can start after even a single treatment and typically within a few days. The mechanism is unknown but thought to be related to the probable mobilization of neurotransmitters caused by the seizure; thus ECT could be considered a type of trimonoaminergic modulator. In experimental animals, ECT downregulates beta

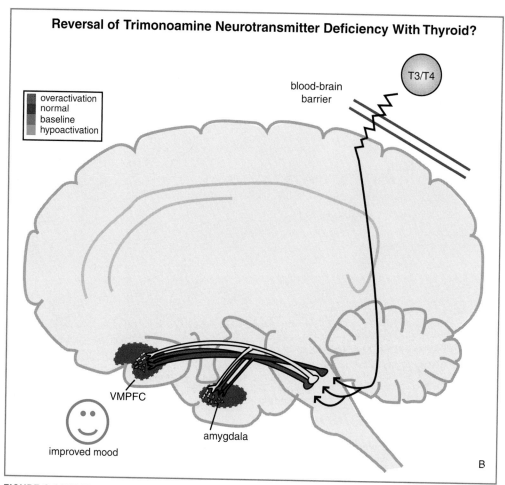

Reversal of Trimonoamine Neurotransmitter Deficiency With Thyroid?

overactivation
normal
baseline
hypoactivation

T3/T4

blood-brain
barrier

VMPFC

amygdala

improved mood

B

FIGURE 2-112B Thyroid hormone as an augmenting agent. Administration of thyroid hormone (T3/T4) in patients with thyroid deficiency may boost monoamine levels and thus contribute to improved mood in patients with depression.

1 receptors (analogous to antidepressants) but upregulates 5HT2A receptors (opposite of antidepressants). Memory loss and social stigma are the primary problems associated with ECT, which limit its use. There can also be striking regional differences across the various nations of the world in the frequency of ECT use and in ECT techniques. For example, ECT is often more commonly used in Europe and the United Kingdom and on the East Coast of the United States; it is less commonly used on the West Coast.

If the mechanism of therapeutic action of ECT could be unraveled, it might lead to new antidepressant treatments capable of rapid onset of antidepressant effects or with special value for refractory patients. More recently, at least three newer forms of therapeutic brain stimulation have emerged. These are mentioned here only in brief, as it is not the intent of this chapter, which focuses on psychopharmacological treatments, to review these promising new treatments in depth. However, these three new forms of therapeutic brain stimulation treatments are listed here as potential "trimonoaminergic modulators," and their hypothetical mechanisms of action are shown in Figures 2-114 to 2-116.

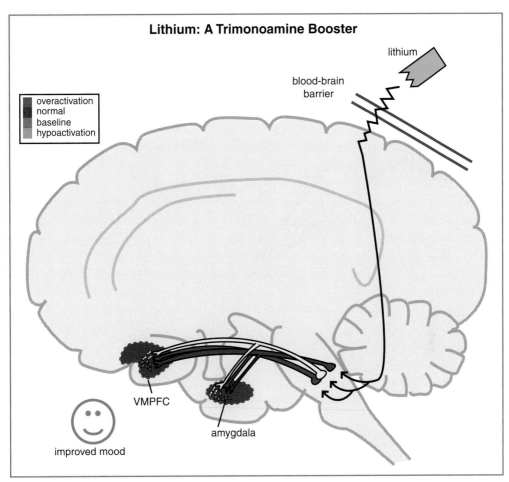

FIGURE 2-113 Lithium in depression. Although the mechanism of action of lithium is not clear, it does seem to boost the actions of monoamines, which may make it an efficacious augmenting agent in depression.

Vagus nerve stimulation, or VNS, is an approved treatment for depression in the United States and some other countries; it provides a continuous train of electrical pulses delivered from a pacemaker-like device surgically implanted in the left chest wall together with an implanted lead wrapped around the vagus nerve in the left side of the neck. The implanted pulse generator is then programmed with a telemetric wand using a computer to deliver pulses to the vagus nerve, typically for thirty seconds every five minutes twenty-four hours a day. Adjustable parameters include pulse width, signal frequency, output current, signal "on" time, and signal "off" time. The treatment thus requires a surgical implantation procedure, typically under general anesthesia. Battery life of the implanted pulse generator ranges from three to ten years.

The vagus nerve has direct and indirect anatomical connections with the trimonoaminergic neurotransmitter system in the brainstem, especially the noradrenergic locus coeruleus and the serotonergic midbrain raphe (Figure 2-114). It is possible that trans-synaptic excitation of neurotransmitter centers from input received via the vagus nerve is capable of boosting the output of neurotransmitters from these monoamine neurotransmitter centers and thereby boosting the therapeutic action of drugs in depressed patients with insufficient

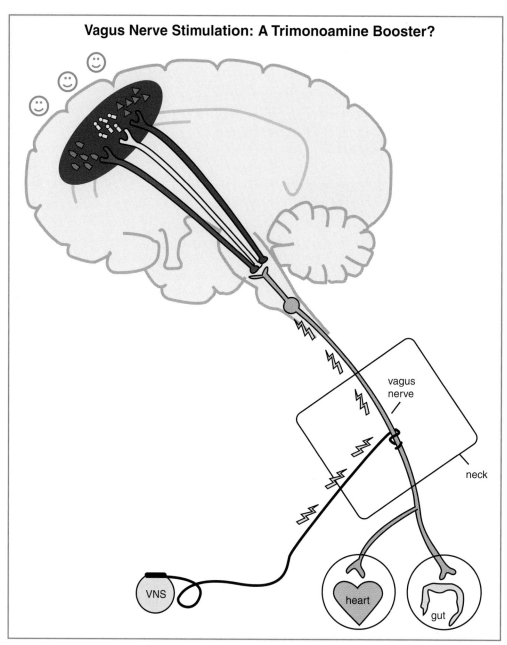

FIGURE 2-114 Vagus nerve stimulation. The vagus nerve has connections with neurotransmitter centers in the brainstem, in particular the midbrain raphe (serotonin) and the locus coeruleus (norepinephrine), and thus can modulate monoamine activity. Vagus nerve stimulation is a treatment in which a pacemaker-like device is surgically implanted in the chest wall with an implanted lead wrapped around the vagus nerve in the neck. This device delivers pulses to the vagus nerve, thus stimulating it to boost monoamine neurotransmission.

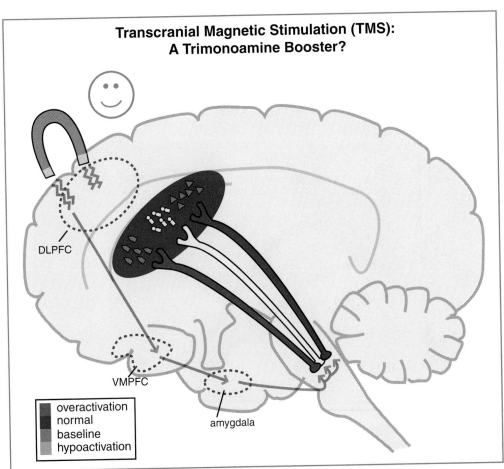

Transcranial Magnetic Stimulation (TMS): A Trimonoamine Booster?

DLPFC

VMPFC

amygdala

overactivation
normal
baseline
hypoactivation

FIGURE 2-115 Transcranial magnetic stimulation. Transcranial magnetic stimulation is a treatment in which a rapidly alternating current passes through a small coil placed over the scalp. This generates a magnetic field that induces an electrical current in the underlying areas of the brain (dorsolateral prefrontal cortex, or DLPFC). The affected neurons then signal other areas of the brain. Presumably, stimulation of brain regions in which there is monoamine deficiency would lead to a boost in monoamine activity and thus alleviation of depressive symptoms.

response to antidepressants (Figure 2-114). Thus vagus nerve stimulation may be a unique form of trimonoaminergic modulator (TMM). The onset of antidepressant action by VNS is generally delayed by several weeks, and the major side effect may be hoarseness from the spread of electrical stimulation in the neck to the vocal cords.

Transcranial magnetic stimulation, or TMS, is another new brain stimulation treatment for depression in the late stages of clinical trials in several different countries; it uses a rapidly alternating current passing through a small coil placed over the scalp. TMS generates a magnetic field that induces an electrical current in the underlying areas of the brain. This electrical current depolarizes the affected cortical neurons, thereby causing nerve impulses to flow out of the underlying brain areas (Figure 2-115). During the treatment, the patient is awake and reclines comfortably in a chair while the magnetic coil is placed snugly against the scalp. There are few if any side effects except headache.

The TMS apparatus is localized so as to create an electrical impulse over the dorsolateral prefrontal cortex (Figure 2-115). Presumably, daily stimulation of this brain area for

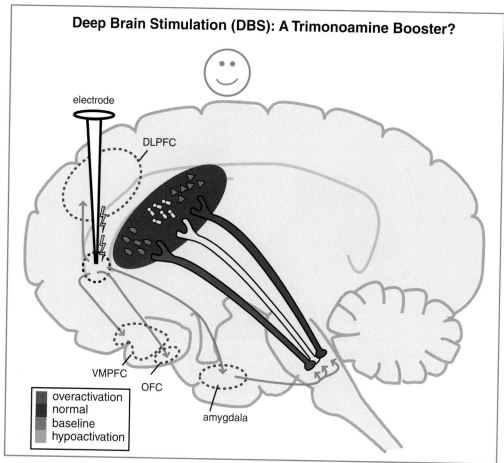

FIGURE 2-116 Deep brain stimulation. Deep brain stimulation involves a battery-powered pulse generator implanted in the chest wall. One or two leads are tunneled directly into the brain. The device then sends brief repeated pulses to the brain, which may have the result of boosting monoamine activity and thus alleviating depressive symptoms.

up to an hour over several weeks causes activation of various brain circuits that leads to an antidepressant effect. If this procedure activates a brain circuit beginning in dorsolateral prefrontal cortex and connecting to other brain areas, such as ventromedial prefrontal cortex and amygdala, with connections to the brainstem centers of the trimonoaminergic neurotransmitter system, the net result could be trimonoaminergic modulation, especially for patients inadequately responsive to treatment with antidepressants (Figure 2-115).

Finally, a highly experimental treatment for the most severe forms of depression is known as **deep brain stimulation** (Figure 2-116). Deep brain stimulation of neurons in some brain areas has proven to be effective for the treatment of motor complications in Parkinson's disease and is now under study for treatment-resistant depression. The stimulation device is a battery-powered pulse generator implanted in the chest wall, like a pacemaker or VNS device. One or two leads are tunneled under the scalp and then into the brain, guided by neuroimaging and brain stimulation recording during the implantation procedure to facilitate the exact placement of the lead in the targeted brain area. The tip of each lead is composed of several contact areas that usually spread sequentially to cover additional parts of the intended anatomic target. The pulse generator delivers brief, repeated pulses of current, which is adjusted based on individual tissue impedance. The most common side effects are from the procedure itself. There is ongoing debate on where to place the stimulating electrodes for the treatment of depression and how such stimulation might work to treat depression in patients inadequately responsive to antidepressants. Currently, a popular location for electrodes in the treatment of depression with deep brain stimulation is in the subgenual area of the anterior cingulate cortex, part of the ventromedial prefrontal cortex (Figure 2-116). This brain area has important connections to other areas of the prefrontal cortex, including other areas of the ventromedial prefrontal cortex, orbitofrontal cortex, and dorsolateral prefrontal cortex as well as the amygdala (Figure 2-116). It is conceivable that electrical stimulation of this brain area results in the activation of circuits that lead back to brainstem monoamine centers, therefore acting as trimonoaminergic modulators in these patients. Some reports of this treatment approach are encouraging.

Psychotherapy

In recent years, modern psychotherapy research has begun to standardize and test selected psychotherapeutic approaches to treatment in a manner analogous to the way in which antidepressants are tested in clinical trials. Thus, psychotherapeutic treatments are now being tested by being administered according to standard protocols by therapists receiving standardized training and using standardized manuals as well as in standard "doses" for a fixed duration. Such uses of psychotherapies are being compared in clinical trials to placebo or antidepressants. The results have shown that brief interpersonal therapy (IPT) and cognitive behavioral therapy (CBT) for depression may be as effective as antidepressants in certain patients. Proof of efficacy of certain psychotherapies is thus beginning to evolve.

Research is only beginning to show how to combine psychotherapy with drugs. Although some of the earliest studies did not indicate any additive benefit of tricyclic antidepressants and interpersonal therapy, recent studies are now demonstrating that there can be an additive benefit of psychotherapy augmentation of antidepressants. One study of nortriptyline suggests additive benefit of interpersonal psychotherapy, particularly when looking at long-term outcomes. Another recent study of nefazodone suggests that nefazodone is particularly effective when combined with cognitive behavioral psychotherapy for patients with chronic depression. In this study, psychotherapy was an especially essential element in the treatment of patients with chronic depression who had a history of childhood trauma. It is not known whether the addition of psychotherapy in antidepressant responders who are not in full remission might lead to remission and recovery, but this is an intuitively attractive possibility, and the usefulness of this approach for selected patients is empirically obvious to practitioners.

Psychotherapy is likely a form of learning that may counteract inefficient information processing in various brain circuits, not unlike the actions attributed to the various antidepressants being discussed in this chapter. Thus, effective forms of psychotherapy may themselves be a form of trimonoaminergic modulator.

Antidepressants in clinical practice

How do you choose an antidepressant?

With so many treatment options, many questions arise not only about how to choose a first-line agent but also what to do when the first-line treatment fails to cause remission. Various treatment options are organized in Figure 2-117 as the "depression pharmacy."

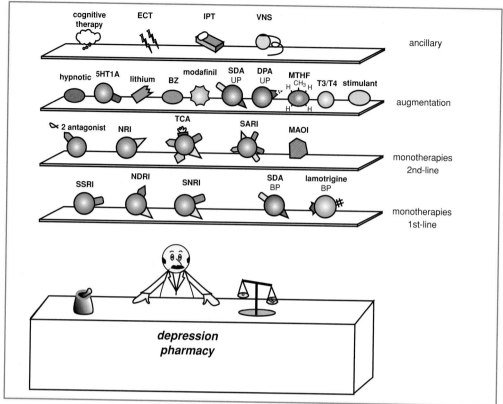

FIGURE 2-117 Depression pharmacy. First-line treatments for unipolar depression include serotonin selective reuptake inhibitors (SSRIs), norepinephrine and dopamine reuptake inhibitors (NDRIs), and serotonin norepinephrine reuptake inhibitors (SNRIs), while first-line treatments for bipolar depression include serotonin dopamine antagonists (SDAs) and lamotrigine. Second-line monotherapies include alpha 2 antagonists, selective norepinephrine reuptake inhibitors (NRIs), tricyclic antidepressants (TCAs), serotonin 2A antagonist/reuptake inhibitors (SARIs), and monoamine oxidase inhibitors (MAOIs). Potentially useful augmenting agents include hypnotics, serotonin 1A (5HT1A) agonists, lithium, benzodiazepines, modafinil, SDAs, dopamine partial agonists (DPAs), L-5-methyl-tetrahydrofolate (MTHF), thyroid hormone (T3/T4), and stimulants. Ancillary treatments to medications may include cognitive therapy, electroconvulsive therapy (ECT), interpersonal therapy (IPT), and vagus nerve stimulation (VNS).

The choices for first-line treatments for unipolar depression generally include an SSRI, SNRI, or NDRI for unipolar depression and lamotrigine or an atypical antipsychotic for bipolar depression. The treatment of bipolar depression is discussed in greater detail in Chapter 3, on mood stabilizers. Here the focus is on unipolar depression.

Generally, because of the greater side effect burden, treatments relegated to second-line choices include many of the older antidepressants, such as the alpha 2 antagonist mirtazapine, the SARI trazodone, the MAO inhibitors, and the TCAs (Figure 2-117). Selective NRIs such as reboxetine and off-label use of atomoxetine could be considered here. Agents generally used for augmentation of a first- or second-line antidepressant and not as a monotherapy are also indicated in Figure 2-117 and include a multitude of options. Finally, antidepressants can be augmented with ancillary treatments that are not drugs, including psychotherapy (such as cognitive behavior therapy or interpersonal therapy) and currently available electrical stimulation therapies (i.e., ECT and VNS).

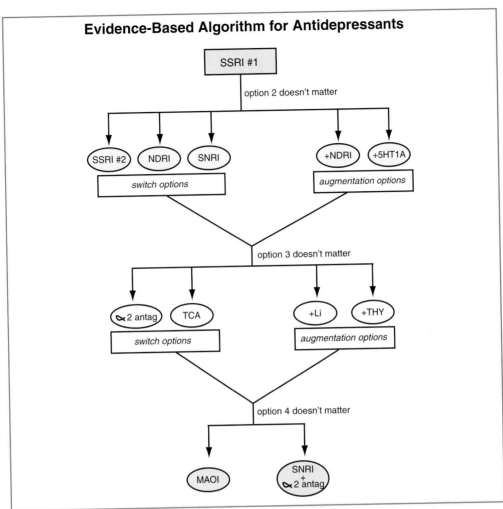

FIGURE 2-118 Evidence-based algorithm for antidepressants. Serotonin selective reuptake inhibitors (SSRIs) are generally considered the first-line treatment for depression. Patients with no response or who do not tolerate the medication may best be switched to another, while those with a partial response may do best with augmentation; however, there is little evidence to suggest which agent to switch to or which to add as an augmenting agent. Current data do not support the superiority of one over another; thus any may be a viable option.

Evidence-based antidepressant selections

One way to organize the various treatment choices for depression is to follow an evidence-based algorithm (e.g., Figure 2-118). Unfortunately there is little evidence for the superiority of one option over another. One general principle on which most patients and prescribers agree is when to switch versus when to augment. Thus there is a preference for switching when the first treatment has intolerable side effects or when there is no response whatsoever but to augment the first treatment with a second treatment when there is a partial response to the first treatment. Other than this guideline, there is little evidence that one treatment option is better than another (Figure 2-118). All treatments subsequent to the first one seem to have diminishing returns in terms of chances to reach remission (Figure 2-8) or chances to remain in remission (Figure 2-10). Thus evidence-based algorithms are not

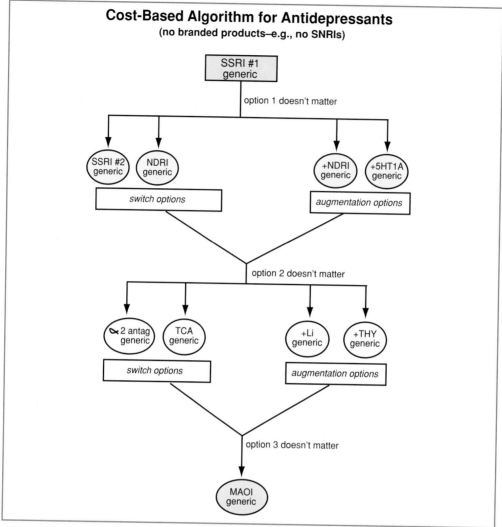

Cost-Based Algorithm for Antidepressants
(no branded products–e.g., no SNRIs)

FIGURE 2-119 Cost-based algorithm for antidepressants. If a cost-based approach were taken for creating an antidepressant algorithm, as some experts and agencies have suggested, many useful options would likely be restricted, making it difficult to tailor treatment to each individual's needs.

able to provide clear guidelines on how to choose an antidepressant and what to do if an antidepressant does not work.

Cost-based antidepressant selections

In the absence of clear evidence of superiority of one option over another, some experts and agencies have suggested that payors should fund only low-cost treatments and thus follow a cost-based algorithm for antidepressants (Figure 2-119). Such an approach would guide prescribers through a series of options of inexpensive generic products and eliminate the use of branded products. That would mean different things in different countries but would essentially rule out the use of SNRIs, some SSRIs, once-daily NDRIs, atypical antipsychotics, modafinil, and most new stimulants from the depression pharmacy (Figure 2-117) until all the less expensive options were tried first and failed (Figure 2-118). This is a rather nihilistic approach to the treatment of depression and does not allow tailoring the best treatment available to an individual.

Symptom-based antidepressant selections

Finally, the neurobiologically informed psychopharmacologist may opt for adapting a symptom-based approach to selecting or combining a series of antidepressants (Figures 2-120 to 2-127). This strategy allows the construction of a portfolio of multiple agents to treat all residual symptoms of unipolar depression until the patient achieves sustained remission (Figures 2-120 to 2-127). This is the approach advocated by this book; it is based on the notion of tailoring treatments for individual patients.

First, symptoms are constructed into a diagnosis and then deconstructed into a list of specific symptoms that the individual patient is experiencing. Next, these symptoms are matched with the brain circuits that hypothetically mediate these symptoms and with the known neuropharmacological regulation of these circuits by neurotransmitters. Finally, available treatment options that target these neuropharmacological mechanisms are chosen to eliminate symptoms one by one. When symptoms persist, a treatment with a different mechanism is added or switched. No evidence proves that this is a superior approach, but it appeals not only to clinical intuition but also to neurobiological reasoning. In the absence of options that have proven superiority, the symptom-based approach is what is advocated here and what has mostly been followed throughout this book.

Reduced positive affect versus increased negative affect

For example, already discussed is how depression can be conceptualized as having symptoms either of reduced positive affect, increased negative affect, or both, with reduced positive affect hypothetically linked to dysregulation of DA (and NE) and with increased negative affect hypothetically linked to dysregulation of 5HT (and NE) (Figure 1-55). Applying this to antidepressant selection, patients with reduced positive affect may benefit from agents that boost DA activity, including NDRIs, SNRIs, selective NRIs, or MAOIs as first-line options, with the possibility of utilizing modafinil or stimulants as augmenting agents (Figure 2-120). On the other hand, patients with increased negative affect may benefit from serotonergic antidepressants such as SSRIs, SNRIs, as well as SARIs, especially in augmentation (Figure 2-120). When patients have both sets of symptoms or when symptoms of reduced positive affect emerge as side effects of SSRIs or SNRIs, putting these options together can make sense (Figure 2-120). The much neglected MAOIs may also be useful here as monotherapy.

Residual symptoms and circuits after first-line treatment of depression

The symptom-based algorithm can be taken several steps further, as most patients have more complicated or unique residual symptoms than indicated in Figure 2-120. Recall that the most common residual symptoms following antidepressant treatment are insomnia, problems concentrating, and fatigue (Figures 2-9 and 2-121). Thus it would be a good idea to have a strategy with several effective tactics available for this commonly encountered situation. The symptom-based algorithm for choosing an antidepressant suggests that one first listen to the patient to determine the specific residual symptoms that are preventing full remission and then match them to hypothetically malfunctioning brain circuits (Figure 2-122). Malfunctioning circuits tied to specific symptoms of depression are discussed extensively in Chapter 1 and illustrated as well in Figures 1-46 through 1-54. Once the specific symptoms and their circuits are determined, the idea at this point is to target the regulatory neurotransmitters for these circuits and their associated symptoms with selected

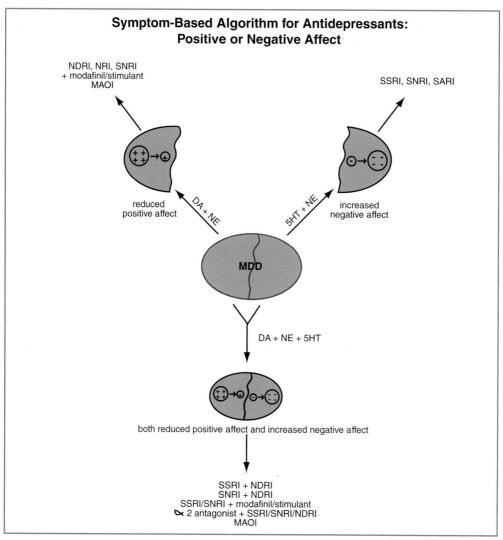

FIGURE 2-120 Symptom-based algorithm for antidepressants. A symptom-based approach to antidepressant selection follows the theory that each of a patient's symptoms is matched with brain circuits and neurotransmitters that hypothetically mediate that symptom; this information is then used to select a corresponding pharmacological mechanism. One way to apply the symptom-based approach is to determine whether symptoms represent reduced positive affect, which is mediated by dopamine (DA) and norepinephrine (NE), or increased negative affect, which is mediated by serotonin (5HT) or NE or both. Treatment options can then be selected based on the hypothetically mediating neurotransmitters. Agents such as norepinephrine dopamine reuptake inhibitors (NDRIs), norepinephrine reuptake inhibitors (NRIs), serotonin norepinephrine reuptake inhibitors (SNRIs), and monoamine oxidase inhibitors (MAOIs) are thus options for treating reduced positive affect. On the other hand, agents such as serotonin selective reuptake inhibitors (SSRIs), SNRIs, and serotonin 2A antagonist/reuptake inhibitors (SARIs) are thus options for increased negative affect. Patients with both sets of symptoms may benefit from combination treatment or an MAOI.

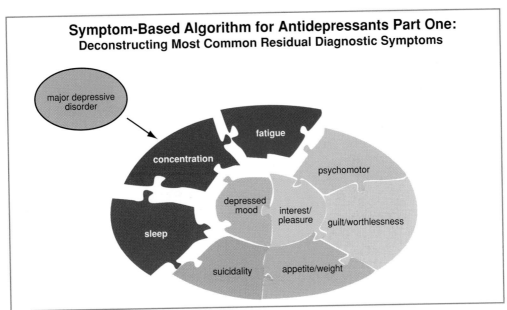

FIGURE 2-121 Symptom-based algorithm for antidepressants, part 1. Shown here is the diagnosis of major depressive disorder deconstructed into its symptoms [as defined by the *Diagnostic and Statistical Manual of Mental Disorders*, fourth edition (DSM-IV)]. Of these, sleep disturbances, problems concentrating, and fatigue are the most common residual symptoms.

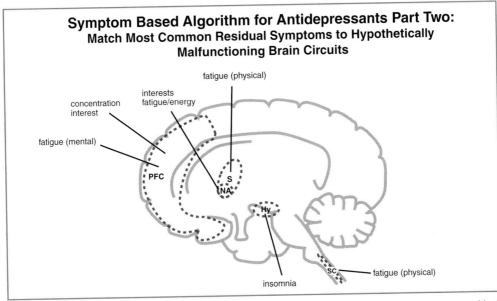

FIGURE 2-122 Symptom-based algorithm for antidepressants, part 2. In this figure the most common residual symptoms of major depression are linked to hypothetically malfunctioning brain circuits. Insomnia may be linked to the hypothalamus, problems concentrating to the dorsolateral prefrontal cortex (PFC), reduced interest to the PFC and nucleus accumbens (NA), and fatigue to the PFC, striatum (S), NA, and spinal cord (SC).

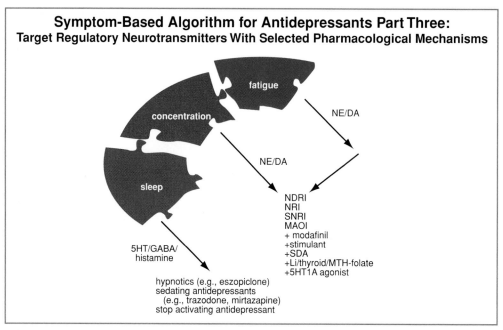

FIGURE 2-123 Symptom-based algorithm for antidepressants, part 3. Residual symptoms of depression can be linked to the neurotransmitters that regulate them and then, in turn, to pharmacological mechanisms. Fatigue and concentration are regulated in large part by norepinephrine (NE) and dopamine (DA), which are affected by many antidepressants, including norepinephrine dopamine reuptake inhibitors (NDRIs), selective norepinephrine reuptake inhibitors (NRIs), serotonin norepinephrine reuptake inhibitors (SNRIs), and monoamine oxidase inhibitors (MAOIs). Augmenting agents that affect NE and/or DA include modafinil, stimulants, serotonin dopamine antagonists (SDAs), lithium, thyroid hormone, L-5-methyl-tetrahydrofolate (MTHF), and serotonin (5HT) 1A agonists. Sleep disturbance is regulated by 5HT, gamma-aminobutyric acid (GABA), and histamine and can be treated with sedative hypnotics, sedating antidepressants such as trazodone or mirtazapine, or by discontinuing an activating antidepressant.

pharmacological mechanisms, as shown specifically for these common residual symptoms in Figure 2-123.

For problems with concentration and interest as well as for fatigue, this approach suggests targeting both NE and DA with first-line antidepressants plus augmenting agents that act on these neurotransmitters, as indicated in Figure 2-123. This can also call for stopping the SSRI if it is partially the cause of these symptoms. On the other hand, for insomnia, this symptom is hypothetically associated with an entirely different malfunctioning circuit regulated by different neurotransmitters (Figure 2-123). Therefore the treatment of this symptom calls for a different approach – namely, the use of hypnotics that act on the GABA system or sedating antidepressants that work to block rather than boost the serotonin or histamine system (Figure 2-123). It is possible that any of the symptoms shown in Figure 2-123 would respond to whatever drug is administered, but this symptom-based approach can tailor the treatment portfolio to the individual patient, possibly finding a faster way of reducing specific symptoms with more tolerable treatment selections for each patient than a purely random approach.

The symptom-based approach for selecting antidepressants may be even more important when targeting symptoms that are not components of the formal diagnostic criteria for depression but are common, bothersome, and likely to interfere with attaining remission

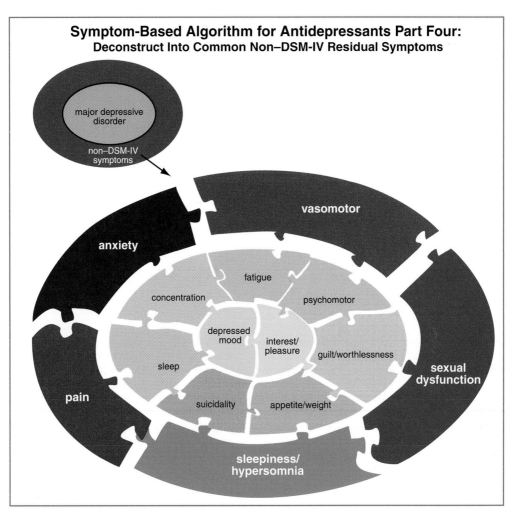

FIGURE 2-124 Symptom-based algorithm for antidepressants, part 4. There are several common symptoms of depression that are nonetheless not part of the formal diagnostic criteria for major depressive disorder. These include painful physical symptoms, excessive daytime sleepiness/hypersomnia with problems of arousal and alertness, anxiety, vasomotor symptoms, and sexual dysfunction.

if they persist (Figure 2-124). Five such symptoms commonly associated with depression which, however, are not formal components of the major depressive disorder symptom profile are highlighted in Figures 2-124 through 2-127 and include anxiety, pain, excessive daytime sleepiness/hypersomnia/problems with arousal and alertness, sexual dysfunction, and vasomotor symptoms (in women) (Figures 2-124 to 2-126).

Comorbid psychiatric illnesses distinct from major depression can also occur with a major depressive episode (Figure 2-127). Each of these comorbid conditions will likely require the elimination of all symptoms if a patient with major depression is to achieve a true remission.

In taking a history of symptoms before and after treatment with each antidepressant intervention, it is a good idea to solicit whether any of these comorbid conditions exist as

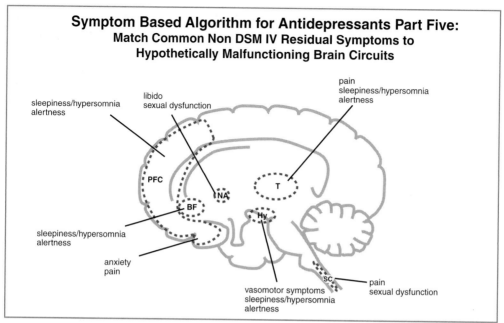

FIGURE 2-125 Symptom-based algorithm for antidepressants, part 5. In this figure common residual symptoms of major depression that are not part of formal diagnostic criteria are linked to hypothetically malfunctioning brain circuits. Painful physical symptoms are linked to the spinal cord (SC), thalamus (T), and ventral portions of the prefrontal cortex (PFC), while anxiety is associated with the ventral PFC. Vasomotor symptoms are mediated by the hypothalamus (Hy) and sexual dysfunction by the SC and nucleus accumbens (NA). Sleep symptoms that are part of the diagnostic criteria of depression involve mostly insomnia, linked to the hypothalamus; however, shown here are problems with hypersomnia and excessive daytime sleepiness, which may be beyond those symptoms included in the diagnostic criteria and be linked to problems with arousal and alertness and to arousal pathways not only in the hypothalamus but also the thalamus (T), basal forebrain (BF), and prefrontal cortex (PFC).

well as whether any of the nondiagnostic symptoms of depression are present along with the nine formal diagnostic symptoms of major depression (Figure 1-44). Each patient should have his or her major depressive episode deconstructed not only into diagnostic symptoms but also into all associated symptoms and comorbid conditions on each visit (Figure 2-124). Each and every symptom can then be mapped onto hypothetically malfunctioning brain circuits (Figure 2-125).

The pathways for the five additional nondiagnostic symptoms shown in Figure 2-126 obviously involve some differences from the pathways for the nine diagnostic symptoms shown in Figures 1-45 to 1-54 and thus often require different treatment approaches based on the unique pharmacological regulatory mechanisms that must be targeted to relieve these symptoms of depression as well. Sometimes it is said that for a good clinician to get patients with major depression into remission, he or she must target at least fourteen of the nine symptoms of depression!

Fortunately psychiatric drug treatments do not respect psychiatric disorders. Treatments that target pharmacological mechanisms in specific brain circuits do so no matter what psychiatric disorder is associated with the symptom linked to that circuit. Thus symptoms of one psychiatric disorder may be treatable with a proven agent that is known to treat the same symptom in another psychiatric disorder.

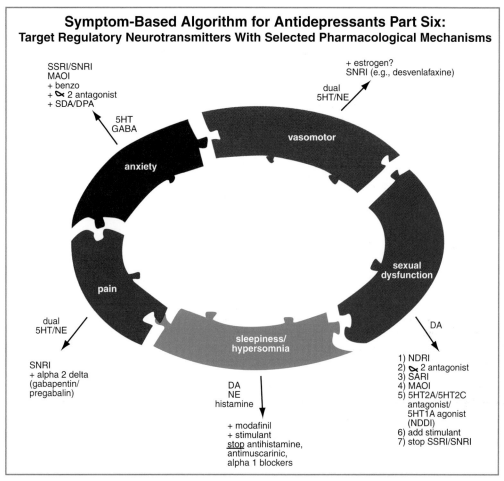

Symptom-Based Algorithm for Antidepressants Part Six:
Target Regulatory Neurotransmitters With Selected Pharmacological Mechanisms

FIGURE 2-126 Symptom-based algorithm for antidepressants, part 6. Residual symptoms of depression can be linked to the neurotransmitters that regulate them and then, in turn, to pharmacological mechanisms. Painful physical symptoms are mediated by norepinephrine (NE) and to a lesser extent serotonin (5HT) and may be treated with serotonin norepinephrine reuptake inhibitors (SNRIs) or alpha 2 delta ligands (pregabalin, gabapentin). Anxiety is related to 5HT and gamma-aminobutyric acid (GABA); it can be treated with serotonin selective reuptake inhibitors (SSRIs), SNRIs, or monoamine oxidase inhibitors (MAOIs) as monotherapies as well as by augmentation with benzodiazepines, alpha 2 antagonists, serotonin dopamine antagonists (SDAs), or dopamine partial agonists (DPAs). Vasomotor symptoms may be modulated by NE and 5HT and treated with SNRIs; augmentation with estrogen therapy is also an option. Sexual dysfunction is regulated primarily by dopamine (DA) and may be treated with norepinephrine dopamine reuptake inhibitors (NDRIs), alpha 2 antagonists, serotonin 2A antagonist/reuptake inhibitors (SARIs), MAOIs, 5HT2A/5HT2C antagonists, 5HT1A agonists, addition of a stimulant, or by stopping an SSRI or SNRI. Hypersomnia and problems with arousal and alertness are regulated by DA, NE, and histamine and can be treated with activating agents such as modafinil or stimulants or by stopping sedating agents with antihistamine, antimuscarinic, and/or alpha 1 blocking properties.

For example, anxiety can be reduced in patients with major depression who do not meet full criteria for an anxiety disorder with the same serotonin and GABA mechanisms proven to work in anxiety disorders (Figure 2-126).

Sleepiness/hypersomnia is a common associated symptom of depression but not all that frequently detected because patients who have this problem surprisingly do not often

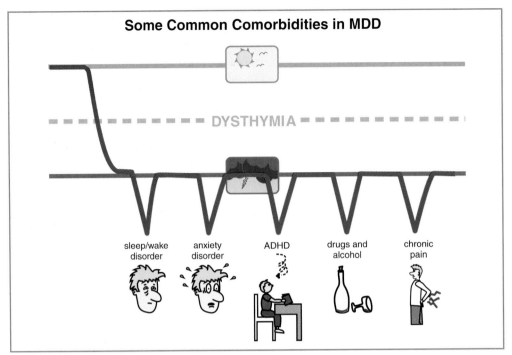

FIGURE 2-127 Common comorbidities in major depressive disorder (MDD). Some common comorbidities in MDD include sleep/wake disorders, anxiety disorders, attention deficit hyperactivity disorder (ADHD), substance use disorders, and chronic painful conditions.

complain about it. Although sleep disturbance in general is one of the diagnostic criteria for a major depressive episode (Figures 1-44 and 2-121), the specific sleep disturbance is usually insomnia. "Hypersomnia" can less commonly be one of the diagnostic criteria for a major depressive episode, but in this instance generally means oversleeping in the form of prolonged sleep episodes at night or increased daytime sleep. What is emphasized in Figures 2-124 and 2-126 is a type of hypersomnia that is frequently missed in patients with a major depressive episode because they often fail to complain about it: namely, excessive daytime sleepiness but not necessarily oversleeping. This type of hypersomnia/sleepiness is hypothetically linked to problems with arousal mechanisms and alertness as well as to problems with cognitive and executive functioning and is hypothetically linked with a different set of brain circuits (see Figure 2-125) than insomnia (Figure 2-122). Thus, excessive daytime sleepiness/hypersomnia/alertness is included here as one of the non–DSM-IV residual symptoms in Figures 2-124 and 2-125. Mechanisms to be targeted for sleepiness and hypersomnia in major depression are the same mechanisms proven effective for these same symptoms when they occur in various sleep/wake disorders, including agents that can boost DA, NE, and/or histamine (Figure 2-126).

Painful physical symptoms are present in many if not most depressed patients yet are not considered part of the diagnostic criteria for a major depressive episode. Nevertheless, it is important to relieve painful symptoms to attain remission of depression; approaches include a dual 5HT/NE strategy with possible augmentation by alpha 2 delta ligands, which is the same approach utilized in patients with chronic pain disorders (Figure 2-126).

Vasomotor symptoms that can accompany depression in perimenopausal and menopausal women have already been discussed. As mentioned, vasomotor symptoms in depressed women can be targeted with the same medications utilized to treat vasomotor symptoms in patients who are not depressed – namely, SNRIs.

Finally, sexual dysfunction can be a complicated problem of many causes and can range from lack of libido to problems with arousal of peripheral genitalia to lack of orgasm/ejaculation. Increasing DA or decreasing 5HT are the usual approaches to this set of problems whether the patient has major depression or not (Figure 2-126).

In summary, the symptom-based algorithm for selecting and combining antidepressants and for building a portfolio of mechanisms until each diagnostic and associated symptom of depression is abolished is the modern psychopharmacologist's approach to major depression. This approach follows contemporary notions of neurobiological disease and drug mechanisms. The symptom-based approach to treating major depression is not the only way to select treatments for this disorder, and it is important to remember that no matter what approach is chosen, the goal of treatment is remission.

Should antidepressant combinations be the standard for treating unipolar major depressive disorder?

Given the disappointing number of patients who attain remission from a major depressive episode even after four consecutive treatments (Figure 2-8) and who can maintain that remission over the long run (Figure 2-10), the paradigm of monotherapy for major depression is rapidly changing to one of multiple simultaneous pharmacological mechanisms, often with two or more therapeutic agents. In this respect, the pattern is following that of the treatment of bipolar disorder, which usually requires administration of more than one agent, as discussed in Chapter 3, on mood stabilizers. Rather than have a simple regimen of one antidepressant and a patient who is not in remission, it now seems highly preferable to have a patient in remission without symptoms no matter how many agents this takes. Several specific suggestions of antidepressant combinations are shown in Figures 2-128 to 2-134. Many others can be constructed, but these particular combinations or "combos" have enjoyed widespread use even though there is not much in the way of actual evidence-based data from clinical trials to show that their combination results in superior efficacy. Nevertheless, these suggestions may be useful for practicing clinicians to use in some patients.

Single-action and multiple-action monotherapies have already been extensively discussed in this chapter, as have combos containing lithium, thyroid, serotonin 2A antagonists and dopaminergic agents (Figure 2-128). Several additional combos are shown in Figure 2-128; they are discussed here and illustrated as well in Figures 2-129 through 2-134.

5HT1A Combo

The serotonin 1A partial agonist (SPA) buspirone is an approved treatment for anxiety but is more commonly used to augment patients with major depressive episodes who are partial responders to SSRIs (Figures 2-128 and 2-129). The beta blocker pindolol is also a partial agonist at 5HT1A receptors and has been utilized experimentally as an augmenting agent to SSRIs (Figure 2-128). Gepirone, a new 5HT1A partial agonist, is in late clinical testing in depression and may be useful not only as an augmenting agent for partial responders to SSRIs, but also as a monotherapy for major depression.

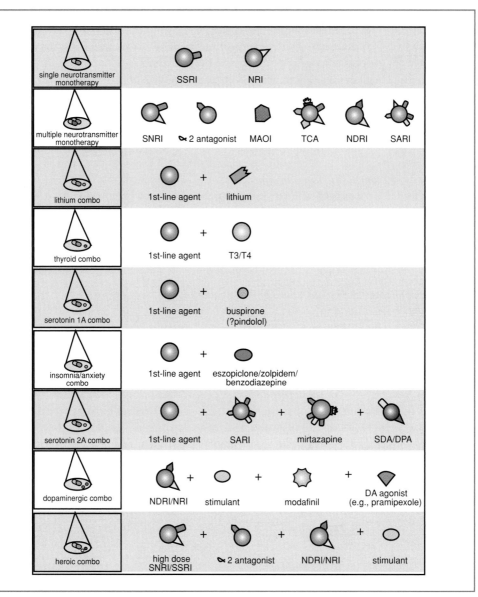

FIGURE 2-128 Combination treatments for unipolar depression. The treatment of depression generally begins with a single agent, called a first-line agent, as monotherapy. If single agents acting by a single neurotransmitter mechanism fail, then single agents acting by multiple neurotransmitter mechanisms may be effective. If these monotherapies also fail, antidepressants are often used in combination with other drugs or hormones or even other antidepressants. For example, a first-line agent can be paired with lithium (lithium combo). Another strategy is to augment a first-line agent with thyroid hormone (thyroid combo). Yet another approach is addition of the serotonin 1A (5HT1A) partial agonist buspirone or possibly the 5HT1A antagonist pindolol to a first-line antidepressant, especially a serotonin selective reuptake inhibitor (serotonin 1A combo). Short-term use of sedative–hypnotics or anxiolytics may be necessary if insomnia or anxiety is persistent and cannot be managed by other strategies (insomnia/anxiety combo). Another multimechanism option is to add a serotonin 2A antagonist such as a serotonin 2 antagonist/reuptake inhibitor (SARI), mirtazapine, or a serotonin dopamine antagonist (SDA) or dopamine partial agonist (DPA) (serotonin 2A combo). Patients with fatigue or cognitive symptoms may benefit from the addition of an agent that enhances dopamine neurotransmission (dopaminergic combo). Finally, patients who are not responding may need to be treated with high doses of a first-line agent in combination with an alpha 2 antagonist, norepinephrine dopamine reuptake inhibitor, or stimulant.

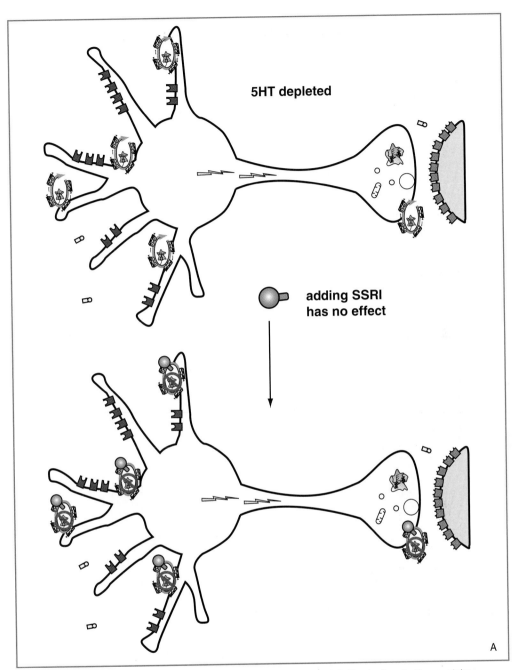

FIGURE 2-129A Mechanism of action of buspirone augmentation, part 1. Serotonin selective reuptake inhibitors (SSRIs) act indirectly by increasing synaptic levels of serotonin (5HT) that have been released there. If 5HT is depleted, there is no 5HT release and SSRIs are ineffective. This has been postulated to be the explanation for the lack of SSRI therapeutic actions or loss of therapeutic action of SSRI ("poop out") in some patients.

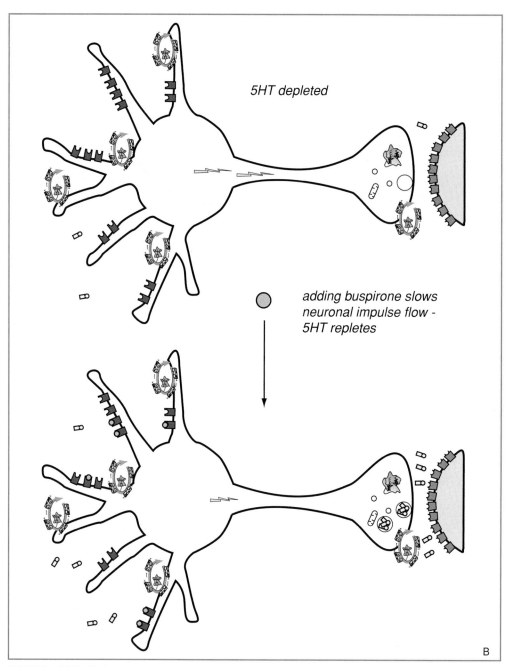

5HT depleted

adding buspirone slows neuronal impulse flow - 5HT repletes

B

FIGURE 2-129B Mechanism of action of buspirone augmentation, part 2. Shown here is how buspirone may augment the action of serotonin selective reuptake inhibitors (SSRIs) both by repleting serotonin (5HT) and directly desensitizing 5HT1A receptors. One theoretical mechanism of how 5HT is allowed to reaccumulate in the 5HT-depleted neuron is the shutdown of neuronal impulse flow. If 5HT release is essentially turned off for a while so that the neuron retains all the 5HT it synthesizes, this may allow repletion of 5HT stores. A 5HT partial agonist such as buspirone acts directly on somatodendritic autoreceptors to inhibit neuronal impulse flow, possibly allowing repletion of 5HT stores. Also, buspirone could boost actions directly at 5HT1A receptors to help the small amount of 5HT available in this scenario accomplish the targeted desensitization of 5HT1A somatodendritic autoreceptors that is necessary for antidepressant actions.

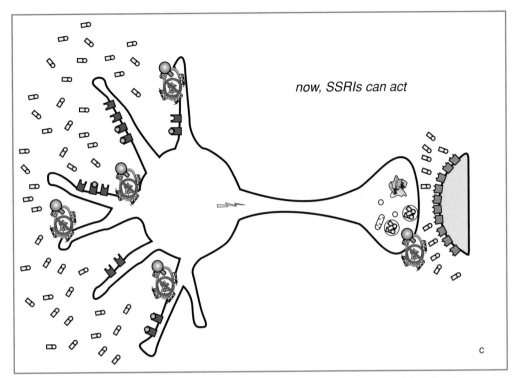

now, SSRIs can act

c

FIGURE 2-129C Mechanism of action of buspirone augmentation, part 3. Shown here is how buspirone potentiates ineffective serotonin selective reuptake inhibitor (SSRI) action at serotonin 1A (5HT1A) somatodendritic autoreceptors, resulting in the desired disinhibition of the 5HT neuron. This combination of 5HT1A agonists plus SSRIs may be more effective, not only in depression but also in other disorders treated by SSRIs, such as obsessive compulsive disorder and panic.

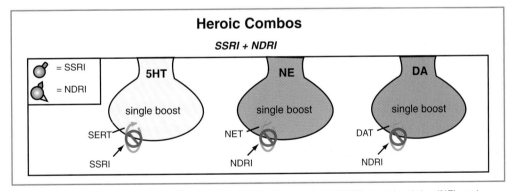

FIGURE 2-130 Heroic combos, part 1: SSRI plus NDRI. Here serotonin (5HT), norepinephrine (NE), and dopamine (DA) are all single-boosted.

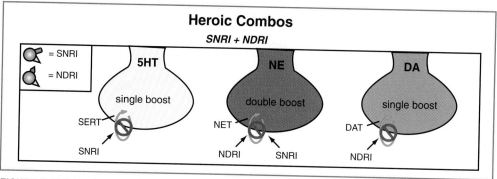

FIGURE 2-131 Heroic combos, part 2: SNRI plus NDRI. Serotonin norepinephrine reuptake inhibitor (SNRI) plus a norepinephrine dopamine reuptake inhibitor (NDRI) leads to a single boost for serotonin (5HT), a double boost for norepinephrine (NE), and a single boost for dopamine (DA).

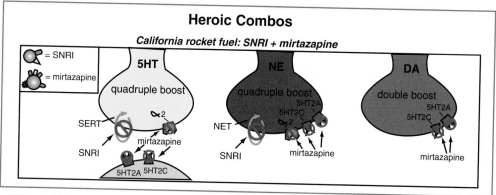

FIGURE 2-132 Heroic combos, part 3: California rocket fuel (SNRI plus mirtazapine). Serotonin norepinephrine reuptake inhibitor (SNRI) plus mirtazapine is a combination that has a great degree of theoretical synergy: norepinephrine reuptake blockade plus alpha 2 blockade, serotonin (5HT) reuptake plus 5HT2A and 5HT2C antagonism, and thus many 5HT actions plus norepinephrine (NE) actions. Specifically, 5HT is quadruple-boosted (with reuptake blockade, alpha 2 antagonism, 5HT2A antagonism, and 5HT2C antagonism), NE is quadruple-boosted (with reuptake blockade, alpha 2 antagonism, 5HT2A antagonism, and 5HT2C antagonism), and there may even be a double boost of dopamine (with 5HT2A and 5HT2C antagonism).

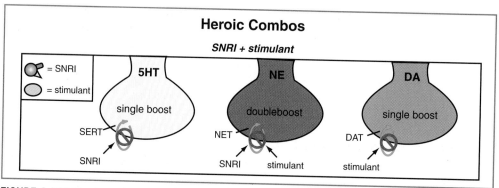

FIGURE 2-133 Heroic combos, part 4: SNRI plus stimulant. Here serotonin (5HT) and dopamine (DA) are single-boosted and norepinephrine (NE) is double-boosted.

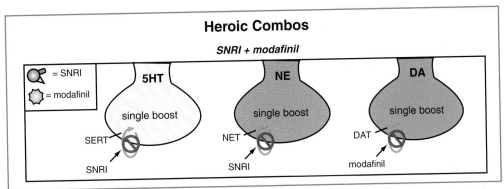

FIGURE 2-134 Heroic combos, part 5: SNRI plus modafinil. Here serotonin (5HT) and norepinephrine (NE) are single-boosted by the serotonin norepinephrine reuptake inhibitor (SNRI) while dopamine (DA) is single-boosted by modafinil.

Buspirone is a short-acting compound requiring twice- or thrice-daily administration; its peak-dose side effects of nausea and dizziness have interfered with its wide use as a monotherapy. Gepirone is being tested in a controlled-release formulation as gepirone ER and thus requires only once-daily administration, with lesser peak-dose side effects than buspirone. Possible additional advantages of gepirone ER over buspirone include being a "fuller" or "less partial" agonist than buspirone and possibly being metabolized to active metabolites, including a 5HT1A full agonist as well as another active metabolite with alpha 2 antagonist properties. The antidepressant actions of alpha 2 antagonism are discussed above, in the section on mirtazapine (see Figures 2-51 to 2-54). Unlike SSRIs and SNRIs, neither buspirone nor gepirone is associated with sexual dysfunction.

One theory for how the combination of a 5HT1A partial agonist with an SSRI can have enhanced efficacy is the notion that an SSRI monotherapy added to the regimen of a patient with severely depleted serotonin levels would have no therapeutic actions, since there is no serotonin released whose reuptake can be blocked by the SSRI (Figure 2-129A). However, adding a 5HT1A partial agonist like buspirone (or gepirone ER) would act at somatodendritic 5HT1A autoreceptors, and this would be predicted to allow serotonin levels to be repleted (Figure 2-129B). Now SSRIs would be able to act because serotonin would again be released and its reuptake could again be blocked (Figure 2-129C).

Triple-action combo: SSRI/SNRI ± NDRI

If boosting one neurotransmitter is good and two is better, maybe boosting three is best (one of the heroic combos in Figure 2-128 and also illustrated in Figures 2-130 and 2-131). Triple-action antidepressant therapy with modulation of all three of the trimonoamine neurotransmitter systems would be predicted to occur by combining either an SSRI with an NDRI, perhaps the most popular combination in U.S. antidepressant psychopharmacology (Figure 2-130), or combining an SNRI with an NDRI, providing even more noradrenergic and dopaminergic action (Figure 2-131).

California rocket fuel: SNRI plus mirtazapine

This potentially powerful combination utilizes the pharmacological synergy attained by adding the enhanced serotonin and norepinephrine release from inhibition of both dual serotonin and norepinephrine reuptake by an SNRI to the disinhibition of both

TABLE 2-14 Antidepressants in development: various monoaminergic mechanisms

---

Atypical antipsychotics as antidepressants for unipolar major depression
- quetiapine
- ziprasidone
- aripiprazole
- olanzapine
- risperidone
- paliperidone
- bifeprunox
- asenapine
- SX 313, 314

Triple reuptake inhibitors (TRIs): serotonin, norepinephrine and dopamine reuptake inhibitors (SNDRIs)
- DOV 216303
- DOV 21947
- GW 372475 (NS2359)
- Boehringer/NS2330
- NS2360
- Sepracor SEP 225289

TRI plus
- SRI>NRI>DRI/5HT2C, 5HT3, 5HT2A, alpha 1A
  - Lu AA24530
- SRI>NRI>DRI/5HT6
  - Lu AA37096
- SRI>NRI/5HT2A/alpha 1A/5HT6
  - Lu AA34893

NDDIs – norepinephrine dopamine disinhibitors
- agomelatine (Valdoxan) – 5HT2C antagonist/melatonin 1/2 agonist
- flibanserin (Ectris) – 5HT2A/2C antagonist/5HT1A agonist – (for HSDD, hypoactive sexual desire disorder)

Beta 3 agonist
- amibegron (SR58611A)

---

serotonin and norepinephrine release by the alpha 2 antagonist actions of mirtazapine (Figure 2-132). It is even possible that additional pro-dopaminergic actions result from the combination of norepinephrine reuptake blockade in prefrontal cortex due to SNRI actions with 5HT2A/2C actions disinhibiting dopamine release (Figure 2-132). This combination can provide very powerful antidepressant action for some patients with unipolar major depressive episodes.

Arousal combos

The frequent complaints of residual fatigue, loss of energy, motivation, sex drive, and problems concentrating/problems with alertness may be approached by combining either a stimulant with an SNRI (Figure 2-133) or modafinil with an SNRI (Figure 2-134) to recruit triple monoamine action and especially enhancement of dopamine.

TABLE 2-15 Antidepressants in development: novel serotonin-linked mechanisms

5HT1A partial agonists
    gepirone ER
    PRX 00023
    MN 305
5HT6 agonists/antagonists
5HT1B/D antagonist
    elzasonan
SSRI plus 5HT1A PA
    vilazodone (SB 659746A)
Sigma 1/5HT1A PA>SRI
    VPI 013 (OPC 14523)
SSRI/5HT3>5HT1A
    Lu AA21004
5HT1A agonist/5HT2A antagonist
    TGW-00-AD/AA
SRI/5HT2/5HT1A/5HT1D
    TGBA-01-AD

Future treatments for mood disorders

An explosion of potential new treatments with novel mechanisms are in testing for major depression (Tables 2-14 to 2-17). This includes the use of **atypical antipsychotics** for unipolar major depression and for treatment-resistant unipolar depression (Table 2-14).

Atypical antipsychotics are discussed in greater detail in the following chapter on mood stabilizers and bipolar depression. Whether these same agents will be proven effective with a sufficiently favorable side effect and cost profile for unipolar depression is still under intense investigation.

A large number of **novel serotonin targets** are in testing and are listed in Table 2-15. One particularly interesting novel serotonin target is the **5HT2C receptor**. This receptor was extensively discussed earlier in this chapter in relation to the SSRI fluoxetine (Figure 2-25) and to the SARI trazodone (Figure 2-64). Blockade of 5HT2C receptors causes release of both norepinephrine and dopamine, which is why these agents can be called **norepinephrine dopamine disinhibitors or NDDIs**. A novel antidepressant **agomelatine** (Valdoxan; Table 2-14) combines this property of 5HT2C antagonism and thus NDDI actions with additional agonist actions at melatonin receptors (MT1 and MT2) (Figure 2-135). Agomelatine also has 5HT2B antagonist properties. This portfolio of pharmacological actions predicts not only antidepressant actions due to the NDDI mechanism of 5HT2C antagonism but also sleep-enhancing properties due to MT1 and MT2 agonist actions (Figure 2-135). Another NDDI with 5HT2C antagonist properties is **flibanserin** (Ectris). This agent also has 5HT2A antagonist and 5HT1A agonist properties and, owing to its robust NDDI properties, is under investigation for sexual dysfunction linked to deficient dopamine activity, including conditions such as hypoactive sexual desire disorder (HSDD).

TABLE 2-16 Antidepressants in development: targeting neurokinins

NK2 antagonists
    saredutant (SR48968)
    SAR 1022279
    SSR 241586 (NK2 and NK3)
    SR 144190
    GR 159897
NK3 antagonists
    osanetant (SR142801)
    talnetant (SB223412)
    SR 146977
Substance P antagonists
    aprepitant/MK869/L-754030 (Emend)
    L-758,298; L-829–165; L-733,060
    CP122721; CP99994; CP96345
    casopitant GW679769
    vestipitant GW 597599 +/− paroxetine
    LY 686017
    GW823296
    nolpitantium SR140333
    SSR240600; R-673
    NKP-608/AV608
    CGP49823
    SDZ NKT 34311
    SB679769
    GW597599
    vafopitant GR205171

TABLE 2-17 Antidepressants in development: targeting novel sites of action

MIF-1 pentapeptide analogs
    nemifitide (INN 00835)
    5-hydroxy-nemifitide (INN 01134)
Glucocorticoid antagonists
    mifepristone (Corlux)
    Org 34517; Org 34850 (glucocorticoid receptor II antagonists)
CRF1 antagonists
    R121919
    CP316,311
    BMS 562086
    GW876008
    ONO-233M
    JNJ19567470/TS041
    SSR125543
    SSR126374
Vasopressin 1B antagonists
    SSR149415

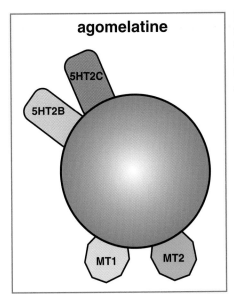

FIGURE 2-135 Icon of agomelatine. The novel antidepressant agomelatine, in testing, combines the property of serotonin (5HT) 2C antagonism (and thus indirect enhancement of norepinephrine and dopamine) with actions at melatonin 1 (M1) and melatonin 2 (M2) receptors. Agomelatine is also an antagonist at 5HT2B receptors.

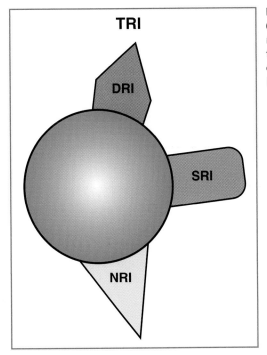

FIGURE 2-136 Icon of triple reuptake inhibitor (TRI). Several triple reuptake inhibitors (serotonin norepinephrine dopamine reuptake inhibitors) are in testing. Different agents may have different balances of serotonin to norepinephrine to dopamine reuptake blockade.

Triple reuptake inhibitors (TRIs) or serotonin-norepinephrine-dopamine-reuptake inhibitors (SNDRIs) (Figure 2-136)

These drugs are testing the idea that if one mechanism is good (i.e., SSRI) and two mechanisms are better (i.e., SNRI), then maybe targeting all three mechanisms of the tri-monoamine neurotransmitter system would be the best in terms of efficacy. Several different

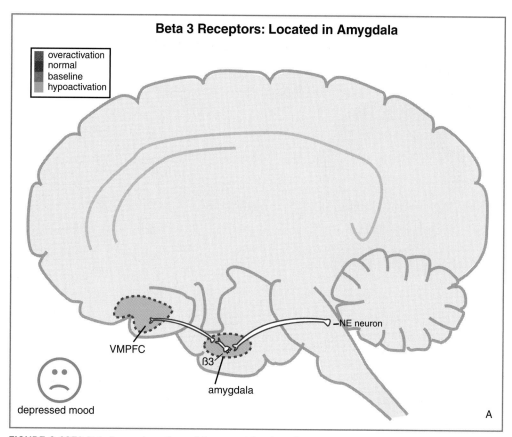

FIGURE 2-137A Beta 3 receptors. Some data suggest that beta 3 receptors, located in the amygdala, may be related to depressed mood. Decreased efficiency of these receptors could lead to hypoactivation of the amygdala as well as brain regions closely connected to the amygdala, such as the ventromedial prefrontal cortex (VMPFC).

triple reuptake inhibitors (or serotonin-norepinephrine-dopamine reuptake inhibitors) are listed in Table 2-14. Some of these agents have additional pharmacological properties as well ("TRI plus" in Table 2-14). The question for TRIs is how much blockade of each monoamine transporter is desired, especially for the dopamine transporter or DAT. This was also discussed extensively in the section on NDRIs above. Too much dopamine activity can lead to a drug of abuse, and not enough means that the agent is essentially an SNRI. Perhaps the desirable profile is robust inhibition of the serotonin transporter and substantial inhibition of the norepinephrine transporter, like the known SNRI, plus a little frosting on the cake of 10% to 25% inhibition of DAT. Some testing suggests that DRI action also increases acetylcholine release, so TRIs may modulate a fourth neurotransmitter system and act as multitransmitter modulators. Further testing will determine whether the available TRIs will represent an advance over SSRIs or SNRIs in the treatment of depression.

Beta 3 agonist

A very novel mechanism for an antidepressant is posed by **amibegron**, an agonist of beta 3 receptors (Table 2-14). The role of beta 3 receptors in the brain is still being clarified, but it

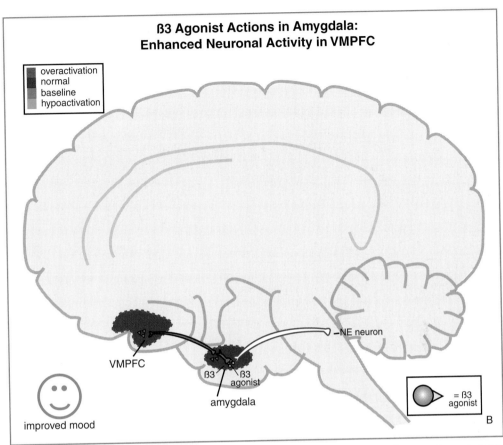

ß3 Agonist Actions in Amygdala: Enhanced Neuronal Activity in VMPFC

overactivation
normal
baseline
hypoactivation

VMPFC

ß3   ß3
agonist

amygdala

—NE neuron

improved mood

= ß3
agonist

B

FIGURE 2-137B Beta 3 agonists. Agonists of beta 3 receptors in the amygdala may restore neurotransmission in that region, thus also restoring neurotransmission in the ventromedial prefrontal cortex (VMPFC). This may lead to improved mood. Amibegron is a beta 3 agonist currently in testing.

appears that they may be localized in high density in the amygdala, where they may regulate neuronal activity in ventromedial prefrontal cortex and thereby exert their antidepressant actions (Figure 2-137). Extensive testing in animal models of depression demonstrates the antidepressant actions of amibegron, and human testing is currently in progress.

Also, a large number of agents that act at several other novel targets are listed in Tables 2-16 and 2-17. Many of the agents listed in Table 2-17 are low-molecular-weight drugs that target stress hormone release from the hypothalamic-pituitary-adrenal (HPA) axis, including **glucocorticoid antagonists, corticotrophin releasing factor 1 (CRF1) antagonists, and vasopressin 1B antagonists**. These agents are in testing not only for depression but also for various stress-related conditions. **Nemifitide** is itself a novel pentapeptide modeled on the structure of melanocyte inhibitory factor (MIF-1), a tripeptide shown to be active in animal models of depression and in small clinical studies of depressed patients (Table 2-17 and Figure 2-138). MIF-1 (also known as L-prolyl-L-leucy-L-glycinamide, or PLG) is also the tripeptide tail of oxytocin and its precursor neurophysin. Nemifitide is a pentapeptide analog not only of the tripeptide MIF-1 but also of the tripeptide tail of vasopressin (Figure 2-138). Nemifitide is administered by subcutaneous injection and has been shown to be active in animal models of depression; it is in testing in depressed patients,

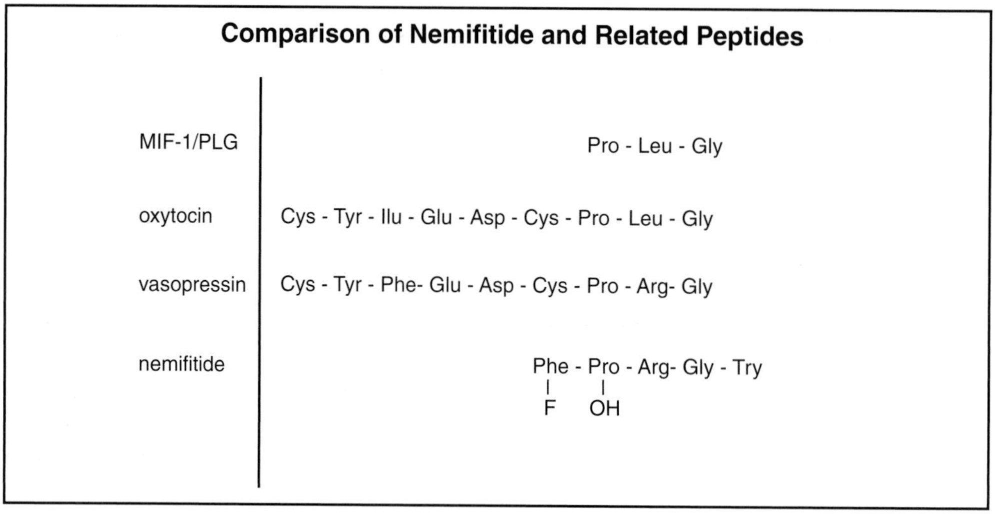

Comparison of Nemifitide and Related Peptides

MIF-1/PLG	Pro - Leu - Gly
oxytocin	Cys - Tyr - Ilu - Glu - Asp - Cys - Pro - Leu - Gly
vasopressin	Cys - Tyr - Phe- Glu - Asp - Cys - Pro - Arg- Gly
nemifitide	Phe - Pro - Arg- Gly - Try
	F OH

FIGURE 2-138 Novel peptides. Novel peptides in testing for depression include nemifitide, an analog of melanocyte inhibitory factor (MIF-1; also known as L-prolyl-L-leucine-L-glycinamide, or PLG). PLG is also the tripeptide tail of oxytocin and its precursor neurophysin. Nemifitide's structure shows that it is also structurally related to the tripeptide tail of vasopressin. Nemifitide has shown antidepressant actions in animal models and in early clinical testing in depression.

where early findings suggest possible efficacy with rapid onset, including effectiveness in treatment-resistant patients. Further testing in patients with major depressive episodes is ongoing.

Another class of peptide antagonists is the **neurokinin antagonists** (Table 2-16). Neurokinins belong to the family of peptides known as tachykinins (Table 2-18). Tachykinins include not only neurokinins but also newly discovered endokinins and tachykinin

TABLE 2-18 Human tachykinins

Neurokinins
    SP (substance P; neurokinin 1; NK1)
    NKA (neurokinin A)
    NPK (neuropeptide K; extended form of NKA)
    NP gamma (neuropeptide gamma; another extended form of NKA)
    NKA 3-10 (shortened form of NKA)
    NKB (neurokinin B)
Endokinins
    EKA (endokinin A)
    EKB (endokinin B)
    hHK 1 (human hemokinin 1)
    hHK 4-11 (shortened form of hHK1)
Tachykinin gene–related peptides
    EKC (endokinin C)
    EKD (endokinin D)

TABLE 2-19 Neurokinin receptors

Neurokinin 1 receptors
    Also called substance P receptors
    In brain, agonist is substance P
    In periphery, agonist is either substance P, or one of the endokinins
Neurokinin 2 receptors
    Agonist is NKA (neurokinin A, and its extended and shortened versions)
Neurokinin 3 receptors
    Agonist is NKB (neurokinin B)

gene–related peptides that act mostly outside the brain but at the same receptors where the tachykinins act (especially the NK1 receptor) (Table 2-18). Low-molecular-weight antagonists (Table 2-16) have been identified for each of the three known neurokinin receptors, NK1, NK2, and NK3 (Table 2-19). **NK1 antagonists, also known as substance P antagonists**, have been hotly pursued for many years as treatments not only for depression but also for pain, schizophrenia, and other psychiatric disorders. To date, the clinical results with substance P antagonists, from testing in major depression and in pain-related conditions, have been disappointing. However, recent evidence suggests that **saredutant**, an **NK2 antagonist**, may be effective not only in animal models of depression but also in patients with major depressive episodes (Table 2-16). Hypothetically, conditions associated with excessive release of endogenous NKA (or its extended or shortened versions (see Tables 2-18 and 2-19), especially under conditions of stress or major depression, benefit from the blocking of NK2 receptors; that could explain why this mechanism may produce an antidepressant effect. **NK3 antagonists** are also in testing for various psychiatric disorders.

Summary

This extensive chapter began with an overview of antidepressant response, remission, relapse, and residual symptoms after treatment with antidepressants. The leading hypothesis for major depression for the past forty years, namely the monoamine hypothesis, was discussed and critiqued. The mechanisms of action of the major antidepressant drugs, including dozens of individual agents working by many unique mechanisms, were also covered. The acute pharmacological actions of these agents on receptors and enzymes were described, as well as the major hypothesis – trimonoamine modulation of serotonin, dopamine, and norepinephrine – which attempts to explain how all current antidepressants ultimately work. Pharmacokinetic concepts relating to the metabolism of antidepressants and mood stabilizers by the cytochrome P450 enzyme system were also introduced.

Specific antidepressant agents that the reader should now understand include the serotonin selective reuptake inhibitors (SSRIs), serotonin norepinephrine reuptake inhibitors (SNRIs), norepinephrine dopamine reuptake inhibitors (NDRIs), selective norepinephrine reuptake inhibitors (selective NRIs), alpha 2 antagonists, serotonin antagonist/reuptake inhibitors (SARIs), MAO inhibitors, and tricyclic antidepressants. We have also covered numerous trimonoamine modulators (TMMs) that either have antidepressant action or boost the antidepressant action of other agents, including estrogen, 5-L-methyl-tetrahydrofolate, S-adenosyl-methionine, thyroid, lithium, therapeutic electrical modulation therapies such as electroconvulsive therapy (ECT), vagus nerve stimulation (VNS), transcranial magnetic stimulation (TMS), and deep brain stimulation (DBS) and, briefly, psychotherapy. Also provided was some guidance for how to select and combine antidepressants by following a symptom-based algorithm for patients who do not remit on their first antidepressant. Some options for combining drugs to treat such patients were illustrated and a glimpse into the future was provided by mentioning numerous novel antidepressants on the horizon.

Mood Stabilizers

This chapter reviews pharmacological concepts underlying the use of mood stabilizers. There are many definitions of a mood stabilizer and various drugs that act by distinctive mechanisms. The goal of this chapter is to acquaint the reader with current ideas about how different mood stabilizers work. The mechanisms of action of these drugs will be explained by building on general pharmacological concepts introduced in earlier chapters. Also to be discussed are concepts about how these drugs are best used in clinical practice, including strategies for what to do if initial treatments fail and how to rationally combine one mood stabilizer with another, as well as whether and when to combine a mood stabilizer with an antidepressant. Finally, the reader is introduced to some novel mood stabilizers in clinical development that may become available in the future.

The treatment of mood stabilizers in this chapter is at the conceptual level, not at the pragmatic level. The reader should consult standard drug handbooks (such as the companion *Essential Psychopharmacology: Prescriber's Guide*) for details of doses, side effects, drug interactions, and other issues relevant to the prescribing of these drugs in clinical practice.

Definition of a mood stabilizer: a labile label

"There is no such thing as a mood stabilizer."
- FDA

"Long live the mood stabilizers."
– Prescribers

What is a mood stabilizer? Originally, a mood stabilizer was a drug that treated mania and prevented its recurrence, thus "stabilizing" the manic pole of bipolar disorder. More recently, the concept of "mood stabilizer" has been defined in a wide-ranging manner, from "something that acts like lithium" to "an anticonvulsant used to treat bipolar disorder" to "an atypical antipsychotic used to treat bipolar disorder," with antidepressants being considered as "mood destabilizers." With all this competing terminology and the number of drugs for the treatment of bipolar disorder exploding, the term "mood stabilizer" has become so confusing that regulatory authorities and some experts now suggest that it would be best to use another term for agents that treat bipolar disorder.

Rather than using the term "mood stabilizers," some would argue that there are drugs that can treat any or all of four distinct phases of bipolar disorder (Figures 3-1 and 3-2). Thus, a drug can be "mania-minded" and "treat from above" to reduce symptoms of mania and/or "stabilize from above" to prevent relapse and the recurrence of mania (Figure 3-1). Furthermore, drugs can be "depression-minded" and "treat from below" to reduce symptoms of bipolar depression and/or "stabilize from below" to prevent relapse and the recurrence of depression (Figure 3-2). This chapter discusses agents that have one or more of these actions in bipolar disorder; for historical purposes and simplification, any of these agents may be referred to as a "mood stabilizer."

Lithium, the classic mood stabilizer

Bipolar disorder has been treated with lithium for at least 50 years. Lithium is an ion whose mechanism of action is not certain. Candidates for its mechanism of action are various signal transduction sites beyond neurotransmitter receptors (Figure 3-3). This includes second messengers, such as the phosphatidyl inositol system, where lithium inhibits the enzyme inositol monophosphatase; modulation of G proteins; and, most recently, regulation of gene expression for growth factors and neuronal plasticity by interaction with downstream signal

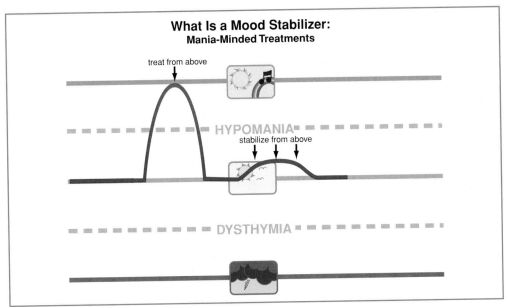

FIGURE 3-1 Mania-minded treatments. Although the ideal "mood stabilizer" would treat both mania and bipolar depression while also preventing episodes of either pole, in reality there is as yet not evidence to suggest that any single agent can achieve this consistently. Rather, different agents may be efficacious for different phases of bipolar disorder. As shown here, some agents seem to be "mania-minded" and thus able to "treat from above" and/or "stabilize from above" – in other words, to reduce and/or prevent symptoms of mania.

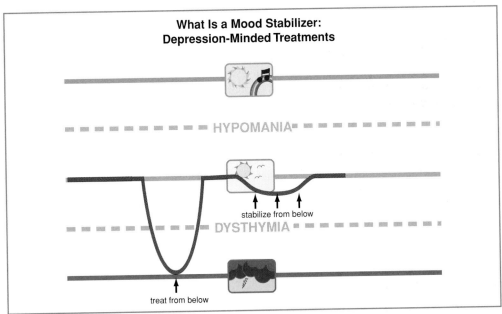

FIGURE 3-2 Depression-minded treatments. Although the ideal "mood stabilizer" would treat both mania and bipolar depression while also preventing episodes of either pole, as mentioned for the previous illustration, in reality there is as yet not evidence to suggest that any single agent can achieve this consistently. Rather, different agents may be efficacious for different phases of bipolar disorder. As shown here, some agents seem to be "depression-minded" and thus able to "treat from below" and/or "stabilize from below" – in other words, to reduce and/or prevent symptoms of bipolar depression.

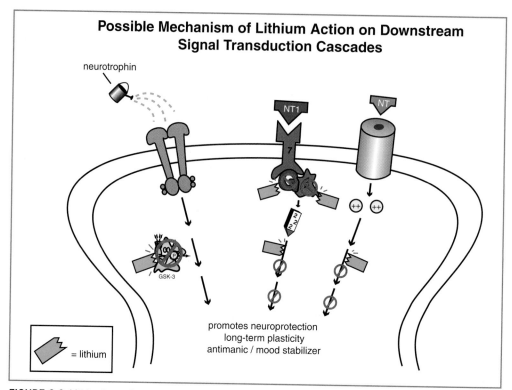

Possible Mechanism of Lithium Action on Downstream Signal Transduction Cascades

neurotrophin

NT1

NT

GSK-3

promotes neuroprotection
long-term plasticity
antimanic / mood stabilizer

= lithium

FIGURE 3-3 Lithium's mechanism of action. Although lithium is the oldest treatment for bipolar disorder, its mechanism of action is still not well understood. Several possible mechanisms exist and are shown here. Lithium may work by affecting signal transduction, perhaps through its inhibition of second messenger enzymes such as inositol monophosphatase (right), by modulation of G proteins (middle), or by interaction at various sites within downstream signal transduction cascades (left).

transduction cascades, including inhibition of glycogen synthetase kinase 3 (GSK3) and protein kinase C (illustrated in Figure 3-3).

However lithium works, it is proven effective in manic episodes and in the prevention of recurrence, especially for manic episodes and perhaps to a lesser extent for depressive episodes (Figure 3-4). In fact, lithium is the first psychotropic drug to be proven effective in maintenance treatment for any psychiatric disorder, and it has opened the way for maintenance claims for many other psychotropic agents over the past decades. Lithium is less well established as a robust treatment for acute bipolar depression but probably has some efficacy for this phase of the illness and certainly is well established as preventing suicide, deliberate self-harm, and death from all causes in patients with mood disorders (Figure 3-4).

Lithium was once popular as an augmenting agent to antidepressants for unipolar depression, as discussed in Chapter 2 and illustrated in Figure 2-113. In retrospect, some of the patients categorized in past decades as having unipolar depression who were treated with lithium augmentation would today be considered as fitting into the bipolar spectrum; therefore it should not be surprising that such patients have responded favorably to lithium augmentation of antidepressants (Figure 1-12). Lithium's putative mechanism as a tri-monoamine modulator to boost antidepressant action is discussed in Chapter 2 (Figure 2-113).

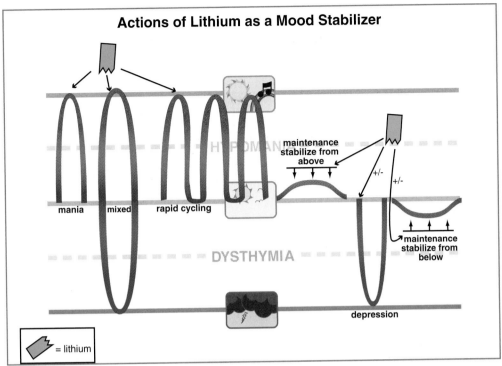

FIGURE 3-4 Actions of lithium as a mood stabilizer. Lithium has proven efficacy in mania, particularly for euphoric mania, although some experts suggest that it may not be as effective for rapid cycling or mixed episodes. Lithium is also efficacious for the prevention of manic episodes and of suicide. Lithium's efficacy for treating and preventing the depressed phase of bipolar disorder is less well established.

For many reasons, the use of lithium has declined in recent years, particularly among younger psychopharmacologists. This is due to many factors, including the entry of multiple new treatment options into the therapeutic armamentarium for bipolar disorder, to the side effects and monitoring burdens of lithium, and also to the lack of promotional marketing efforts for lithium, which is now a generic drug. Also, some experts feel that lithium is not as effective for rapid cycling and mixed episodes of bipolar disorder; they recommend it preferentially for euphoric mania but not for rapid cycling or mixed episodes. However, this selective use of lithium may not be justified, since response can be very individualized no matter what types of bipolar symptoms are being experienced.

Furthermore, lithium today is no longer used as high-dose monotherapy but rather as one member of a portfolio of treatments. Thus modern psychopharmacologists can now, in many cases, utilize lithium by treating patients with doses toward the bottom of the therapeutic range, often giving it only once daily and combining it with other mood stabilizers. This strategy of using lithium as an augmenting agent may provide incremental efficacy with acceptable tolerability.

Well-known side effects of lithium include gastrointestinal symptoms such as dyspepsia, nausea, vomiting, and diarrhea as well as weight gain, hair loss, acne, tremor, sedation, decreased cognition, and incoordination. There are also long-term adverse effects on the thyroid and kidney. Lithium has a narrow therapeutic window, requiring monitoring of plasma drug levels. Because of possible weight gain and metabolic complications, modern treatment with lithium also requires metabolic monitoring, just like that recommended for atypical antipsychotics. This includes body mass index, fasting triglycerides, and other parameters. Keeping lithium doses above threshold therapeutic levels yet below side effect levels may be one of the best ways to utilize this important therapeutic agent in the modern era, rather than neglecting it.

Anticonvulsants as mood stabilizers

Based on the theory that mania may "kindle" further episodes of mania, a logical parallel with seizure disorders was drawn, since seizures can kindle more seizures. Thus trials of several anticonvulsants in bipolar disorder have been conducted (Table 3-1). Since the first anticonvulsants tested, namely carbamazepine and valproate, proved effective in treating the manic phase of bipolar disorder, this has led to the idea than any anticonvulsant would be a mood stabilizer, especially for mania. However, this has not proven to be the case. Numerous anticonvulsants are discussed below, including not only those with proven efficacy in different phases of bipolar disorder but also those with dubious efficacy (Table 3-1).

Anticonvulsants are among the most interesting psychotropic agents, as some of them are effective for bipolar disorder while others are also effective for various pain syndromes (Table 3-1) and for other clinical uses, especially anxiety (Table 3-2). Differences in efficacy (and side effects) for the various anticonvulsants undoubtedly arise because of differences in mechanisms of action (Tables 3-3 and 3-4). Although the mechanisms of action of anticonvulsants and other mood stabilizers are being rapidly clarified, especially their actions on voltage-sensitive ion channels (Table 3-3), it is not yet known with certainty which specific pharmacological action is linked to which specific clinical action, including side effects. Various putative mechanisms are given in Tables 3-3 and 3-4 and discussed in more detail for several individual agents later in this chapter. In reality, anticonvulsants have complex, multiple, and as yet not well characterized mechanisms specifically linked to their various clinical actions. The known actions and their hypothesized links to mood-stabilizing effects are discussed here.

Valproic acid

As is the case for all anticonvulsants, the exact mechanism of action of valproic acid (also valproate sodium, or valproate) is uncertain; however, even less may be known about the mechanism of valproate than for many other anticonvulsants. Various hypotheses are discussed here and summarized in Figures 3-5 through 3-8. At least three possibilities exist for how valproic acid works: inhibiting voltage-sensitive sodium channels (Figure 3-6), boosting the actions of the neurotransmitter gamma-aminobutyric acid (GABA) (Figure 3-7), and regulating downstream signal transduction cascades (Figure 3-8). It is not known whether these actions explain the mood-stabilizing actions, the anticonvulsant actions, the antimigraine actions, or the side effects of valproic acid. Obviously this simple molecule has multiple and complex clinical effects; current research is aimed at determining which of the various possibilities explains the mood-stabilizing effects of valproic acid, so that new agents with more efficacy and fewer side effects can be developed by targeting the relevant pharmacological mechanism for bipolar disorder.

One hypothesis to explain mood-stabilizing antimanic actions is the possibility that valproate acts to diminish excessive neurotransmission by diminishing the flow of ions through voltage-sensitive sodium channels (VSSCs) (Figure 3-6). No specific molecular site of action

TABLE 3-1 Putative clinical actions of mood stabilizers with anticonvulsant and pain actions

Agent	Epilepsy	Mania-minded		Depression-minded		Pain		
		Treat from above	Stabilize from above	Treat from below	Stabilize from below	Neuropathic	Fibromyalgia	Migraine
valproate	++++	++++	++	+	+/-	+		++++
carbamazepine	++++	++++	++	+	+/-	++++	+	+
oxcarbazepine/licarbazepine	++++	++	+	+/-	+/-	++	+	
lamotrigine	++++	+/-	++++	+++	++++	+/-		
riluzole	+			+	+/-			
memantine			+/-	+	+/-			
amantadine				+				
ketamine				+				
topiramate	++++	+/-	+/-			+/-		++++
zonisamide	++++	+/-	+/-					
gabapentin	++++	+/-	+/-			+++	++	
pregabalin	++++	+/-	+/-			++++	+++	
levetiracetam	++++	+/-	+/-			+/-		
calcium channel blockers		+	+/-					

TABLE 3-2 Putative clinical actions of mood stabilizers with additional clinical actions

Agent	Parkinson's	Anesthesia	ALS	Alzheimer's	Substance abuse	Anxiety	BP/arrhythmia
valproate						+	
carbamazepine						+/−	
oxcarbazepine/ licarbazepine						+/−	
lamotrigine						+	
riluzole			++++			+	
memantine				++++			
amantadine	++++						
ketamine		++++					
topiramate					+	+	
zonisamide							
gabapentin						++	
pregabalin						++	
levetiracetam						+/−	
calcium channel blockers							++++

ALS, amyotrophic lateral sclerosis; BP, blood pressure.

for valproate has been clarified, but it is possible that valproate may change the sensitivity of sodium channels by altering phosphorylation of VSSCs either by binding directly to the VSSC or its regulatory units or by inhibiting phosphorylating enzymes (Figure 3-6). If less sodium is able to pass into neurons, it may lead to diminished release of glutamate and therefore less excitatory neurotransmission, but this is only a theory. There may be additional effects of valproate on other voltage-sensitive ion channels, but these are poorly characterized and may relate to side effects as well as to therapeutic effects (Tables 3-3 and 3-4).

Another idea is that valproate enhances the actions of GABA, either by increasing its release, decreasing its reuptake, or slowing its metabolic inactivation (Figure 3-7). The direct site of action of valproate which causes the enhancement of GABA remains unknown, but there is good evidence that the downstream effects of valproate ultimately do result in more GABA activity and thus more inhibitory neurotransmission, possibly explaining its antimanic actions.

Finally, a number of downstream actions on complex signal transduction cascades have been described in recent years (Figure 3-8). Like lithium, valproate may inhibit GSK3, but it may also target many other downstream sites, from blockade of phosphokinase C (PKC) and myristolated alanine rich C kinase substrate (MARCKS) to activating various signals that promote neuroprotection and long-term plasticity, such as extracellular signal-regulated kinase (ERK kinase), cytoprotective protein B-cell lymphoma/leukemia-2 gene (BCL2), GAP43, and others (Figure 3-8). The effects of these signal transduction cascades are only now being clarified, and which of these possible effects of valproate might be relevant to mood-stabilizing actions is not yet understood.

There is a unique and patented pharmaceutical formulation of valproic acid called divalproex (Depakote), also available in a once-daily extended-release formulation

TABLE 3-3 Putative mechanisms of action of mood stabilizers on voltage-sensitive ion channels, synaptic vesicles, and carbonic anhydrase

Agent	Alpha unit VSSC	Nonspecific VSSC	Alpha 2 delta VSCC	L-channel VSCC	Nonspecific VSCC	Nonspecific potassium channel	Synaptic vesicle SV2A	Carbonic anhydrase
valproate		++			+			
carbamazepine	++++	++			++	++		
oxcarbazepine/ licarbazepine	++++	+			+	+		
lamotrigine	++++	+			+	+		
riluzole	++	+			+	+		
memantine								
amantadine								
ketamine								
topiramate		++			++			+++
zonisamide		++			++			
gabapentin			++++					
pregabalin			++++					
levetiracetam							++++	
calcium channel blockers				++++				

VSSC, voltage-sensitive sodium channel; VSCC, voltage-sensitive calcium channel.

TABLE 3-4 Mechanisms of action of mood stabilizers on GABA, glutamate, sigma, and dopamine

Agent	Nonspecific GABA	Nonspecific glutamate	Glutamate release	NMDA open channel	NMDA magnesium	Sigma 1	Dopamine
valproate	++	+	+/−				
carbamazepine	+	+/−					
oxcarbazepine/ licarbazepine	+						
lamotrigine		++	++++				
riluzole		++	+++				
memantine					++++	++	+/−
amantadine					++++	++	++
ketamine				++++		+++	
topiramate	+	+					
zonisamide	+	+					
gabapentin			+++				
pregabalin			+++				
levetiracetam							
calcium channel blockers							

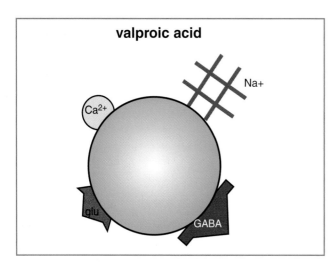

valproic acid

FIGURE 3-5 Valproic acid. Shown here is an icon of the pharmacological actions of valproic acid, an anticonvulsant used in the treatment of bipolar disorder. Valproic acid (also valproate) may work by interfering with voltage-sensitive sodium channels, enhancing the inhibitory actions of gamma-aminobutyric acid (GABA), and regulating downstream signal transduction cascades, although which of these actions may be related to mood stabilization is not clear. Valproate may also interact with other ion channels, such as voltage-sensitive calcium channels, and also indirectly block glutamate actions.

(divalproex ER; Depakote ER). This formulation reduces gastrointestinal side effects and other peak-dose side effects such as sedation and possibly alopecia. Valproate is proven effective for the acute manic phase of bipolar disorder (Figure 3-9). It is also commonly used long term to prevent the recurrence of mania, although its prophylactic effects have not been as well established. The antidepressant actions of valproate have not been well established nor has it been convincingly shown to stabilize against recurrent depressive episodes (Figure 3-9). Some experts believe that valproic acid is more effective than lithium for rapid cycling and mixed episodes of mania. In reality, such episodes are very difficult to

Possible Sites of Action of Valproate on VSSCs

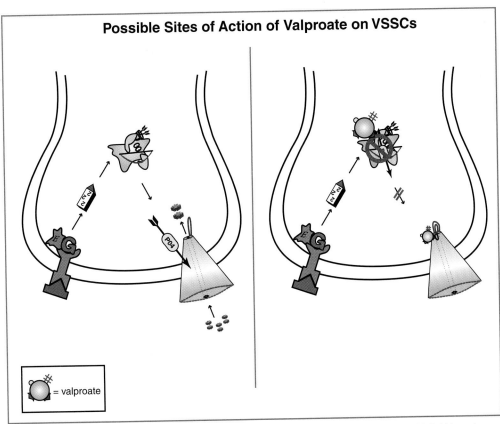

FIGURE 3-6 Possible sites of action of valproate on voltage-sensitive sodium channels (VSSCs). Valproate may exert antimanic effects by changing the sensitivity of VSSCs, perhaps by directly binding to channel subunits or inhibiting phosphorylating enzymes that regulate the sensitivity of these ion channels. Inhibition of VSSCs would lead to reduced sodium influx and, in turn, potentially to reduced glutamate excitatory neurotransmission, which is a possible mechanism for mania efficacy.

treat, and combinations of two or more mood stabilizers, including lithium plus valproate, are usually in order.

Oral loading of valproate can lead to rapid stabilization, and plasma levels are monitored to keep drug levels within the therapeutic range. Although most studies of valproate are done with monotherapy, pushing toward the top of the therapeutic range, the side effects of this dosing strategy are often unacceptable. As mentioned for lithium, valproate can also be utilized once a day in doses that are toward the bottom of the therapeutic range, in combination with other mood stabilizers, to improve tolerability and compliance. For efficacy, it may be ideal to push the dose, but no drug works if your patient refuses to take it, and valproic acid often has unacceptable side effects such as hair loss, weight gain, and sedation. Certain problems can be avoided by lowering the dose, but this will generally lower efficacy; thus, when valproate is given in lower doses, there may be a requirement to combine it with other mood stabilizers. Some side effects may be related more to chronicity of exposure rather than to dose and thus may not be avoided by reducing the dose. This includes warnings for liver, pancreatic, and fetal toxicities such as neural tube defects as well as concerns about weight gain, metabolic complications, and possible risk of

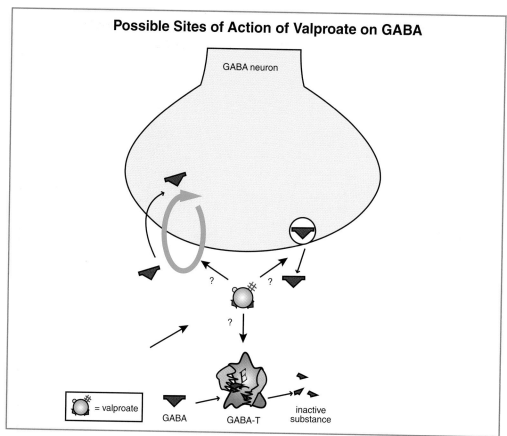

FIGURE 3-7 Possible sites of action of valproate on gamma-aminobutyric acid (GABA). Valproate's antimanic effects may be due to enhancement of GABA neurotransmission, perhaps by inhibiting GABA reuptake, enhancing GABA release, or interfering with the metabolism of GABA by GABA-T (GABA transaminase).

amenorrhea and polycystic ovaries in women of childbearing potential. A syndrome of menstrual disturbances, polycystic ovaries, hyperandrogenism, obesity, and insulin resistance may be associated with valproic acid therapy in such women. Thus, as mentioned for lithium, the modern psychopharmacologist must provide metabolic monitoring for patients taking valproate.

Carbamazepine

This anticonvulsant was actually the first to be shown effective in the manic phase of bipolar disorder, but it did not receive FDA approval until recently as a once-daily controlled-release formulation (Equetro). Although carbamazepine and valproate both act on the manic phase of bipolar disorder (Table 3-1), they appear to have different pharmacological mechanisms of action (Tables 3-3 and 3-4) and also different clinical actions (Tables 3-1 and 3-2), including different side effect profiles. Thus carbamazepine is hypothesized to act by blocking voltage-sensitive sodium channels (VSSCs), perhaps at a site within the channel itself, also known as the alpha subunit of VSSCs (Figure 3-10; Table 3-3). The action of

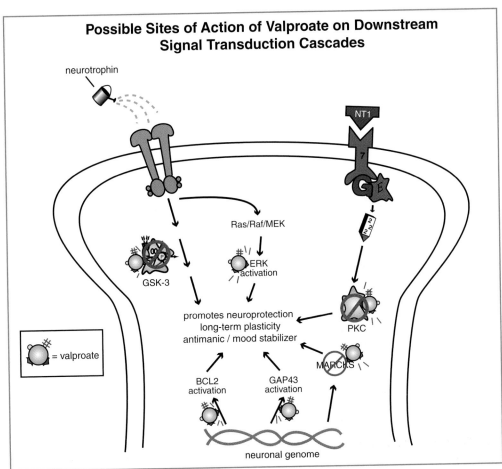

Possible Sites of Action of Valproate on Downstream Signal Transduction Cascades

neurotrophin

NT1

Ras/Raf/MEK

GSK-3

ERK
activation

PKC

promotes neuroprotection
long-term plasticity
antimanic / mood stabilizer

= valproate

MARCKS

BCL2
activation

GAP43
activation

neuronal genome

FIGURE 3-8 Possible sites of action of valproate on downstream signal transduction cascades. Valproate has been shown to have multiple downstream effects on signal transduction cascades, which may be involved in its antimanic effects. Valproate inhibits glycogen synthetase kinase 3 (GSK3), phosphokinase C (PKC), and myristolated alanine rich C kinase substrate (MARCKS). In addition, valproate activates signals that promote neuroprotection and long-term plasticity, such as extracellular signal-regulated kinase (ERK), cytoprotective protein B-cell lymphoma/leukemia-2 gene (BCL2), and GAP43.

carbamazepine on the alpha subunit of VSSCs is different from the hypothesized actions of valproate, but it is shared with the anticonvulsants oxcarbazepine and eslicarbazepine, the active metabolite of oxcarbazepine (Table 3-3; Figures 3-11 and 3-12). Although both carbamazepine and valproate are anticonvulsants and are used to treat mania from above, there are many differences between these two agents. For example, valproate is proven effective in migraine, but carbamazepine is proven effective in neuropathic pain (Table 3-1). Furthermore, carbamazepine has a different side effect profile than valproate, including suppressant effects on the bone marrow, requiring blood counts to be monitored, and notable induction of the cytochrome P450 enzyme 3A4. Carbamazepine is sedating and can cause fetal toxicity such as neural tube defects. Generally, this agent is considered a second-line mood stabilizer. It is proven effective in bipolar mania and is often utilized as maintenance treatment for preventing manic recurrences, but it has not been as extensively studied in the depressed phase of bipolar disorder (Figure 3-13).

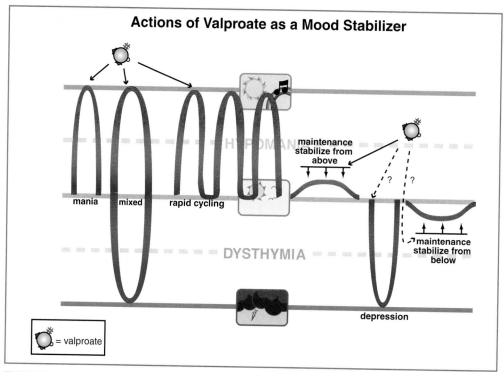

FIGURE 3-9 Actions of valproate as a mood stabilizer. Valproate has proven efficacy for the manic phase of bipolar disorder and may also prevent recurrence of mania. Valproate does not have established efficacy for treating or preventing the depressed phase of bipolar disorder, although it may be effective for the depressed phase in some patients.

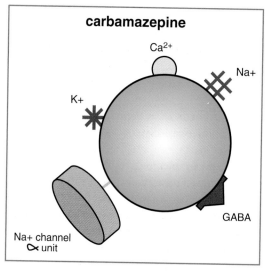

FIGURE 3-10 Carbamazepine. Shown here is an icon of the pharmacological actions of carbamazepine, an anticonvulsant used in the treatment of bipolar disorder. Carbamazepine may work by binding to the alpha subunit of voltage-sensitive sodium channels (VSSCs) and could perhaps have actions at other ion channels for calcium and potassium. By interfering with voltage-sensitive channels, carbamazepine may enhance the inhibitory actions of gamma-aminobutyric acid (GABA).

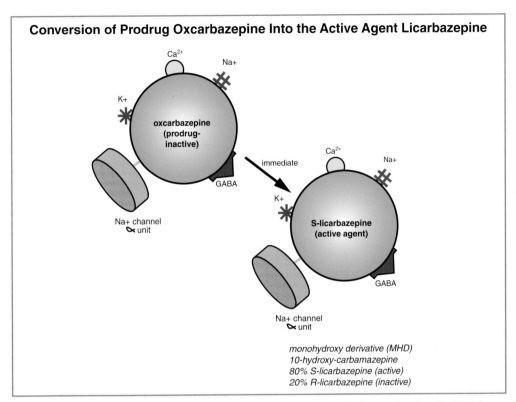

Conversion of Prodrug Oxcarbazepine Into the Active Agent Licarbazepine

monohydroxy derivative (MHD)
10-hydroxy-carbamazepine
80% S-licarbazepine (active)
20% R-licarbazepine (inactive)

FIGURE 3-11 Conversion of oxcarbazepine into licarbazepine. Oxcarbazepine is a prodrug (inactive) that is converted into the active drug 10-hydroxy derivative (monohydroxyderivative), which is called licarbazepine. Licarbazepine has two enantiomers, R and S; it is specifically the S enantiomer that is active.

Oxcarbazepine/eslicarbazepine

Oxcarbazepine is structurally related to carbamazepine, but it is not a metabolite of carbamazepine. Oxcarbazepine is actually not the active form of the drug but a prodrug that is immediately converted into a 10-hydroxy derivative, also called the monohydroxyderivative; most recently it has been named licarbazepine (Figure 3-12). The active form of licarbazepine is the S enantiomer, known as eslicarbazepine. Thus oxcarbazepine really works via conversion to eslicarbazepine.

Oxcarbazepine is well known as an anticonvulsant with a presumed mechanism of anticonvulsant action the same as that for carbamazepine, namely, binding to the open channel conformation of the VSSC at a site within the channel itself on the alpha subunit (Table 3-3 and Figure 3-12). However, oxcarbazepine seems to differ in some important ways from carbamazepine, including being less sedating, having less bone marrow toxicity, and also having fewer CYP450 3A4 interactions, making it a more tolerable agent that is easier to dose. On the other hand, oxcarbazepine has never been proven to work as a mood stabilizer. Nevertheless, because of its similar postulated mechanism of action (Table 3-3 and Figure 3-2) but a better tolerability profile, oxcarbazepine has been utilized "off label" by many clinicians, especially for the manic phase of bipolar disorder (Figure 3-13). Because the patent protection has expired, the active moiety eslicarbazepine as a potential mood stabilizer is now being investigated, particularly for the manic phase and possibly for maintenance against the relapse of mania. Eslicarbazepine is not yet marketed.

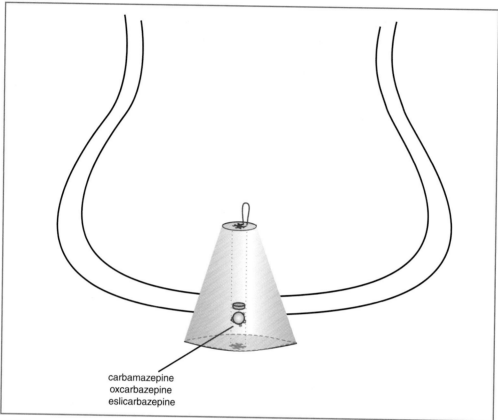

FIGURE 3-12 Binding site of carbamazepine, oxcarbazepine, and licarbazepine. Carbamazepine, oxcarbazepine, and licarbazepine are believed to share a common binding site, located within the open channel conformation of the voltage-sensitive sodium channel (VSSC) alpha subunit.

Lamotrigine

Lamotrigine (Figure 3-14) is approved as a mood stabilizer to prevent the recurrence of both mania and depression. There are many curious things about lamotrigine as a mood stabilizer. First, the FDA has not approved its use for bipolar depression, yet most experts believe lamotrigine to be effective for this indication. In fact, given the growing concern about antidepressants inducing mania, causing mood instability, and increasing suicidality in bipolar disorder, lamotrigine has largely replaced antidepressants and found its way to first-line treatment of bipolar depression. In that regard, lamotrigine has transformed the treatment of this difficult phase of bipolar disorder as one of the very few agents that seem to be effective for bipolar depression based on results seen in clinical practice rather than on evidence derived from clinical trials.

A second interesting thing about lamotrigine is that even though it has some over-lapping mechanistic actions with carbamazepine – namely, binding to the open channel conformation of VSSCs (Table 3-1 and Figure 3-15) – lamotrigine is not approved for bipolar mania. Perhaps its actions at VSSCs are not potent enough (Figure 3-15), or per-haps the long titration period required in starting this drug makes it difficult to show any useful effectiveness for mania, which generally requires treatment with drugs that can work quickly.

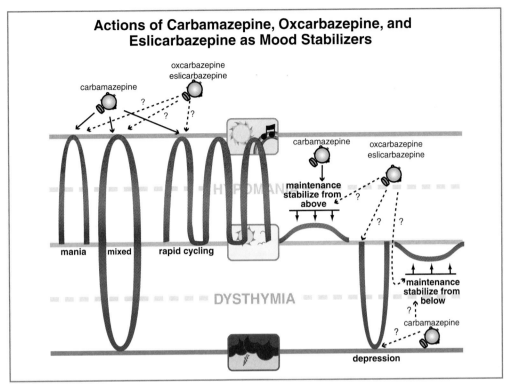

FIGURE 3-13 Actions of carbamazepine, oxcarbazepine, and eslicarbazepine as mood stabilizers.
Carbamazepine has proven efficacy in the manic phase of bipolar disorder and may also be useful for preventing the recurrence of mania. Carbamazepine's efficacy for treating and/or preventing depression is not well established. The mood-stabilizing effects of oxcarbazepine and eslicarbazepine are also not established, but the similarity in proposed mechanism of action to carbamazepine's suggests they would have similar effects.

A third aspect of lamotrigine that is unusual for an antidepressant mood stabilizer is its tolerability profile. Lamotrigine is generally well tolerated for an anticonvulsant, except for its propensity to cause rashes, including (rarely) the life-threatening Stevens–Johnson syndrome (toxic epidermal necrolysis). Rashes caused by lamotrigine can be minimized by very slow uptitration of drug during the initiation of therapy, avoiding or managing drug interactions such as those with valproate that raise lamotrigine levels, and understanding how to identify and manage serious rashes, including being able to distinguish them from benign rashes (see the discussion of lamotrigine in the *Essential Psychopharmacology Prescriber's Guide*).

Finally, lamotrigine seems to have some unique aspects to its mechanism of action (Tables 3-3 and 3-4). That is, it may act to reduce the release of the excitatory neurotransmitter glutamate (Figure 3-16 and Table 3-4). It is not clear whether this action is secondary to blocking the activation of VSSCs (Figure 3-15) or to some additional synaptic action (Figure 3-16). Reduction of excitatory glutamatergic neurotransmission, especially if this is excessive in bipolar depression, may be a unique action of lamotrigine and could explain why it has such a different clinical profile as a treatment and stabilizer from below (Figure 3-17). That is, it shares some actions on VSSCs with anticonvulsants such as carbamazepine and eslicarbazepine (compare Figures 3-12 and 3-15; also Table 3-3) that are apparently effective for the manic phase of bipolar disorder (Table 3-1); yet

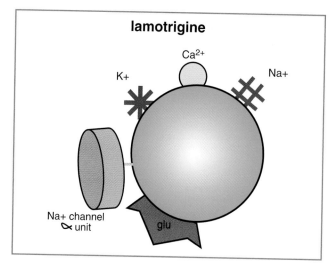

FIGURE 3-14 Lamotrigine. Shown here is an icon of the pharmacological actions of lamotrigine, an anticonvulsant used in the treatment of bipolar disorder. Lamotrigine may work by blocking the alpha subunit of voltage-sensitive sodium channels (VSSCs) and could perhaps also have actions at other ion channels for calcium and potassium. Lamotrigine is also thought to reduce the release of the excitatory neurotransmitter glutamate.

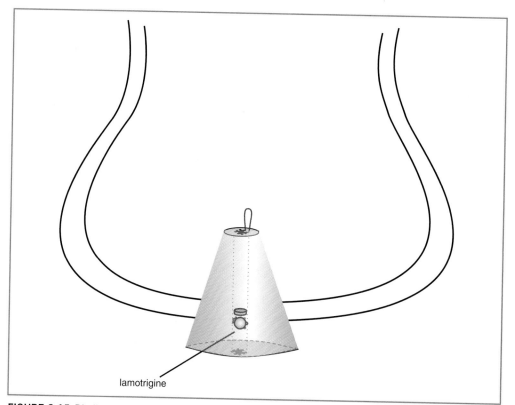

FIGURE 3-15 Binding site of lamotrigine. Lamotrigine is believed to bind to a site within the open channel conformation of the voltage-sensitive sodium channel (VSSC) alpha subunit.

lamotrigine has a relatively unique profile of effectiveness for the depressed phase and for preventing the recurrence of depression (compare Figures 3-13 and 3-17; also Table 3-1). The additional actions that lamotrigine may have upon glutamate release could theoretically account for this difference in clinical profile, but much further research will be necessary in order to understand those pharmacological mechanisms necessary to treat the

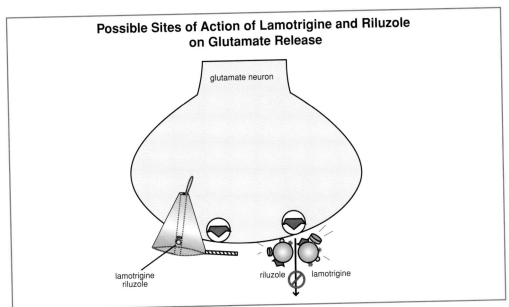

Possible Sites of Action of Lamotrigine and Riluzole on Glutamate Release

glutamate neuron

lamotrigine
riluzole

riluzole   lamotrigine

FIGURE 3-16 Possible sites of action of lamotrigine and riluzole on glutamate release. It is possible that lamotrigine reduces glutamate release through its blockade of voltage-sensitive sodium channels (VSSCs). Alternatively, lamotrigine may have this effect via an additional synaptic action that has not yet been identified. Riluzole, another anticonvulsant approved to treat amyotrophic lateral sclerosis (ALS or Lou Gehrig's disease), also reduces glutamate release and may do so via the same mechanism as lamotrigine, and may thus have therapeutic actions in bipolar disorder.

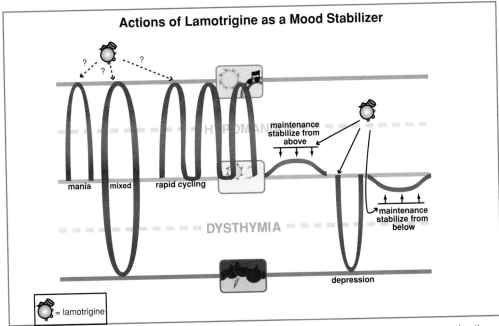

Actions of Lamotrigine as a Mood Stabilizer

HYPOMANIA

maintenance
stabilize from
above

mania   mixed   rapid cycling

DYSTHYMIA

maintenance
stabilize from
below

depression

= lamotrigine

FIGURE 3-17 Actions of lamotrigine as a mood stabilizer. Lamotrigine has proven efficacy for preventing the recurrence of both manic and depressive episodes and has also demonstrated efficacy for treating the depressed phase of bipolar disorder. Lamotrigine has not demonstrated efficacy for treating mania despite a shared binding site with agents that do (e.g., carbamazepine); this may be due to differences in the manner of binding or to the dosing requirements of lamotrigine.

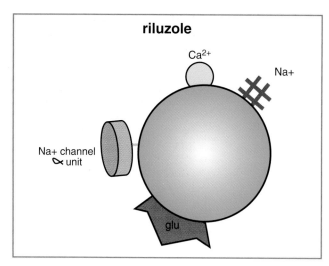

riluzole

Ca²⁺

Na+

Na+ channel
∝ unit

glu

FIGURE 3-18 Riluzole. Shown here is an icon of the pharmacological actions of riluzole, an agent with anticonvulsant properties developed for use in amyotrophic lateral sclerosis (ALS). Riluzole may also be effective in bipolar disorder, as its mechanism of action appears to be similar to that of lamotrigine. Specifically, riluzole is believed to block the alpha subunit of voltage-sensitive sodium channels (VSSCs) and also to reduce the release of the excitatory neurotransmitter glutamate.

manic phase versus those necessary to treat the depressed phase of bipolar disorder. In the meantime, lamotrigine is a mainstay of treating and stabilizing recurrences of the depressed phase of bipolar disorder, and the elucidation of its mechanism of action will be critical to discovering additional agents with clinical efficacy for bipolar depression.

Riluzole

Riluzole (Figure 3-18) has anticonvulsant actions in preclinical models but was developed to slow the progression of amyotrophic lateral sclerosis (ALS, or Lou Gerhig's disease) (Table 3-2). Theoretically, riluzole binds to VSSCs and prevents glutamate release in an action similar to that postulated for lamotrigine (Figure 3-16 and Table 3-4). The idea is that diminishing glutamate release in ALS would prevent the postulated excitotoxicity that might be causing death of motor neurons in ALS. If ALS is caused by glutamate-mediated excitotoxicity, an agent that prevents glutamate release would theoretically prevent or slow disease progression. Excessive glutamate activity may not only be occurring in ALS but is also a leading hypothesis for the dysregulation of neurotransmission during bipolar depression, although not necessarily so severe as to cause widespread neuronal loss.

Owing to riluzole's putative action in preventing glutamate release, it has been tested in case series in a number of treatment-resistant conditions hypothetically linked to excessive glutamate activity, including not only bipolar depression but also treatment-resistant unipolar depression and anxiety disorders, with some promising results. Further research with riluzole is in progress, as it is for other agents that interfere with glutamate neurotransmission (discussed later in this chapter). There is great need for another agent that has the same clinical effects as lamotrigine. The problem with riluzole is that it is quite expensive, and has frequent liver function abnormalities associated with its use.

Topiramate

Topiramate (Figure 3-19) is another compound approved as an anticonvulsant and for migraine; it has also been tested in bipolar disorder, but with ambiguous results

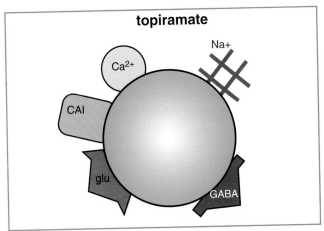

topiramate

Na+

Ca²⁺

CAI

glu

GABA

FIGURE 3-19 Topiramate. Shown here is an icon of the pharmacological actions of topiramate, an anticonvulsant that has been tested, with varying results, in the treatment of bipolar disorder. Its exact binding site is not known, but it may interfere with voltage-sensitive sodium and/or calcium channels and thereby enhance the function of gamma-aminobutyric acid (GABA) and reduce glutamate function. Topiramate is also a weak inhibitor of carbonic anhydrase.

(Table 3-1). It does seem to be associated with weight loss and is sometimes given as an adjunct to mood stabilizers that cause weight gain, but it can cause unacceptable sedation in some patients. Topiramate is also being tested in various substance abuse disorders, including stimulant abuse and alcoholism (Table 3-2). However, topiramate is not clearly effective as a mood stabilizer, either from evidence-based randomized controlled trials (which are not consistently positive) or from clinical practice.

The reason that topiramate may not have the robust efficacy of valproate or carbamazepine in the manic phase or of lamotrigine in the depressed and maintenance phases of bipolar disorder is that it has a different mechanism of action from any of these agents (Tables 3-3 and 3-4). The exact binding site for topiramate is not known, but this agent seems to enhance GABA function and reduce glutamate function by interfering with both sodium and calcium channels, but in a different way and at a different site than the previously discussed anticonvulsants (Tables 3-3 and 3-4). In addition, topiramate is a weak inhibitor of carbonic anhydrase (Figure 3-19; Table 3-3). Topiramate is now considered an adjunctive treatment for bipolar disorder, perhaps helpful for weight gain, insomnia or anxiety, or possibly for comorbid substance abuse but not necessarily as a mood stabilizer per se.

Zonisamide

Zonisamide (Figure 3-20) is another anticonvulsant that is not approved for bipolar disorder but is sometimes used to treat this condition (Table 3-1). Its mechanism of action is also unknown, as is its binding site, but its mechanism seems to be different from that of the other anticonvulsants that are proven mood stabilizers (Tables 3-3 and 3-4). Like topiramate, zonisamide may enhance GABA function and reduce glutamate function by interfering with both sodium and calcium channels. Interestingly, like topiramate, zonisamide may also cause weight loss. As a sulfonamide derivative, zonisamide can be associated with rashes, including (rarely) a serious rash (Stevens–Johnson syndrome, or toxic epidermal necrolysis). Zonisamide is considered an adjunctive treatment without, as yet, convincing evidence of efficacy in bipolar disorder.

Gabapentin and pregabalin

Gabapentin and pregabalin (Figure 3-21) seem to have little or no action as mood stabilizers, yet they are robust treatments for various pain conditions, from neuropathic pain

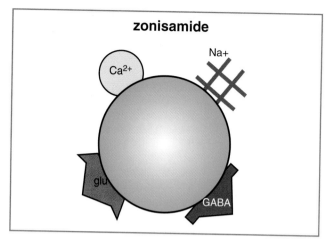

FIGURE 3-20 Zonisamide. Shown here is an icon of the pharmacological actions of zonisamide, an anticonvulsant that is not well tested in the treatment of bipolar disorder. Its mechanism of action is not known, but it may interfere with voltage-sensitive sodium and/or calcium channels and thereby enhance the function of gamma-aminobutyric acid (GABA) and reduce glutamate function.

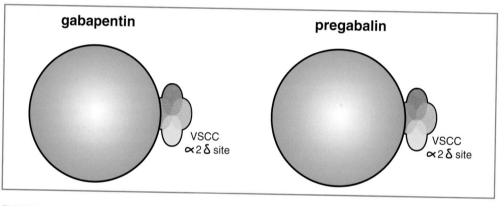

FIGURE 3-21 Gabapentin and pregabalin. Shown here are icons of the pharmacological actions of gabapentin and pregabalin, two anticonvulsants that do not appear to have efficacy in bipolar disorder. These agents bind to the alpha 2 delta subunit of voltage-sensitive calcium channels (VSCCs) and, rather than being efficacious as mood stabilizers, instead seem to have efficacy in chronic pain and anxiety.

to fibromyalgia, and for various anxiety disorders (Tables 3-1 and 3-2). Gabapentin and pregabalin may also be useful treatments for some sleep disorders. However, these agents are not currently considered to be effective mood stabilizers.

Gabapentin and pregabalin are now classified as "alpha 2 delta ligands" since they are known to bind selectively and with high affinity to the alpha 2 delta site of voltage-sensitive calcium channels (VSCCs) (Table 3-3). It appears that blocking these VSCCs when they are open and in use causes improvement of pain but not stabilization of mood (Table 3-1). That is, "use-dependent" blockade of VSCCs prevents the release of neurotransmitters such as glutamate (Table 3-4) in pain and anxiety pathways and also prevents seizures, but it does not appear to affect the mechanism involved in bipolar disorder, since clinical trials of these agents in bipolar disorder show unconvincing mood stabilization (Tables 3-1 and 3-2). However, many bipolar patients do experience chronic pain, anxiety, and insomnia, and gabapentin and pregabalin may be useful adjunctive treatments to effective mood stabilizers, even though they do not appear to be robustly effective as mood stabilizers

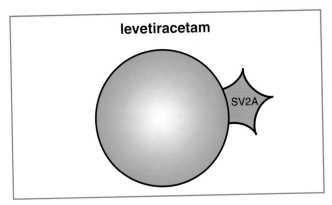

FIGURE 3-22 Levetiracetam. Shown here is an icon of the pharmacological actions of levetiracetam, an anticonvulsant that is not well tested in the treatment of bipolar disorder. Levetiracetam binds to the SV2A protein on synaptic vesicles, which should affect neurotransmitter release.

themselves. This is not surprising, given the very different mechanism of action of these compounds as selective alpha 2 delta ligands, compared to the mechanisms of proven mood stabilizers such as valproate, carbamazepine, and lamotrigine discussed above (Tables 3-3 and 3-4).

Levetiracetam

Levetiracetam (Figure 3-22) is an anticonvulsant with a very novel mechanism of action: it binds to the SV2A protein on synaptic vesicles (Table 3-3). SV2A is a type of transporter. Levetiracetam selectively and potently binds to this site on synaptic vesicles, presumably changing neurotransmission by altering neurotransmitter release, thereby providing anticonvulsant actions (Figure 3-23). Anecdotal use and case studies suggest some utility in bipolar disorder, but this is not yet well established. Since this is a quite different mechanism of action, there is no assurance that this agent will be an effective mood stabilizer, but its unique actions also suggest the possibility of helping some bipolar patients resistant to the other mechanisms of mood stabilization discussed here. Further research is necessary to clarify the value of this mechanism at SV2A synaptic vesicle transporter sites.

Atypical antipsychotics: not just for psychotic mania

When atypical antipsychotics were approved for schizophrenia, it was not surprising that these agents would work for psychotic symptoms associated with mania, since the D2 antagonist actions predict efficacy for psychosis in general. However, it was somewhat surprising that these agents proved effective for the core nonpsychotic symptoms of mania and for maintenance treatment to prevent the recurrence of mania. These latter actions are consistent with those of mood stabilizers such as lithium and various anticonvulsants, which act by very different mechanisms than do the antipsychotics. Furthermore, evolving data now suggest that at least certain atypical antipsychotics are effective for bipolar depression and in preventing the recurrence of depression. The question that arises is how do atypical antipsychotics work as mood stabilizers? Also, do they act by the same pharmacological mechanism as mood stabilizers as they do as antipsychotics? Finally, do they work for the symptoms of mania by the same pharmacological mechanisms as they do for bipolar depression?

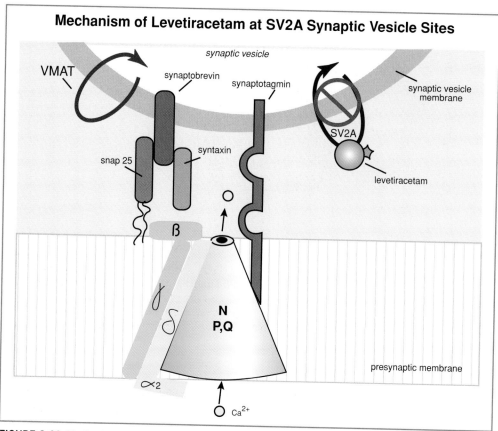

Mechanism of Levetiracetam at SV2A Synaptic Vesicle Sites

FIGURE 3-23 **Mechanism of action of levetiracetam at SV2A synaptic vesicle sites.** Levetiracetam selectively binds to SV2A, a type of transporter on synaptic vesicles. Actions at sites on these vesicles could have downstream effects on neurotransmitter release. VMAT, vesicular monoamine transporter.

Putative pharmacological mechanism of atypical antipsychotics in mania and bipolar depression

The answer to the question of how atypical antipsychotics work in mania is that we do not really know. In fact, theories about atypical antipsychotic pharmacological actions in bipolar disorder are less well developed than they are for schizophrenia. Indeed, it is still a mystery how bipolar disorder itself can create seemingly opposite symptoms during various phases of the illness as well as the combination of both manic and depressive symptoms simultaneously. Ideas about dysfunctional circuits in the depressed phase of bipolar disorder (discussed in Chapter 1 and illustrated in Figures 1-45 through 1-56 and 1-65) are contrasted with different dysfunctions in both overlapping and distinctive circuits during the manic phase of the illness (discussed in Chapter 1 and illustrated for the manic phase in Figures 1-57 through 1-62 and 1-66). Rather than being conceptualized as having activity that is simply "too low" in depression and "too high" in mania, the idea is that dysfunctional circuits in bipolar disorder are "out of tune" and chaotic. According to this notion, mood stabilizers have the ability to "tune" dysfunctional circuits, increasing the efficiency of information processing in symptomatic circuits and thus decreasing symptoms, whether they are manic or depressed.

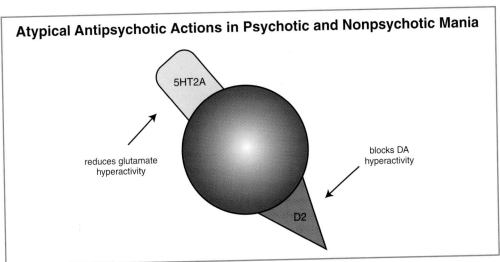

Atypical Antipsychotic Actions in Psychotic and Nonpsychotic Mania

5HT2A

reduces glutamate
hyperactivity

blocks DA
hyperactivity

D2

FIGURE 3-24 Atypical antipsychotic actions in psychotic and nonpsychotic mania. Atypical antipsychotics have established efficacy not only for psychotic mania but also for nonpsychotic mania. Antagonism or partial agonism of dopamine 2 receptors, which block dopamine hyperactivity, may account for the reduction of psychotic symptoms in mania, just as these actions do for psychotic symptoms in schizophrenia. Antagonism of serotonin 2A receptors, which can indirectly reduce glutamate hyperactivity, may account for the reduction of manic symptoms.

If so, the D2 antagonist or partial agonist properties of atypical antipsychotics as well as conventional antipsychotics may account for reduction of psychotic symptoms in mania (Figure 3-24), but the 5HT2A antagonist properties of atypical antipsychotics may account for the reduction of nonpsychotic manic and depressive symptoms. This could occur via reduction of glutamate hyperactivity from overly active pyramidal neurons by 5HT2A antagonist actions. This could reduce symptoms associated with glutamate hyperactivity, which could include both manic and depressive symptoms, depending on the circuit involved (Figures 1-45 through 1-56). Anti-glutamate actions of atypical antipsychotics (Figure 3-24) are consistent with the known pharmacological mechanisms of several anticonvulsants that are also mood stabilizers, as discussed above (Figures 3-12, 3-15, and 3-16 and Table 3-4). The combination of different mechanisms that decrease excessive glutamate activity could explain the observed therapeutic benefits of combining atypical antipsychotics with proven anticonvulsant mood stabilizers.

Several other mechanisms are feasible explanations for how certain atypical antipsychotics work to improve symptoms in the depressed phase of bipolar disorder (Figures 3-25 and 3-26). Numerous mechanisms of different atypical antipsychotics can increase the availability of the trimonoamine neurotransmitters serotonin, dopamine, and norepinephrine, known to be critical in the action of antidepressants in unipolar depression (Figure 3-25). Such actions would be predicted to have favorable effects not only on mood but also on cognition (Figure 3-25). Furthermore, some pharmacological actions of atypical antipsychotics predict favorable effects on sleep and also on neurogenesis (Figure 3-25), but by different yet potentially complementary neurotrophic mechanisms than those proposed for the actions of lithium (Figure 3-3) or valproate (Figure 3-8).

There are very different pharmacological properties of one atypical antipsychotic compared to another, which could potentially explain not only why some atypical antipsychotics

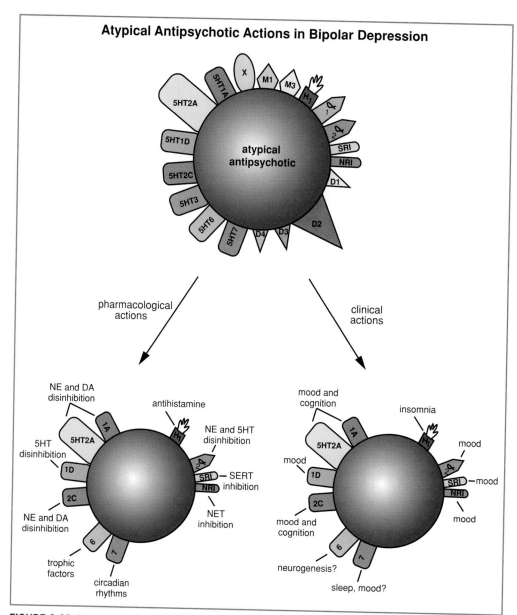

FIGURE 3-25 Atypical antipsychotic actions in bipolar depression. Atypical antipsychotics have multiple mechanisms that lead to increased availability of serotonin (5HT), norepinephrine (NE), and/or dopamine (DA), which could account for the efficacy of some of these agents in bipolar depression. Actions at 5HT2A, 5HT2C, and 5HT1A receptors indirectly lead to NE and DA disinhibition, which may improve mood and cognition. Mood may also be improved by increasing NE and 5HT via actions at alpha 2 receptors, by increasing NE via blockade of the NE transporter, and by increasing 5HT via actions at 5HT1D receptors and blockade of the 5HT transporter. Antihistamine actions could improve insomnia associated with bipolar depression. Actions at other 5HT receptors may also play a role in treating bipolar depression.

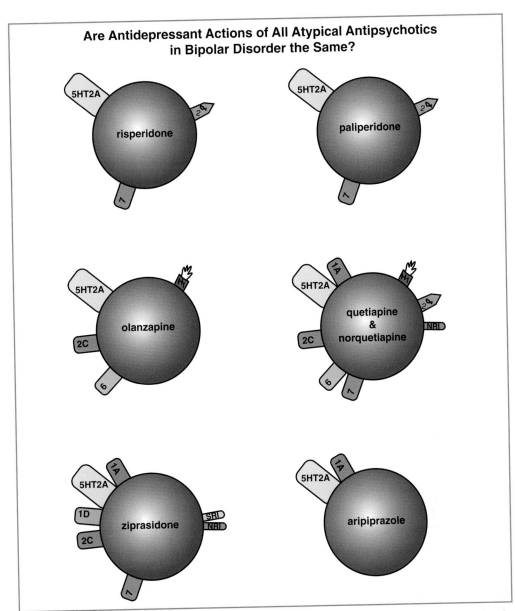

FIGURE 3-26 Atypical antipsychotics: differing portfolios of pharmacological actions for bipolar depression. As shown here, each atypical antipsychotic has a unique portfolio of pharmacological actions, which may contribute to its antidepressant actions. This may explain why these agents differ in their ability to treat the depressed phase of bipolar disorder and also why some patients respond to one of these drugs and not to another.

have different actions in bipolar disorder than other atypical antipsychotics but also why some bipolar patients respond to one atypical antipsychotic and not another (Figure 3-26). Thus, all atypical antipsychotics are approved for schizophrenia and most for mania but only a few for bipolar depression. This may be somewhat of an artifact of commercial considerations and lack of completion of clinical trials for some of the newer agents, but it may also reflect differing portfolios of pharmacological actions (Figure 3-26) among those properties that might have antidepressant effects (Figure 3-25). Much further research

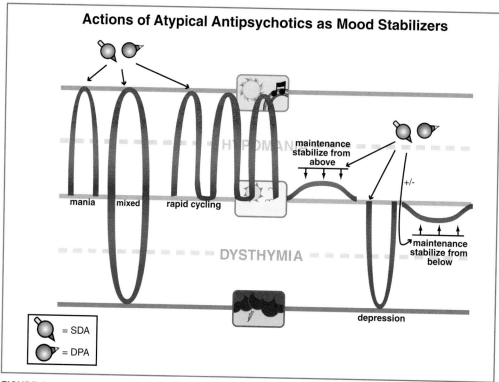

FIGURE 3-27 Actions of atypical antipsychotics as mood stabilizers. The atypical antipsychotics risperidone, olanzapine, quetiapine, ziprasidone, and aripiprazole all have established efficacy for treating the manic phase of bipolar disorder, and some (particularly aripiprazole and olanzapine) have also demonstrated efficacy for preventing the recurrence of mania. Quetiapine and olanzapine are efficacious for treating bipolar depression; other atypical antipsychotics may be effective as well but are not currently well studied. Atypical antipsychotics are not well studied in the prevention of depression recurrence.

must be completed before we will know the reason why atypical antipsychotics may work in mania or in bipolar depression. In the meantime, these agents as a class provide some of the broadest efficacy in bipolar disorder available (Figure 3-27) – indeed, broader than that for most anticonvulsants (Figures 3-9, 3-13, and 3-17; also Table 3-1) and comparable or better than that for lithium (Figure 3-4). Increasingly therefore, bipolar disorder is not only treated with two or more agents but with one of those agents as an atypical antipsychotic.

Other agents used in bipolar disorder

Benzodiazepines

Although benzodiazepines are not formally approved as mood stabilizers, they are anti-convulsants, anxiolytics, and sedative hypnotics and therefore provide valuable adjunctive treatment to proven mood stabilizers. In emergent situations, intramuscular or oral administration of benzodiazepines can have a calming action immediately and provide valuable time for mood stabilizers with a longer onset of action to begin working. Also, benzodiazepines are quite valuable for patients on an as-needed basis for intermittent agitation, insomnia, and incipient manic symptoms. Skilled intermittent use can leverage the mood-stabilizing actions of concomitant mood stabilizers and prevent eruption of more severe symptoms,

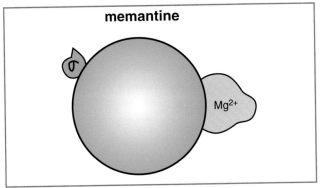

FIGURE 3-28 Memantine. Shown here is an icon of the pharmacological actions of memantine, an N-methyl-d-aspartate (NMDA) antagonist at the magnesium site that is used in Alzheimer's disease. By blocking NMDA receptors, memantine can prevent the excitatory actions of glutamate, which could potentially lead to efficacy in bipolar disorder, although such use is not established. Memantine also has actions at sigma receptors, but the significance of this is not known.

possibly also avoiding rehospitalization. Of course benzodiazepines should be administered with caution, especially to patients with comorbid substance abuse.

Memantine

Memantine is a weak NMDA glutamate receptor antagonist (Figure 3-28) approved for the treatment of Alzheimer's disease but not for bipolar disorder. Notions that bipolar disorder can be associated with glutamate hyperactivity, particularly in the depressed phase, coupled with observations that some anticonvulsants that reduce glutamate actions may be mood stabilizers, particularly for bipolar depression, have led to the hypothesis that agents that can reduce glutamate actions might be useful for bipolar depression. This has already been discussed above for riluzole, an agent which, like lamotrigine, may block glutamate release (Figure 3-16; Table 3-4). It is conceivable that agents like memantine, which can block the synaptic actions of glutamate at NMDA receptors, could exert therapeutic actions in bipolar disorder as well; this has led to the testing of several such compounds, including memantine. The role of any possible sigma receptor actions of memantine in bipolar depression is unknown (Figure 3-28). Early case reports and open trials with memantine in unipolar, treatment-resistant, and bipolar depression have not yielded consistent results. Future trials may require higher dosing or new formulations of memantine.

Amantadine

Amantadine is structurally related to memantine and shares its actions at NMDA receptors, where it has weaker actions than memantine but also has additional actions as a releaser of dopamine by an unknown mechanism that may be linked in part to sigma receptor properties (Figure 3-29). Amantadine was originally approved as an antiviral agent, acting by yet another mechanism. With its pro-dopaminergic actions, amantadine was later approved for Parkinson's disease and for drug-induced parkinsonism. Pro-dopaminergic actions and NMDA antagonist actions are mechanisms suggestive of amantadine's possible efficacy for depression; some case series and anecdotal observations are consistent with this, although activation of mania can be a problem in some patients. Further research is necessary to clarify whether amantadine will prove consistently useful for bipolar depression.

Ketamine

Ketamine (Figure 3-30) is an approved anesthetic that acts by binding to the open channel conformation of the NMDA receptor at a site inside the calcium channel associated with

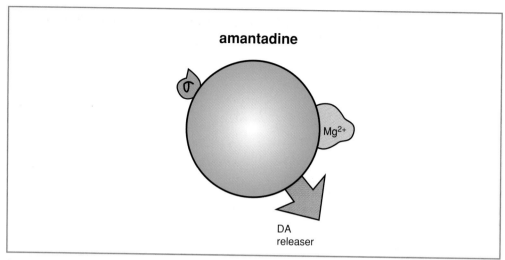

amantadine

FIGURE 3-29 Amantadine. Shown here is an icon of the pharmacological actions of amantadine, an agent approved to treat Parkinson's disease and drug-induced parkinsonism. Amantadine, like memantine, is an antagonist at the magnesium site of N-methyl-d-aspartate (NMDA) receptors and has actions at sigma receptors. In addition, amantadine causes release of dopamine through an unknown mechanism. Amantadine has not been well studied in bipolar disorder but may be effective in treating the depressed phase in some patients, yet it increases the chance of triggering mania, especially in the absence of a concomitantly administered antimanic agent.

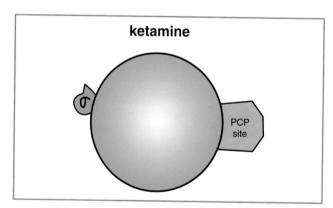

ketamine

FIGURE 3-30 Ketamine. Shown here is an icon of the pharmacological actions of the anesthetic ketamine. Ketamine binds to N-methyl-d-aspartate (NMDA) receptors at the same site as phencyclidine (PCP) but with different effects. Ketamine also has actions at sigma receptors.

this receptor (Figure 3-31 and Tables 3-1, 3-2, and 3-4). This is the same site where phencyclidine (PCP) acts. However, for reasons that are not clear, ketamine is not as psychotomimetic as PCP but blocks NMDA receptors more effectively than memantine. Investigators have recently shown that a low single dose of ketamine administered to patients with treatment-resistant depression creates a rapid-onset antidepressant effect sustained for several days, theoretically by blocking hyperactive glutamate actions. It is not known whether a practical approach to blocking NMDA receptors in unipolar, treatment-resistant, or bipolar depression utilizing a ketamine-like drug will become available, but such results are provocative and may help to identify therapeutic targets for future treatments of bipolar disorder, especially the depressed phase. The possible therapeutic actions in bipolar disorder for various agents that block glutamate are shown in Figure 3-32.

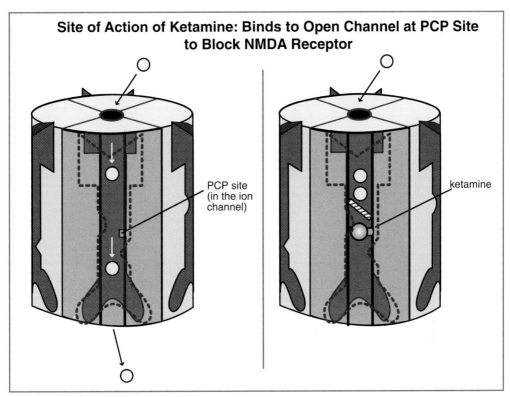

Site of Action of Ketamine: Binds to Open Channel at PCP Site to Block NMDA Receptor

PCP site (in the ion channel)

ketamine

FIGURE 3-31 Site of action of ketamine. The anesthetic ketamine binds to the open channel conformation of the N-methyl-d-aspartate (NMDA) receptor. Specifically, it binds to a site within the calcium channel of this receptor, which is often termed the PCP site because it is also where phencyclidine (PCP) binds. Blockade of NMDA receptors may prevent the excitatory actions of glutamate.

Calcium channel blockers (L-type)

As reviewed above, a number of anticonvulsants that are proven mood stabilizers have actions at voltage-sensitive ion channels, mostly with actions described at voltage-sensitive sodium channels (VSSCs; see Figures 3-12, 3-15, and Table 3-3). Anticonvulsant mood stabilizers may also have various poorly characterized nonspecific actions at a wide variety of other ion channels, including voltage-sensitive calcium channels (VSCCs), voltage-sensitive potassium channels, and others (Table 3-3). One VSCC that is well known is the so-called L-channel. L-type VSCCs should be contrasted with N and P/Q VSCCs. These N and P/Q VSCCs are the ones that are targeted by the alpha 2 delta ligands gabapentin and pregabalin, which have anticonvulsant, pain-reducing, and anxiolytic actions. On the other hand, L-type channels are located on neurons, where their function is still being debated, and also on vascular smooth muscle, where they can be blocked by drugs known as calcium channel blockers, especially the dihydropyridine-type calcium channel blockers used to treat hypertension and arrhythmias (Figure 3-33). Some investigators have targeted these same L-type VSCCs on neurons, and some results from anecdotal observations and case series suggest possible mood-stabilizing actions. However, these actions are not yet proven and further research is needed.

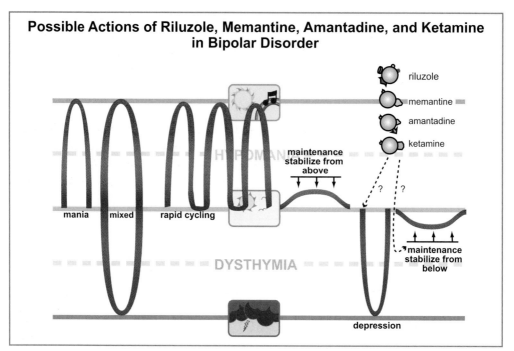

FIGURE 3-32 Possible actions of riluzole, memantine, amantadine, and ketamine in bipolar disorder. Agents that block glutamate – such as riluzole, memantine, amantadine, and ketamine – may be efficacious for treating the depressed phase of bipolar disorder and perhaps also for preventing the recurrence of depression.

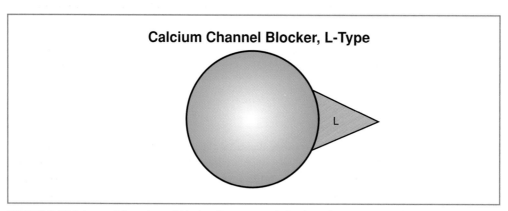

FIGURE 3-33 L-type calcium channel blocker. Some agents being investigated for use in bipolar disorder have actions that block a particular type of voltage-sensitive calcium channel (VSCC) known as the L-type channel. This is a different type of calcium channel than the one targeted by the anticonvulsants pregabalin and gabapentin. L-type channels are located on neurons and also on smooth vascular muscle and are blocked by the calcium channel blockers used to treat hypertension. The role, if any, of L-type calcium channels in bipolar disorder is not yet determined.

Omega-3 fatty acids

The omega-3 fatty acids eicosapentanoic acid (EPA) and docosahexanoic acid (DHA) have been proposed as mood stabilizers or as natural products that may boost the actions of proven mood stabilizers with few if any side effects. EPA is an essential fatty acid that can be metabolized to DHA; it is a normal component of a diet that contains fish. Both EPA and DHA are found in large quantities in the brain, especially in cell membranes. Recent investigations suggest that omega-3 fatty acids may inhibit phosphokinase C (PKC), not unlike the actions described earlier for valproate and illustrated in Figure 3-8. Studies of omega-3 fatty acids are ongoing, but these agents have not yet been proven effective in bipolar disorder.

Inositol

Inositol is a natural product linked to second messenger systems and signal transduction cascades, especially for the phosphatidyl inositol signals related to various neurotransmitter receptors such as the 5HT2A receptor. Inositol has been studied in bipolar disorder and in treatment-resistant bipolar depression, where it may be as effective an augmenting agent to antidepressants as approved mood stabilizers such as lamotrigine and risperidone. Further studies of inositol are necessary.

L-methylfolate (6-(S)-5-methyl-tetrahydrofolate, or MTHF)

The centrally active form of the vitamin folate is L-methylfolate (MTHF), discussed extensively in Chapter 2 and illustrated in Figures 2-107 though 2-111. To boost trimonoamine neurotransmitter function in bipolar disorder, particularly in bipolar depression, MTHF may also be useful, but it has not been studied in bipolar depression as an augmenting agent to antidepressants as extensively as it has been studied in unipolar depression (Figure 2-110). However, there is additional rationale for utilizing MTHF in bipolar disorder because several anticonvulsants interfere with folate absorption or folate metabolism. Thus bipolar patients who are partial responders to mood-stabilizing anticonvulsants (especially lamotrigine, valproate, and carbamazepine but perhaps other anticonvulsants as well) or who lose their response may be considered candidates for taking MTHF supplements.

Thyroid hormone

Some investigators note that thyroid hormone, especially T3, may stabilize mood in some patients with bipolar disorder. This is not well researched and is somewhat controversial, especially for long-term use. Thyroid as a trimonoamine modulator for depression is discussed in Chapter 2 and illustrated in Figure 2-112.

Do antidepressants make you bipolar?

Clinicians are now reexamining the use of antidepressants in patients with bipolar disorder. Increasingly it seems that antidepressants either do not work or may worsen the situation for some of these patients, causing destabilization of mood with induction of mania or hypomania, rapid cycling or mixed states, or even suicidality. There is even an ongoing debate about whether antidepressants can cause someone to develop bipolar disorder who does not have this condition prior to taking an antidepressant. In other words, is bipolar disorder ever a complication of antidepressant treatment? Although this possibility is still under investigation, there is now little debate about the possibility that antidepressants can activate bipolar disorder in patients known to have a bipolar spectrum disorder.

Based on current evidence, it seems likely that someone who develops bipolar disorder after taking an antidepressant would already have had bipolar disorder, but the condition might either have been undiagnosed or wrongly diagnosed and then "unmasked" but not caused by antidepressant treatment. This is a particularly problematic issue for young patients who may present with unipolar depressive symptoms before they express any manic or hypomanic symptoms and who may therefore be particularly vulnerable both to misdiagnosis and to antidepressant-induced activation and suicidality.

How, then, is one to know to whom an antidepressant may be given? Recommendations for the use of antidepressants in patients with known bipolar disorder, who are at risk for bipolar disorder, or who have had activation of mania only on antidepressants are still evolving. Currently, use of antidepressants for individuals in these situations must be considered on a case-by-case basis. Most experts agree that antidepressant monotherapy is generally to be avoided in such individuals and that treatment of depression in bipolar disorder should start with other options, such as lamotrigine, lithium, and/or atypical antipsychotics as monotherapies or in combination. Whether one can add an antidepressant to these agents in patients with bipolar depression who do not have robust treatment responses to these first-line agents is currently being debated. Many treatment guidelines do provide for use of antidepressants in combination with mood stabilizers, but when to do this remains controversial, depending somewhat on the results of ongoing studies and on where one's practice is located and where one was trained. Thus, common sense, integration of one's clinical experience, and keeping up with this evolving area of psychopharmacology is now considered the best practice.

Mood stabilizers in clinical practice

How does one choose a mood stabilizer?

Although many monotherapies are proven effective for one or more phases of bipolar disorder, few patients with a bipolar spectrum disorder can be maintained on monotherapy. Unfortunately for the practicing psychopharmacologist, almost all of the evidence for the efficacy of mood stabilizers is based on studies of monotherapies, whereas almost all patients with bipolar disorder are on combinations of therapeutic agents. Thus evidence-based treatments for the real-world management of bipolar disorder with combinations of mood stabilizers are relatively poorly researched. The options for the treatment of bipolar disorder are shown in the "mood stabilizer pharmacy" in Figure 3-34. This includes not only approved and proven first-line treatments but also numerous other treatments, some of which are considered for second-line or adjunctive treatment, several options aimed specifically at the depressed phase, and ancillary treatments including nondrug therapies (Figure 3-34).

In spite of numerous evidence-based monotherapies and all the lessons from empiric practice-based combinations of these treatments, bipolar disorder remains a highly recurrent, predominantly depressive illness with frequent comorbidities and residual symptoms. How, then, does one obtain the best outcomes for a bipolar patient? The answer proposed here is to learn the mechanisms of action of the known and putative mood stabilizers and their ancillary and adjunctive treatments, familiarize oneself with the evidence for their efficacy and safety in monotherapy trials, and then construct a unique portfolio of treatments for one patient at a time based on the specific symptoms that remain following each successive treatment. This is called the symptom-based treatment algorithm and is also the strategy discussed in Chapter 2 for difficult cases of unipolar depression and illustrated in Figures 2-121 through 2-126.

Symptom-based treatment algorithm for sequential treatment choices and drug combinations in bipolar disorder

Not all bipolar patients are complicated, especially at the onset of the illness and when presenting in primary care in the depressed phase. Therefore, before looking for complicated solutions, the best treatment choice for uncomplicated bipolar patients would first be to do no harm and thus to avoid prescribing antidepressant monotherapy no matter what the current symptoms are. This begins with a prudent determination of when depressive

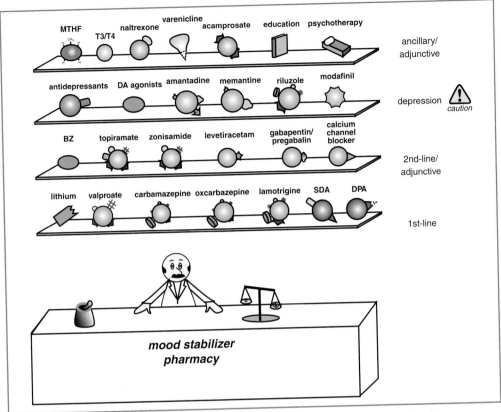

FIGURE 3-34 Mood pharmacy. First-line treatments for bipolar disorder include lithium, valproate, carbamazepine, oxcarbazepine, lamotrigine, serotonin dopamine antagonists (SDAs), and dopamine partial agonists (DPAs). Adjunctive treatment options may include benzodiazepines for agitation; topiramate or zonisamide for weight loss; and gabapentin or pregabalin for anxiety, sleep, or pain. Other potential augmenting agents that may be of benefit include levetiracetam and calcium channel blockers. Cautious augmentation with antidepressants, dopamine agonists, amantadine, memantine, riluzole, or modafinil may be useful for bipolar depression. Additional possible augmenting agents for bipolar disorder include L-methylfolate (MTHF), thyroid hormone, naltrexone, varenicline, and acamprosate. Patient education and psychotherapy can also be beneficial.

symptoms are due to bipolar versus unipolar depression; if bipolar, this may lead to the decision to use lamotrigine or an atypical antipsychotic, or their combination, while avoiding antidepressants.

Also, when a patient presents in the manic phase, it should be appreciated that "mild mania" is not an oxymoron. Some bipolar patients present in this state, which suggests treatment with either valproate, lithium, or an atypical antipsychotic monotherapy or their combination, which may reduce manic symptoms substantially. In primary care, there may be a wish to avoid valproate and lithium and even lamotrigine owing to a lack of familiarity with these agents and to start with an atypical antipsychotic (while avoiding an antidepressant), with referral to a specialist if treatment results are not satisfactory.

That is the easy part. What about the majority of patients who present to psychopharmacologists with severe, recurrent, mixed, rapid cycling symptoms, abundant comorbidity, and inadequate treatment responses with multiple residual symptoms after receiving all the treatments described above? Here it may be prudent to follow the course discussed earlier in Chapter 2 and illustrated in Figures 2-121 through 2-126; that is, to choose combinations

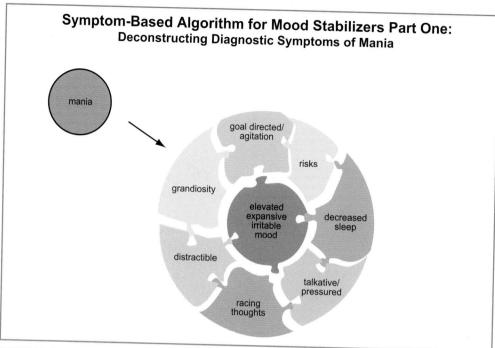

FIGURE 3-35 Symptom-based algorithm for mood stabilizers, part 1. A symptom-based approach to the selection of a mood stabilizer follows the theory that each of a patient's symptoms can be matched with malfunctioning brain circuits and neurotransmitters that hypothetically mediate those symptoms; this information is then used to select a corresponding pharmacological mechanism for treatment. Shown here is the diagnosis of a manic episode deconstructed into its core symptom of elevated, expansive, or irritable mood plus the other seven diagnostic symptoms of mania [as defined by the *Diagnostic and Statistical Manual of Mental Disorders*, fourth edition (DSM-IV)].

of treatment based on the specific symptoms a patient is experiencing, attempting to relieve all residual symptoms, and to achieve full remission. This is called the "symptom-based algorithm" and is outlined in Figures 3-35 through 3-41.

The symptom-based strategy begins with the construction of a diagnosis and then deconstructing this into a list of specific symptoms that the individual patient is experiencing. Next, these symptoms are matched with the brain circuits that hypothetically mediate these symptoms and with the known neuropharmacological regulation of these circuits by neurotransmitters. Finally, available treatment options that target these neuropharmacological mechanisms are chosen to eliminate the symptoms one by one. When symptoms persist, a treatment with a different mechanism is added or switched to. No evidence proves that this is a superior approach, but it appeals not only to clinical intuition but also to neurobiological reasoning. In the absence of options that have proven superiority, the symptom-based approach is advocated here and is what we have mostly followed throughout this book.

Residual symptoms and circuits after first-line treatment of bipolar disorder

Malfunctioning circuits tied to specific symptoms of depression are discussed extensively in Chapter 1 and illustrated as well in Figures 1-46 through 1-54. Once the specific depressive symptoms and the hypothetically malfunctioning circuits have been determined, the next step is to target the regulatory neurotransmitters for these circuits with selected pharmacological mechanisms in order to enhance the efficiency of information processing in these

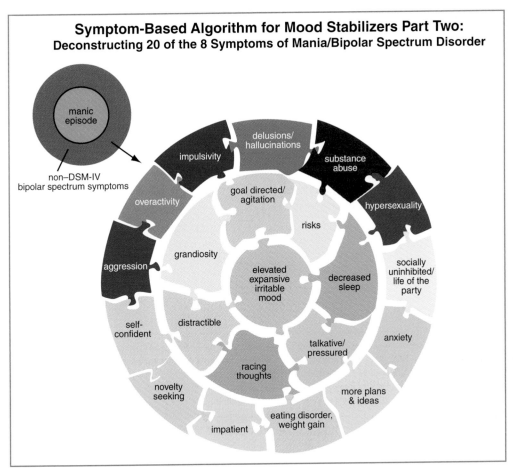

Symptom-Based Algorithm for Mood Stabilizers Part Two:
Deconstructing 20 of the 8 Symptoms of Mania/Bipolar Spectrum Disorder

FIGURE 3-36 Symptom-based algorithm for mood stabilizers, part 2. Several common symptoms associated with mania can be disabling and prevent remission but are nonetheless not part of the formal diagnostic criteria for a manic episode. These are shown here as the outer ring.

circuits and thereby reduce symptoms. This is shown specifically for the common residual symptoms of fatigue, loss of concentration, and insomnia in depression in Figure 2-123 along with the recommended treatments; this is also the same approach taken for depression in bipolar disorder as long as it is done while augmenting a mood stabilizer that protects against the possible emergence of mania, which is associated with some of the treatments suggested.

How about residual symptoms of mania that continue after treatment with a mood stabilizer? Core diagnostic symptoms of mania are shown in Figure 3-35 and discussed extensively in Chapter 1 and illustrated in Figures 1-56 through 1-62. The circuits hypothetically associated with each of these symptoms are summarized in Figure 1-57, and the regulation of numerous specific circuits by monoamine neurotransmitters is shown in Figures 1-58 through 1-62.

If this is not complicated enough, there are many other symptoms associated with a manic or mixed episode that are not considered core diagnostic criteria; these are illustrated as the outer ring in Figure 3-36. The postulated circuits associated with each of these nondiagnostic symptoms of mania are summarized in Figure 3-37. Similarly, the nondiagnostic

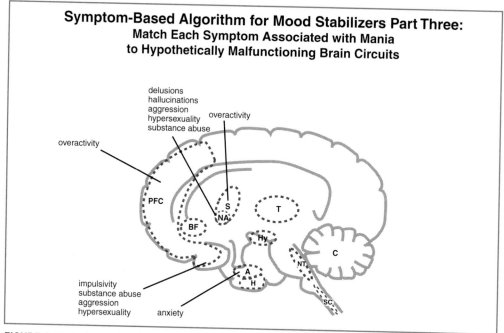

FIGURE 3-37 Symptom-based algorithm for mood stabilizers, part 3. In this figure common associated but not diagnostic symptoms of mania are linked to hypothetically malfunctioning brain circuits. Delusions and hallucinations are linked primarily to the nucleus accumbens (NA); while aggression, hypersexuality, and substance abuse are mediated not only by the NA but also by the prefrontal cortex (PFC). The PFC may also play a role in impulsivity and overactivity; overactivity is also associated with the striatum (S). Anxiety may occur in bipolar disorder and is primarily mediated by the amygdala (A).

symptoms associated with depression are discussed in chapter 2 and illustrated in Figure 2-124, with associated circuits shown in Figure 2-125 and suggested treatments in Figure 2-126. These same considerations in Figures 2-124 through 2-126 apply as well for bipolar patients in the depressed or mixed phases of the illness.

Suggested treatments for the nondiagnostic mania-related symptoms are shown in Figures 3-38 through 3-41. Differing mechanisms of action for mood stabilizers, discussed throughout this chapter, are illustrated in Figures 13-39 through 3-41. Since these mechanisms are certainly quite different, act at separate and distinct targets, and may be additive if not synergistic when combined, they provide the rationale for combining drugs with different mechanisms when ongoing treatments are associated with residual symptoms and not with complete remission.

That is, manic symptoms are largely conceptualized as the product of unstable and excessive if not chaotic neurotransmission in specific brain circuits, depending on the exact symptom being expressed (Figure 3-37). This state of unstable and excessive neurotransmission is illustrated in Figure 3-39A with a "bipolar storm" shown brewing between the two neurons in the circuit, conceptualized as too much sodium ion flow through voltage-sensitive sodium channels (VSSCs), too much calcium flow through voltage-sensitive calcium channels (VSCCs), and too much release of excitatory glutamate neurotransmitter. In reality, the problem may be that a bipolar circuit is "out of tune" and therefore acting inconsistently and chaotically in its neurotransmission rather than simply being too active as shown in Figure 3-39A.

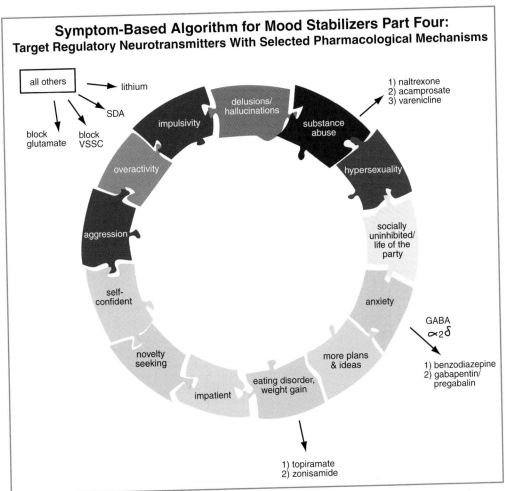

FIGURE 3-38 Symptom-based algorithm for mood stabilizers, part 4. Nondiagnostic symptoms of mania can be linked to the neurotransmitters that regulate them and in turn linked to pharmacological mechanisms for treatment selection. Many of these symptoms may be targeted by first-line treatments that block voltage-sensitive sodium channels (VSSCs), dopamine 2 and serotonin 2A receptors (by atypical antipsychotics), or glutamate; lithium may also treat many of these symptoms. Particular symptoms that may benefit from adjunctive treatment include substance abuse, which may be treated by naltrexone (alcohol), acamprosate (alcohol), or varenicline (smoking); anxiety, which may be related to gamma-aminobutyric acid (GABA) and voltage-sensitive calcium channels (VSCCs) and treated with benzodiazepines or gabapentin/pregabalin; and eating disorders or weight gain, which may be treated by topiramate or zonisamide.

Figures 3-39B and C through 3-41 show the various pharmacological mechanisms of action that can be selected or combined in order to attempt to reduce all symptoms and achieve remission in bipolar disorder. This starts with stabilizing and reducing neurotransmission in targeted and symptomatic circuits by blocking VSSCs with some mood stabilizers (Figure 3-39B), by reducing glutamate release or glutamate actions at NMDA receptors (Figure 3-39C) with other mood stabilizers, and/or by reducing dopamine hyperactivity with atypical antipsychotics or lithium (Figure 3-40), and/or by reducing glutamate hyperactivity by blocking 5HT2A receptors with atypical antipsychotics (Figure 3-41).

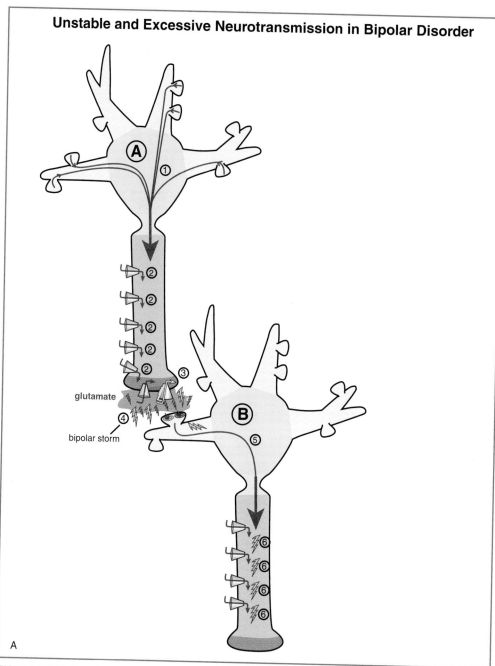

Unstable and Excessive Neurotransmission in Bipolar Disorder

glutamate

bipolar storm

A

FIGURE 3-39A Unstable and excessive neurotransmission in bipolar disorder. Rather than being a function of too much or too little neurotransmission, bipolar disorder may instead occur as a result of unstable and excessive neurotransmission culminating in a "bipolar storm" at synapses. The bipolar storm is conceptualized here as too much activity of neuron A with widespread input from its dendritic tree (1) triggering too much axonal impulse flow, mediated by overly active voltage-sensitive sodium channels (2). When the nerve impulse invades the axon terminal, this, in turn, overly activates the voltage-sensitive calcium channels linked to glutamate release there (3), triggering a "bipolar storm" (4) of excessive, chaotic, or unpredictable neurotransmission from neuron A to neuron B. Postsynaptic NMDA receptors on neuron B detect this bipolar storm (4) and propagate excessive, chaotic, or unpredictable neurotransmission in neuron B (5), which in turn converts this information into its own nerve impulse, its own excessive activation of voltage-sensitive sodium channels (6), and so on.

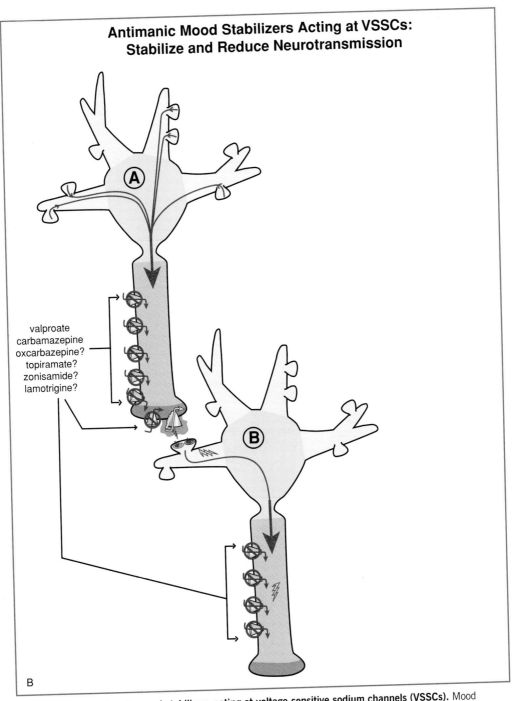

FIGURE 3-39B Antimanic mood stabilizers acting at voltage-sensitive sodium channels (VSSCs). Mood stabilizers that block VSSCs may stabilize and reduce propagation of nerve impulses and neurotransmission and thus reduce symptoms of mania. Examples of antimanic agents that act at VSSCs are valproate and carbamazepine; other VSSC blockers include oxcarbazepine, topiramate, zonisamide, and lamotrigine.

Antidepressant Mood Stabilizers Acting at Glutamate: Stabilize and Reduce Glutamate Hyperactivity

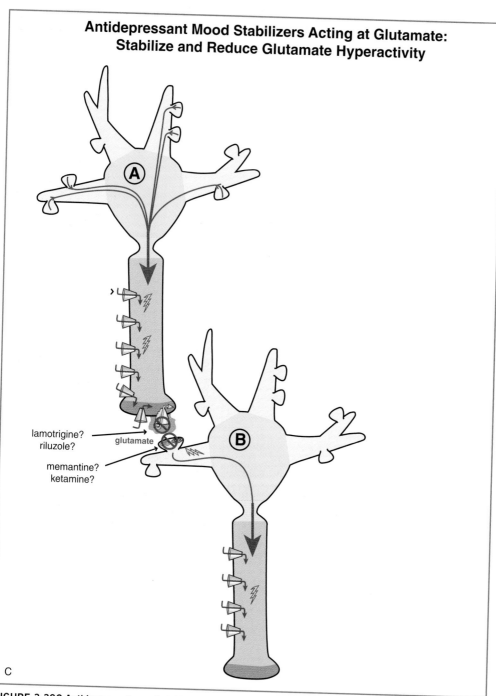

lamotrigine?
riluzole?

glutamate

memantine?
ketamine?

C

FIGURE 3-39C Antidepressant mood stabilizers acting at glutamate. Agents that reduce glutamate release or block glutamate actions at N-methyl-d-aspartate (NMDA) receptors may stabilize and reduce glutamate hyperactivity and thus have efficacy in the depressed phase of bipolar disorder. Lamotrigine and riluzole may reduce glutamate release, while memantine and ketamine act at NMDA receptors.

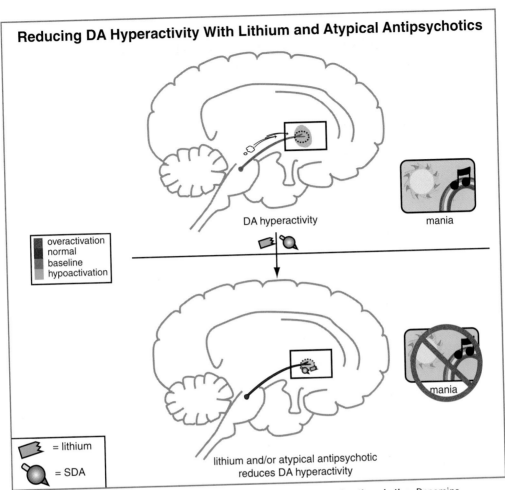

FIGURE 3-40 Reducing dopamine hyperactivity with lithium and atypical antipsychotics. Dopamine hyperactivity could play a role in the development of manic symptoms; therefore the reduction of dopamine hyperactivity, which can be achieved with lithium or atypical antipsychotics, may be an effective antimanic strategy.

If this is not sufficient, other pharmacological mechanisms may need to be recruited to suppress all symptoms. Pain and anxiety are discussed in Chapter 2 and the associated circuits illustrated in Figure 2-125 and treatment recommendations given in Figure 2-126. These concepts also apply when these same symptoms are residual in bipolar disorder. Adjunctive topiramate or zonisamide may be helpful for weight gain, and adjunctive drug abuse treatments may be helpful for substance abuse, including acamprosate and/or naltrexone for alcohol abuse and varenicline for smoking cessation (Figure 3-38).

Finally, bipolar disorder may not only have associated nondiagnostic symptoms but also many comorbid conditions, ranging from various anxiety disorders, psychosis, impulse control disorders, attention deficit hyperactivity disorder, conduct disorder, borderline personality disorder, migraine, bulimia, thyroid disorders, and many more (Figure 3-42). The point is to try to eliminate all such symptoms so as to get the patient to remission. The importance of this approach is difficult to underestimate. It has been estimated that for every residual manic/hypomanic symptom there is a 20% increase in the chance of manic

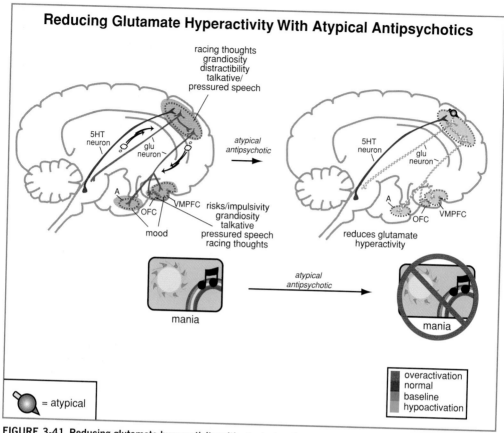

FIGURE 3-41 Reducing glutamate hyperactivity with atypical antipsychotics. Glutamate hyperactivity is proposed to contribute to development of both manic and depressive symptoms in bipolar disorder, perhaps in different pathways. Blockade of serotonin 2A (5HT2A) receptors by atypical antipsychotics can lead to reduced glutamate hyperactivity and thus may treat these symptoms. Potential sites of action for mania are shown here.

relapse, and for every residual depressive symptom a 15% increase in the chance of depressive relapse. This is why psychopharmacologists should consider treating all 20 of the 8 symptoms of a bipolar manic episode (Figure 3-36), all 14 of the 9 symptoms of a depressive episode (Figure 2-124), all comorbidities, and beyond! This requires taking a history that looks for all such symptoms not only before treatment but also after each sequential treatment. Each patient would have his or her bipolar symptoms deconstructed not only into diagnostic symptoms but also into all associated symptoms and comorbid conditions on each visit (Figures 2-124, 2-127, 3-36, and 3-42). Each and every symptom could then be mapped onto hypothetically malfunctioning brain circuits (Figures 2-125 and 3-37). The goal of treatment, of course, is not only sustained remission but also the prevention of more complicated and unstable outcomes, including the development of resistance to known treatments (Figure 1-29).

Bipolar disorder and women

The use of antidepressants in women is extensively discussed in Chapter 2 and illustrated in Figures 2-97 through 2-106. Although gender issues in bipolar disorder are less well investigated than they are in unipolar disorder, a brief discussion is in order for those special considerations known to be relevant to women with bipolar disorder.

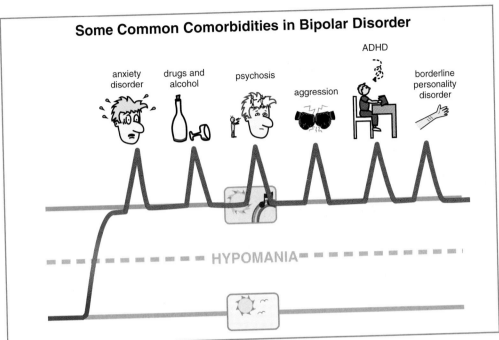

Some Common Comorbidities in Bipolar Disorder

FIGURE 3-42 Common comorbidities in bipolar disorder. Many patients with bipolar disorder also have comorbid conditions. Common comorbidities include anxiety disorders, drug and alcohol abuse, psychosis, attention deficit hyperactivity disorder (ADHD), and borderline personality disorder. Aggression may also be a common symptom in patients with bipolar disorder.

For example, in women, bipolar disorder is even more depressive in nature than it is in men with this condition, with more suicide attempts, mixed mania, and rapid cycling than in men. Women have more thyroid dysfunction than men, and some experts believe that augmentation of bipolar patients with thyroid hormone (T3) – in men but particularly in women – may enhance stability even in the absence of overt thyroid dysfunction (see discussion in Chapter 2; also Figure 2-112 as well as Figure 3-34). Women are more likely than men to report atypical or reverse vegetative symptoms during the depressed phase, especially increased appetite and weight gain. Comorbid anxiety and eating disorders are more frequent in bipolar women; comorbid substance use disorders are more frequent in men.

There is limited evidence that bipolar disorder may worsen during the premenstrual phase in some women, just as unipolar major depression may worsen premenstrually (discussed in Chapter 2 as menstrual magnification and illustrated in Figure 2-100). Pregnancy is not protective against bipolar mood episodes, and the postpartum period is a very high risk time for experiencing first onset and recurrence of depressive, manic, mixed, and psychotic episodes (postpartum depressive episodes are discussed in Chapter 2 and illustrated in Figures 2-100 and 2-103).

There is little empirical study of bipolar disorder in perimenopausal or postmenopausal women, but there are suggestions that bipolar recurrence is more common during perimenopause and that estrogen may stabilize mood in perimenopausal women with bipolar disorder. No research shows what specific interventions to make for a perimenopausal bipolar woman with vasomotor symptoms or for perimenopausal or postmenopausal women who have unstable mood symptoms and do not take estrogen replacement therapy. Vasomotor symptoms in unipolar depression are discussed in Chapter 2 and illustrated in Figures 2-104 through 2-106.

No major gender differences have been consistently reported for mood stabilizers in terms of efficacy, but there are differences in side effects, including the possible risk of polycystic ovarian syndrome with amenorrhea, hyperandrogenism, weight gain, and insulin resistance from valproate in women.

During pregnancy, most anticonvulsant mood stabilizers and lithium are associated with risk for various fetal toxicities. Some may be mitigated by coadministration of folate. However, at this writing it may be prudent to consider stabilizing bipolar women with atypical antipsychotics during pregnancy. If mood stabilizers are discontinued for pregnancy, this should not be done abruptly, or it may increase the chance of recurrence. Of course, nontreatment of bipolar illness has its consequences, too, as discussed for nontreatment of unipolar depression during pregnancy in Chapter 2 with the problems outlined in Table 2-13. Many of the same considerations apply as well to the treatment of bipolar women during pregnancy, including the decision whether to continue or discontinue mood stabilizers during pregnancy, postpartum periods, and breast-feeding. Such decisions should be made on an individual basis after weighing the risks and benefits for a particular patient. Generally speaking, breast-feeding while taking lithium is not recommended, whereas breast-feeding while taking valproate, lamotrigine, carbamazepine, or atypical antipsychotics can be cautiously considered, with careful monitoring of the infant and, if necessary, obtaining infant blood drug levels.

Children, bipolar disorder, and mood stabilizers

This is one of the great controversial areas of psychopharmacology today. As this book is not focused on child psychopharmacology, only a few key issues will be mentioned here. Controversies in the treatment of unipolar depression in children and adolescents with antidepressants are mentioned in Chapter 2 and illustrated in Figure 2-11. For bipolar disorder, there is debate about whether children even get this illness and whether symptoms attributable to bipolar disorder should be treated at all with powerful psychotropic medications.

In reality, it is increasingly clear that prepubertal and adolescent manias do exist and are more common than had been appreciated in the past; however, the symptoms are different from those of "classic" adult mania. That is, prepubertal mania is characterized by severe irritability, absence of discrete episodes yet periodic "affective storms" with severe, persistent, and often violent outbursts, attacking behavior and anger. Symptoms tend to be chronic and continuous rather than episodic and acute. Moods are only rarely euphoric, but there are high levels of hyperactivity and overactivity. It seems increasingly clear that pediatric mania may not be rare so much as it is difficult to diagnose and to distinguish from attention deficit hyperactivity disorder and conduct disorder. Thus, an atypical picture of a chronic course characterized by predominantly irritable mood and mania mixed with depression looks much different than euphoric mania with a biphasic and episodic course.

Adolescent-onset mania may more frequently include euphoria but otherwise has the symptom characteristics of childhood-onset rather than adult-onset mania. In fact, "mixed mania," affecting 20% to 30% of adults with bipolar mania, may often have its onset in retrospect in childhood or adolescence, with the additional characteristics of chronic course, high rate of suicide, poor response to treatment, and early history of cognitive symptoms highly suggestive of ADHD. Thus, pediatric mania may develop into adult mixed mania.

In children, mania has considerable symptomatic overlap with ADHD, and it has been estimated that over half (and possibly up to 90%) of patients with pediatric mania also have ADHD. This is not just due to "distractibility, motoric hyperactivity, and talkativeness," diagnostic symptoms that overlap with both mania and ADHD, but to true comorbidity. In such patients, it seems to be necessary to stabilize the mania before treating the ADHD to get best results, and also to combine mood stabilizers with ADHD treatments.

In children, conduct disorder is also strongly associated with mania. Most patients with mania qualify for the diagnosis of conduct disorder, making this association quite controversial if it leads to antipsychotic treatment of essentially all children with conduct disorder. However, there are differences in symptoms between the two groups, with physical restlessness and poor judgment more common in comorbid cases of conduct disorder and mania than in cases with mania alone. Finally, anxiety disorders, especially panic disorder and agoraphobia, are frequently comorbid for mania in children.

For treatment, the best options are to use what has been proven in adults, but there is a striking paucity of evidence for how to treat bipolar disorder in children and adolescents. Much further study of mood stabilizers is required in children and adolescents.

Combinations of mood stabilizers are the standard for treating bipolar disorder

Given the disappointing number of patients who attain remission from any phase of bipolar disorder after any given monotherapy or sequence of monotherapies, who can maintain that remission over the long run, and who can tolerate the treatment, it is not surprising that the majority of bipolar patients require treatment with several medications. Rather than have a simple regimen of one mood stabilizer at high doses and a patient with side effects but who is not in remission, it now seems highly preferable to have a patient in remission without symptoms no matter how many agents this takes. Furthermore, sometimes the doses of each agent can be lowered to tolerable levels while the synergy among their therapeutic mechanisms provides more robust efficacy than single agents even in high doses.

Several specific suggestions of mood stabilizer combinations are shown in Figures 3-43 through 3-45. Many others can be constructed, but these particular combinations or "combos" have enjoyed widespread use even though for many of them there are few actual evidence-based data from clinical trials that their combination results in superior efficacy. Because of the strong role of "eminence-based medicine" (with sometimes conflicting recommendations by different experts) rather than "evidence-based medicine" for combination treatments, some of the options are discussed with whimsy and humor below and in Figures 3-43 through 3-45. Nevertheless, treatment of bipolar disorders with rational and empirically useful combinations is serious business and the reader may find that several of these suggestions are useful for practicing clinicians in the treatment of some patients.

The best evidence-based combinations are the addition of lithium or valproate to an atypical antipsychotic, especially antipsychotics such as risperidone, olanzapine, and quetiapine, which have been on the market the longest. Thus these are atypical lithium and atypical valproate combos, as shown in Figure 3-43. Probably clozapine as well as somewhat newer agents such as ziprasidone, aripiprazole, and paliperidone are generally useful as well in combination with either lithium or valproate.

Although lithium, lamotrigine, and valproate have all been available for a long time, there are remarkably few controlled studies of their use together. Nevertheless, they all have different mechanisms of action and have different clinical profiles in the various phases of bipolar illness; they can therefore usefully be combined in clinical practice due to practice-based evidence as li-do (lithium-Depakote/divalproex/valproate), la-li

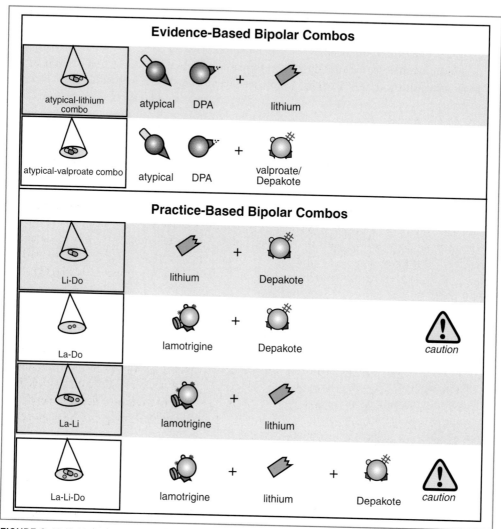

FIGURE 3-43 Evidence- and practice-based bipolar combos. Most patients with bipolar disorder will require treatment with two or more agents. The combinations with the most evidence include addition of an atypical antipsychotic to either lithium (atypical-lithium combo) or valproate/Depakote (atypical-valproate combo). Combinations that are not well studied in controlled trials but that have some practice-based evidence include lithium plus Depakote (li-do), cautious use of lamotrigine plus Depakote (la-do), lamotrigine plus lithium (la-li), and cautious combination of lamotrigine, lithium, and Depakote (la-li-do).

(lamotrigine-lithium), la-do (lamotrigine-Depakote) or even la-li-do (lamotrigine-lithium-Depakote) (Figure 3-43). Combinations of lamotrigine and valproate need to be carefully monitored for the consequences of the drug interactions between the two, especially for elevations of lamotrigine levels and the possible increased risk of rashes, including serious rash, unless the lamotrigine dose is decreased by as much as half.

Various natural products can also be added as adjuncts to any proven mood stabilizer, but these are not expected to have sudden and robust efficacy, including T3, L-methylfolate (MTHF), inositol, omega-3 fatty acids, SAMe, and others (Figure 3-34). Adjuncts are expected to help associated symptoms but not to be mood stabilizing per se, including agents for substance abuse (naltrexone, acamprosate, varenicline); weight loss (zonisamide, topiramate); pain, anxiety, and sleep (gabapentin, pregabalin); agitation (benzodiazepines); and many others (Figure 3-34).

Some of the more innovative if "eminence-based" combos are the most frequently used; several of these are shown in Figures 3-44 and 3-45.

Boston bipolar brew

Several experts, including many trained or working in Boston, are proponents of essentially *never* utilizing an antidepressant for bipolar patients. Thus, a "Boston bipolar brew" is any combination of mood stabilizers that does *not* include an antidepressant (Figure 3-44).

California careful cocktail

On the other hand, some experts in California are more laid back and are proponents of "earning" the right to add an antidepressant, carefully, once having exhausted other options for a bipolar depressed patient whose depression is not in remission. A "California careful cocktail" is the addition of an antidepressant to one or more mood stabilizers, particularly including one or more that has robust efficacy against mania and recurrence of mania (Figure 3-44).

Tennessee mood shine

Yet another option for treating bipolar depression occurs when giving an antidepressant and discovering that the patient either has activating side effects or treatment resistance or that the diagnosis is changing from unipolar to bipolar depression as the condition evolves. In this case, rather than stopping the antidepressant, an atypical antipsychotic is added. Experts in Tennessee came up with the idea to put some shine on depressed mood in patients inadequately responsive or tolerant to antidepressant monotherapy, so this approach is called "Tennessee mood shine" (Figure 3-44).

Buckeye bipolar bullets

Experts working in Ohio, the Buckeye State, have prominently proposed lamotrigine monotherapy as the magic bullet for first-line treatment of bipolar depression as well as for preventing relapse into depression (Figure 3-44). Although this can indeed be highly effective, one must remember that in many ways lamotrigine therapy is the "stealth" approach to treating bipolar depression, given the long titration times (two months or longer) and latency of onset of action once adequate dosing is reached (up to another three months). Thus, efficacy can appear to be clandestine and literally sneak up on the patient over three or four months rather than dramatically boosting mood soon after the initiation of treatment.

Rather than add an antidepressant to lamotrigine when there is inadequate response, an alternative approach would be to avoid that until several other combinations are tried first, including augmentation with an atypical antipsychotic, especially another Buckeye bipolar bullet called quetiapine (the combination is known as "Lami-quel" in Figure 3-44 – i.e., Lamictal/lamotrigine plus Seroquel/quetiapine). Any combination utilizing Seroquel/quetiapine with another mood stabilizer or antidepressant can be called a "Quel kit."

Yet another Buckeye bipolar bullet to combine with lamotrigine rather than augmenting with an antidepressant is the wake-promoting agent modafinil (modafinil combo in Figure 3-44), especially if the patient is "still sleepy after all these cures" and while monitoring for activation of mania.

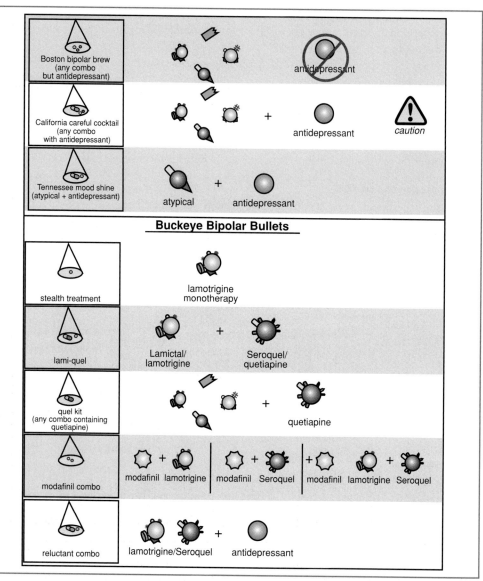

FIGURE 3-44 Bullet combos for bipolar depression. Experts diverge in their opinions of how to treat bipolar depression, particularly when it comes to antidepressants. Some believe that even when combination treatment is required, it should never involve use of an antidepressant (Boston bipolar brew), while others recommend cautious addition of an antidepressant to one or more mood stabilizers (California careful cocktail). For patients who develop symptoms of activation during treatment with an antidepressant for unipolar depression, some experts suggest adding an atypical antipsychotic rather than discontinuing the antidepressant (Tennessee mood shine). Another school of thought (Buckeye bipolar bullets) focuses on lamotrigine as the primary treatment for bipolar depression, with augmentation of other mood stabilizers (as opposed to antidepressants) when lamotrigine monotherapy is not enough. Lamotrigine may be considered a "stealth treatment," as it must be titrated slowly and can have a long latency of onset of action. Reasonable augmenting agents would include an atypical antipsychotic, particularly quetiapine (lami-quel). Quetiapine itself is an established monotherapy for bipolar depression and can be combined with many other agents as well (quel-kit). Another potential agent to add to lamotrigine, quetiapine, or lamotrigine and quetiapine is modafinil, particularly for patients with daytime sleepiness (modafinil combo). If none of these combinations produce a good response, one may consider adding an antidepressant to lamotrigine/quetiapine (reluctant combo).

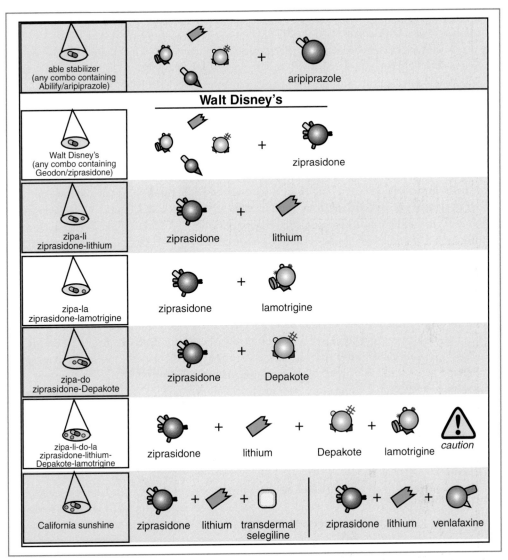

FIGURE 3-45 Atypical combos. Any combination containing the partial dopamine agonist aripiprazole may be referred to as an "able stabilizer," while any combination containing the serotonin dopamine antagonist ziprasidone may be collectively termed a "Walt Disney." These include ziprasidone plus lithium (zipa-li), ziprasidone plus lamotrigine (zipa-la), ziprasidone plus Depakote (zipa-do), and ziprasidone plus lithium, lamotrigine, and Depakote (zipa-li-do-la). California sunshine is a powerful combination for bipolar depression with full-dose ziprasidone and full-dose lithium as well as augmentation with either transdermal selegiline or high-dose venlafaxine.

Finally, after trying all these options, continuing poor response in bipolar depression may require reluctant augmentation of lamotrigine or various of the lamotrigine combos described above with an antidepressant (reluctant combo in Figure 3-44).

"Able stabilizers" include any combo containing the dopamine partial agonist and dopamine system stabilizer Abilify/aripiprazole (Figure 3-45). For depressed patients, it may generally be advisable to use between 2 and 10 mg of aripiprazole and not more for best results in bipolar disorder and in treatment-resistant unipolar depression when combined with antidepressants.

"Walt Disney" combos refer to any mixture containing ziprasidone (Figure 3-45). Thus, this includes zipa-li, zipa-la, zipa-do, zipa-li-do-la. One of the Walt Disneys that may be effective for some of the most resistant of bipolar depressions is called "California sunshine" and includes ziprasidone in combination with lithium, both at full therapeutic doses, with transdermal selegiline or with high-dose venlafaxine.

Future mood stabilizers

Several new possibilities exist for novel mood stabilizers. This includes several new **atypical antipsychotics** in development, from bifeprunox to iloperidone to asenapine and others. Any **new anticonvulsant** is a potential mood stabilizer, and a few are already on the horizon, including eslicarbazepine, the active metabolite of oxcarbazepine discussed above (Figure 3-11) and a compound related to lamotrigine (JZP-4). **Dopamine agonists** such as pramipexole and related agents such as ropinirole may be useful for the depressed phase of bipolar disorder, especially in combination with mood stabilizers that could protect from the possible induction of mania.

New research is also targeting novel ways to **enhance GABA action or to block glutamate action** for new mood stabilizers, although these compounds are generally still in preclinical testing. Another novel site mentioned earlier is the **sigma 1 site**. An interesting set of observations suggests that dextromethorphan, which may act via sigma 1 receptors and secondarily as a weak NMDA antagonist, may be useful in stabilizing affect in involuntary emotional expression disorder (pseudobulbar affect) associated with various neurological conditions. One specific agent combines dextromethorphan with quinidine to enhance dextromethorphan bioavailability (AVP923, or Zenvia) and appears promising for this indication. It is possible that this combination or other agents that target sigma 1 sites may also be useful in stabilizing mood in bipolar disorder, but further research is necessary.

Clearly any antidepressant developed for unipolar depression is a candidate for cautious addition to mood stabilizers in some cases; these agents in development are discussed in Chapter 2. Agents that can reduce stress-related responses by acting at the hypothalamic pituitary adrenal (HPA) axis are also candidates for the treatment of major depressive disorder, bipolar disorder, anxiety disorders, and other conditions. These agents, include **glucocorticoid antagonists, corticotrophin releasing factor (CRF1) antagonists, and vasopressin 1b (V1b) antagonists**.

Scientists are trying to create a future lithium mimetic by targeting actions at the same signal transduction cascades where lithium acts. Such approaches are still highly theoretical and in preclinical testing at this time, including how to activate the formation of **neurotrophic growth factors** such as BDNF or to act at relevant neurotrophic receptors.

Summary

Mood stabilizers have evolved significantly in recent years. They include agents that are mania-minded and treat mania while preventing manic relapse as well as agents that are depression-minded and treat bipolar depression while preventing depressive relapse. Numerous agents of diverse mechanisms of action are mood stabilizers, especially lithium, various anticonvulsants, and atypical antipsychotics. Numerous new agents developed for other uses are also being tested in bipolar disorder. However, because of limits to the efficacy and tolerability of current mood stabilizers, combination therapy is the rule and mood stabilizer monotherapy the exception. Evidence is evolving for how to combine agents to relieve all symptoms of bipolar disorder and prevent relapse, but the treatment of bipolar disorder today remains as much a psychopharmacological art as it does a science. New mood stabilizers of diverse novel mechanisms are also on the horizon.

Suggested Readings

Chapters 1 (Mood Disorders), 2 (Antidepressants), and 3 (Mood Stabilizers)

Agjakamoam GK and Marek GJ. (2000) Serotonin model of schizophrenia: emerging role of glutamate mechanisms. *Brain Res Rev* 31; 302–312.

Akiskal H and Tohen M. (eds) (2006) *Bipolar Psychopharmacotherapy*. West Sussex, England, Wiley and Sons.

Akiskal HS, Akiskal KK, Perugi G, Toni C, Ruffolo G and Tusini G. (2006) Bipolar II and anxious reactive "comorbidity": toward better phenotypic characterization suitable for genotyping. *J Affective Disord* 96; 239–247.

Altshuler LL, Bookheimer SY, Townsend J, Proenza MA, Eisenberger N, Sabb F, Mintz J and Cohen MS. (2005) Blunted activation in orbitofrontal cortex during mania: a functional magnetic resonance imaging study. *Biol Psychiatry* 58; 763–769.

Amargos-Bosch M, Bortolozzi A, Puig MV, Serrats J, Adell A, Celada P, Toth M, Mengod G and Artigas F. (2004) Co-expression in vivo interaction of serotonin 1A and serotonin 2A receptors in pyramidal neurons of prefrontal cortex. *Cereb Cortex* 14; 281–299.

Amargos-Bosch M, Lopez-Gil X, Artigas F and Adell A. (2006) Clozapine and olanzapine, but not haloperidol, suppress serotonin efflux in the medial prefrontal cortex elicited by phencyclidine and ketamine. *Int J Neuropsychopharmacol* 9; 565–573.

Angst J. (2007) The bipolar spectrum. *Br J Psychiatry* 190; 189–191.

Avery DH, Holtzheimer III PE, Fawaz W, Russo J, Neumaier J, Dunner DL, Haynor DR, Claypoole KH, Wajdik C and Roy-Byrne P. (2006) A controlled study of repetitive transcranial magnetic stimulation in medication-resistant major depression. *Biol Psychiatry* 59; 187–194.

Barone P, Scarzella L, Marconi R, Antonini A, Morgante L, Bracco F, Zappia M and Musch B. (2006) Pramipexole versus sertraline in the treatment of depression in Parkinson's disease. *J Neurol* 253; 601–607.

Barsky AJ, Orav EJ and Bates DW. (2005) Somatization increases medical utilization and costs independent of psychiatric and medical comorbidity. *Arch Gen Psychiatry* 62; 903–910.

Baumer FM, Howe M, Gallelli K, Simeonova DI, Hallmayer J and Chang KD. (2006) A pilot study of antidepressant-induced mania in pediatric bipolar disorder: characteristics, risk factors, and the serotonin transporter gene. *Biol Psychiatry* 60; 1005–1012.

Berman RM, Marcus RN, Swanink R, McQuade RD, Carson WH, Corey-Lisle PK and Khan A. (2007) The efficacy and safety of aripiprazole as adjunctive therapy in major depressive disorder: a multicenter, randomized, double-blind, placebo-controlled study. *J Clin Psychiatry* 68; 843–853.

Biederman J. (2006) The evolving face of pediatric mania. *Biol Psychiatry* 60; 901–902.

Biederman J, Mick E, Hammerness P, Harpold T, Aleardi M, Dougherty M and Wozniak J. (2005) Open-label, 8 week trial of olanzapine and risperidone for the treatment of bipolar disorder in preschool age children. *Biol Psychiatry* 58; 589–594.

Bowden CL, Calabrese JR, Ketter TA, Sachs GS, White RL and Thompson TR. (2006) Impact of lamotrigine and lithium on weight in obese and nonobese patients with bipolar I disorder. *Am J Psychiatry* 163; 1199–1201.

Bridge JA, Iyengar S, Salary CB, Barbe RP, Birmaher B, Pincus HA, Ren L and Brent DA. (2007) Clinical response and risk for reported suicidal ideation and suicide attempts in pediatric antidepressant treatment. *JAMA* 297; 15, 1683–1696.

Calabrese JR, Goldberg JF, Ketter TA, Suppes T, Frye M, White R, DeVeaugh-Geiss A and Thompson TR. (2006) Recurrence in bipolar I disorder: a post hoc analysis excluding relapses in two double blind maintenance studies. *Biol Psychiatry* 59; 1061–1064.

Calabrese JR, Shelton MD, Rapport DJ, Youngstrom EA, Jackson K, Bilali S, Ganocy SJ and Findling RL. (2005) A 20-month, double-blind, maintenance trial of lithium versus divalproex in rapid cycling bipolar disorder. *Am J Psychiatry* 162; 2152–2161.

Carli M, Vaviera M, Invernizzi RW and Balducci C. (2006) Dissociable contribution of 5-HT1A and 5-HT 2A receptors in the medial prefrontal cortex to different aspects of executive control such as impulsivity and compulsive perseveration in rats. *Neuropsychopharmacology* 31; 757–767.

Cavanagh J, Patterson J, Pimlott S, Dewar D, Eersels J, Dempsey MF and Wyper D. (2006) Serotonin transporter residual availability during long term antidepressant therapy does not differentiate responder and nonresponder unipolar patients. *Biol Psychiatry* 59; 301–308.

Cipriani A, Barbui C, Brambilla P, Furukawa TA, Hotopf M and Geddes JR. (2006) Are all antidepressants really the same? The case of fluoxetine: a systematic review. *J Clin Psychiatry* 67; 6, 850–864.

Cipriani A, Pretty H, Hawton K and Geddes JR. (2005) Lithium in the prevention of suicidal behavior and all-cause mortality in patients with mood disorders: a systematic review of randomized trials. *Am J Psychiatry* 162; 1805–1819.

Cooper Kazaz R, Apter JT, Cohen R, Karagichev L, Muhammed-Moussa S, Grupper D, Drori T, Newman ME, Sackeim HA, Glaser B and Lerer B. (2007) Combined treatment with sertraline and liothyronine in major depression. *Arch Gen Psychiatry* 64; 679–688.

Cousins DA and Young AH. (2007) The armamentarium of treatments for bipolar disorder: a review of the literature. *Int J Neuropsychopharmacol* 10; 411–431.

Crossley NA and Bauer M. (2007) Acceleration and augmentation of antidepressants with lithium for depressive disorders: two meta-analyses of randomized, placebo-controlled trials. *J Clin Psychiatry* 68; 935–940.

deBartolomeis A, Fiore G and Iasevoli F. (2005) Dopamine-glutamate interaction and antipsychotics mechanism of action: implication for new pharmacological strategies in psychosis. *Curr Pharm Des* 11; 3561–3594.

DelBello MP, Adler CM, Whitsel RM, Stanford KE and Strakowski SM. (2007) A 12-week single blind trial of quetiapine for the treatment of mood symptoms in adolescents at high risk for developing bipolar I disorder. *J Clin Psychiatry* 68; 5, 789–795.

DelBello MP, Hanseman D, Adler CM, Fleck DE and Strakowski SM. (2007) Twelve-month outcome of adolescents with bipolar disorder following first hospitalization for a manic or mixed episode. *Am J Psychiatry* 164; 582–590.

DelBello MP, Kowwatch RA, Adler CM, Stanford KE, Welge JA, Barzman DH, Nelson E and Strakowski SM. (2006) A double-blind randomized pilot study comparing quetiapine and divalproex for adolescent mania. *J Am Acad Child Adolesc Psychiatry* 45; 3, 305–313.

DeMartinis NA, Yeung PP, Entsuah R and Manley AL. (2007) A double-blind, placebo-controlled study of the efficacy and safety of desvenlafaxine succinate in the treatment of major depressive disorder. *J Clin Psychiatry* 68; 677–688.

Dew MA, Whyte EM, Lenze EJ, Houck PR, Mulsant BH, Pollock BG, Stack JA, Ensasi S and Reynolds III CF. (2007) Recovery from major depression in older adults receiving augmentation of antidepressant pharmacotherapy. *Am J Psychiatry* 164; 892–899.

Dickstein DP, Milham MP, Nugent AC, Drevets WC, Charney DS, Pine DS and Leibenluft E. (2005) Frontotemporal alterations in pediatric bipolar disorder. *Arch Gen Psychiatry* 62; 734–741.

Dording CM, Mischoulon D, Peterson TJ, Kornbluh R, Gordon J, Nierenberg AA, Rosenbaum JE and Fava M. (2002) The pharmacologic management of SSRI-induced side effects: a survey of psychiatrists. *Ann Clin Psychiatry* 14; 3, 143–147.

Drabant EM, Hariri AR, Meyer-Lindenberg A, Munoz KE, Mattay VS, Kolachana BS, Egan MF and Weinberger DR. (2006) Catechol O-methyltransferase Val 158 Met genotype and neural mechanisms related to affective arousal and regulation. *Arch Gen Psychiatry* 63; 12, 1396–1406.

Du J, Suzuki K, Wei Y, Wang Y, Blumental R, Chen Z, Falke C, Zarate Jr CA and Manji HK. (2007) The anticonvulsants lamotrigine, riluzole, and valproate differentially regulate AMPA receptor membrane localization: relationship to clinical effects in mood disorders. *Neuropsychopharmacology* 32; 793–802.

Emslie GJ, Yeung PP and Kunz NR. (2007) Long-term, open-label venlafaxine extended release treatment in children and adolescents with major depressive disorder. *CNS Spectr* 12; 3, 223–233.

Epstein J, Pan H, Kocsis JH, Yang Y, Butler T, Chusid J, Hochberg H, Murrough J, Strohmayer E, Stern E and Silbersweig DA. (2006) Lack of ventral striatal response to positive stimuli in depressed versus normal subjects. *Am J Psychiatry* 163; 1784–1790.

Fava M. (2007) Augmenting antidepressants with folate: a clinical perspective. *Clin Psychiatry* 68; Suppl 10, 4–7.

Fava M, Graves LM, Benazzi F, Scaia MJ, Iosifescu DV, Alpert JE and Papakostas GI. (2006) A cross-sectional study of the prevalence of cognitive and physical symptoms during long-term antidepressant treatment. *J Clin Psychiatry* 67; 11, 1754–1758.

Findling RL, Frazier TW, Youngstrom EA, McNamara NK, Stansbrey RJ, Gracious BL, Reed MD, Demeter CA and Calabrese JR. (2007) Double-blind, placebo-controlled trial of divalproex monotherapy in the treatment of symptomatic youth at high risk for developing bipolar disorder. *J Clin Psychiatry* 68; 5, 781–788.

Frank E, Kupfer DJ, Buysse DJ, Swartz HA, Pilkois PA, Houck PR, Rucci P, Novick DM, Grochocinski VJ and Stapf DM. (2007) Randomized trial of weekly, twice monthly and monthly interpersonal psychotherapy as maintenance treatment for women with recurrent depression. *Am J Psychiatry* 164; 761–767.

Fu CHY, Williams SCR, Brammer MJ, Suckling J, Kim J, Cleawre AJ, Walsh ND, Mitterschiffthaler MT and rew CM, Pich EM and Bullmore ET. (2007) Neural responses to happy facial expressions in major depression following antidepressant treatment. *Am J Psychiatry* 164; 599–607.

Gibbons RD, Hur K, Bhumik DK and Mann JJ. (2006) The relationship between antidepressant prescription rates and rate of early adolescent suicide. *Am J Psychiatry* 163; 1898–1904.

Goodwin FK and Jamison KR. (eds) (1990) *Manic Depressive Illness*. New York, Oxford University Press.

Gould GG, Altamirano AV, Javors MA and Frazer A. (2006) A comparison of the chronic treatment effects of venlafaxine and other antidepressants on serotonin and norepinephrine transporters. *Biol Psychiatry* 59; 408–414.

Guzzetta F, Tondo L, Centorrino F and Baldessarini RJ. (2007) Lithium treatment reduces suicide risk in recurrent major depressive disorder. *J Clin Psychiatry* 68; 380–383.

Hasler G, Drevets WC, Gould TD, Gottesman II and Manji HK. (2006) Toward constructing an endophenotype strategy for bipolar disorders. *Biol Psychiatry* 60; 93–105.

Hedlund PB and Sutcliff JG. (2004) Functional, molecular and pharmacological advances in 5-HT7 receptor research. *Trends Pharmacol Sci* 25; 9, 481–486.

Hedlund PB, Huitron-Resendiz S, Henriksen SJ and Sutcliffe JG. (2005) 5-HT7 receptor inhibition and inactivation induce antidepressant like behavior and sleep pattern. *Biol Psychiatry* 58; 831–837.

Hirschfeld RMA, Weisler RH, Rawines SR and Macfadden W. (2006) Quetiapine in the treatment of anxiety in patients with bipolar I or II depression: a secondary analysis from a randomized, double-blind, placebo-controlled study. *J Clin Psychiatry* 67; 3, 355–362.

Houston JP, Ahl J, Meyers AL, Kaiser CJ, Tohen M and Baldessarini RJ. (2006) Reduced suicidal ideation in bipolar I disorder mixed episode patients in a placebo-controlled trial of olanzapine combined with lithium or divalproex. *J Clin Psychiatry* 67; 8, 1246–1252.

Hoyer D, Hannon JP and Martin GR. (2002) Molecular, pharmacological and functional diversity of 5-HT receptors. *Pharmacol Biochem Behav* 71; 533–554.

Joffe H, Cohen LS, Suppes T, McLaughlin WL, Lavori P, Adams JM, Hwang CH, Hall JE and Sachs GS. (2006) Valproate is associated with new onset oligoamenorrhea with hyperandrogenism in women with bipolar disorder. *Biol Psychiatry* 59; 1078–1086.

Judd LL, Akiskal HS, Schettler PJ, Coryell W, Endicott J, Maser JD, Solomon DA, Leon AC and Keller MB. (2003) A prospective investigation of the natural history of the long-term weekly symptomatic status of bipolar II disorder. *Arch Gen Psychiatry* 60; 261–269.

Keedwell PA, Andrew C, Williams SCR, Brammer MJ and Phillips ML. (2005) The neural correlates of anhedonia in major depressive disorder. *Biol Psychiatry* 58; 843–853.

Keedwell PA, Andrew C, Williams SCR, Brammer MJ and Phillips ML. (2005) A double dissociation of ventromedial prefrontal cortical responses to sad and happy stimuli in depressed and healthy individuals. *Biol Psychiatry* 58; 495–503.

Kellner CH, Knapp RG, Petrides G, Rummans TA, Husain MM, Rasmussen K, Mueller M, Bernstein HJ, O'Connor K, Smith G, Biggs M, Bailine SH, Malur C, Yim E, McClintock S and Sampson S. (2006) Continuation electroconvulsive therapy vs pharmacotherapy for relapse prevention in major depression. *Arch Gen Psychiatry* 63; 1337–1344.

Kennedy SH, Konarski JZ, Segal ZV, Lau MA, Bieling PJ, McIntyre RS and Mayberg HS. (2007) Differences in brain glucose metabolism between responders to CBT and venlafaxine in a 16-week randomized controlled trial. *Am J Psychiatry* 164; 778–788.

Kessing LV, Sondergard L, Kvist K and Andersen PK. (2005) Suicide risk in patients treated with lithium. *Arch Gen Psychiatry* 62; 860–866.

Kruger S, Alda M, Young LLT, Goldapple K, Parikh S and Mayberg HS. (2006) Risk and resilience markers in bipolar disorder: brain responses to emotional challenge in bipolar patients and their healthy siblings. *Am J Psychiatry* 163; 257–264.

Krystal JH, Perry Jr EB, Gueorguieva R, Belger A, Madonick SH, Abi-Dargham AA, Cooper TB, MacDougall L, Abi-Saab W and D'Souza DC. (2005) Comparative and interactive human psychopharmacologic effects of ketamine and amphetamine. *Arch Gen Psychiatry* 62; 985–995.

Kuala A and Sanatoria G. (2005) Beyond monoamines: glutamatergic function in mood disorders. *CNS Spectr* 10; 10, 808–819.

Lemke MR, Brecht HM, Koester J and Reichmann H. (2006) Effects of the dopamine agonist pramipaxole on depression, anhedonia and motor functioning in Parkinson's disease. *J Neurol Sci* 248; 266–270.

Leverich GS, Altshuler LL, Rye MA, Suppes T, Keck Jr. PE, Kupka RW, Denicoff KD, Nolen WA, Grunze H, Martinez MI and Post RM. (2006) Risk of switch in mood polarity to hypomania or mania in patients with bipolar depression during acute and continuation trials of venlafaxine, sertraline, and bupropion as adjuncts to mood stabilizers. *Am J Psychiatry* 163; 232–239.

Levinson DF. (2006) The genetics of depression: a review. *Biol Psychiatry* 60; 84–92.

Lieben CKJ, Blokland AR, Sik A, Sung E, van Nieuwenhuizen P and Schreiber R. (2005) The selective 5-HT6 receptor antagonist Ro4368554 restores memory performance in cholinergic and serotonergic models of memory deficiency in the rat. *Neuropsychopharmacology* 30; 2169–2179.

Mah L, Zarate Jr CA, Singh J, Duan YF, Luckenbaugh DA, Manji HK and Drevets WC. (2007) Regional cerebral glucose metabolic abnormalities in bipolar II depression. *Biol Psychiatry* 61; 765–775.

Marcus MM, Jardemark KE, Wadenberg ML, Langlois X, Hertel P and Svensson TH. (2004) Combined alpha 2 and delta 2/3 receptor blockade enhances cortical glutamatergic transmission and reverses cognitive impairment in the rat. *Int J Neuropsychopharmacol* 8; 315–327.

Marek GJ, Martin-Ruis R, Abo A and Artigas F. (2005) The selective 5-HT2A receptor antagonist M100907 enhances antidepressant-like behavioral effects of the SSRI fluoxetine. *Neuropsychopharmacology* 30; 2205–2215.

Mayberg HS. (2007) Defining the neural circuitry of depression: toward a new nosology with therapeutic implications. *Biol Psychiatry* 61; 729–730.

Mayberg HS, Lozano AM, Von V, McNeely HE, Seminowicz D, Hamani C, Schwalb JM and Kennedy SH. (2005) Deep brain stimulation for treatment resistant depression. *Neuron* 45; 651–660.

McGrath PJ, Stewart JW, Fava M, Trivedi MH, Wisniewski SR, Nierenberg AA, Thase ME, Davis L, Biggs MM, Shores-Wilson K, Luther JF, Niederehe G, Warden D and Rush AJ. (2006) Tranylcypromine versus venlafaxine plus mirtazapine following three failed antidepressant medication trials for depression: a STAR*D report. *Am J Psychiatry* 163; 1531–1541.

McMahon FJ, Buervenich S, Charney D, Lipsky R, Rush AJ, Wilson AF, Sorant AJM, Papanicolaou J, Laje G, Fava M, Trivedi MH, Wisniewski SR and Manji H. (2006) Variation in the gene encoding the serotonin 2A receptor is associated with outcome of antidepressant treatment. *Am J Hum Genetics* 78; 804–814.

Meyer JH, McNeely HE, Sagrati S, Boovariwla A, Martin K, Verhoeff NPLG, Wilson AA and Houle S. (2006) Elevated putamen D2 receptor binding potential in major depression with motor retardation: an [^{11}C] raclopride positron emission tomography study. *Am J Psychiatry* 163; 1594–1602.

Michelson D, Adler LA, Amsterdam JD, Dunner DL, Nierenberg AA, Reimherr FW, Schatzberg AF, Kelsey DK and Williams DW. (2007) Addition of atomoxetine for depression incompletely responsive to sertraline: a randomized, double-blind placebo-controlled study. *J Clin Psychiatry* 68; 4, 582–587.

Millan M. (2004) The role of monoamines in the actions of established and "novel" antidepressant agents: a critical review. *Eur J Pharmacol* 500; 371–384.

Mitchell ES and Neumaier JF. (2005) 5-HT6 receptors: a novel target for cognitive enhancement. *Pharmacol Ther* 108; 320–333.

Mitchell ES, Sexton T and Neumaier JF. (2007) Increased expression of 5-HT6 receptors in the rat dorsomedial striatum impairs instrumental learning. *Neuropsychopharmacology* 32; 1520–1530.

Montgomery SA and Andersen HF. (2006) Escitalopram versus venlafaxine XR in the treatment of depression. *Int J Clin Psychopharmacol* 21; 297–309.

Najt P, Perez J, Sanches M, Peluso MAM, Glahn D and Soares JC. (2006) Impulsivity and bipolar disorder. *Eur Neuropsychopharmacol* 17; 313–320.

Narendran R, Frankle WG, Keefe R, Gil R, Martinez D, Slifsein M, Kegeles LS, Talbot PS, Huang Y, Hwang DR, Khenissi L, Cooper TB, Laruelle M and Abi-Dargham A. (2005) Altered prefrontal dopaminergic function in chronic recreational ketamine users. *Am J Psychiatry* 162; 2352–2359.

Nemeroff CB, Mayberg HS, Krahl SE, McNamara J, Frazer A, Henry TR, George MS, Charney DS and Brannan SK. (2006) VNS therapy in treatment resistant depression: clinical evidence and putative neurobiological mechanisms. *Neuropsychopharmacology* 31; 1345–1355.

Nickel MK, Muehlbacher M, Nickel C, Kettler C, Gil FP, Bachler E, Buschmann W, Rother N and Fartacek R. (2006) Aripiprazole in the treatment of patients with borderline personality disorder: a double-blind, placebo-controlled study. *Am J Psychiatry* 163; 833–838.

Nierenberg A, Bronwyn RK, Leslie VC, Alpert JE, Pava JA, Worthington JJ, Rosenbaum JF and Fava M. (1999) Residual symptoms in depressed patients who respond acutely to fluoxetine. *J Clin Psychiatry* 60; 221–225.

Nierenberg AA, Adler LA, Peselow E, Zornberg G and Rosenthal M. (1994) Trazodone for antidepressant-associated insomnia. *Am J Psychiatry* 151; 7, 1069–1072.

Nierenberg AA, Cole JO and Glass L. (1992) Possible trazodone potentiation of fluoxetine: a case series. *J Clin Psychiatry* 53; 3, 83–85.

Nierenberg AA, Farabaugh AH, Alpert JA, Gordon J, Worthington JJ, Rosenbaum JF and Fava M. (2000) Timing of onset of antidepressant response with fluoxetine treatment. *Am J Psychiatry* 157; 1423–1428.

Nierenberg AA, Fava M, Trivedi MH, Wisniewski SR, Thase ME, McGrath PJ, Alpert JE, Warden D, Luther JF, Niederehe G, Lebowitz B, Shores-Wilson K and Rush AJ. (2006) A comparison of lithium and t3 augmentation following two failed medication treatments for depression: a STAR*D report. *Am J Psychiatry* 163; 1519–1530.

Nierenberg AA, Ostacher M, Calabrese JR, Ketter TA, Marangell LB, Miklowitz DJ, Miyahara S, Bauer MS, Thase ME, Wisniewski SR and Sachs GS. (2006) Treatment-resistant bipolar depression: a STEP-BD equipoise randomized effectiveness trial of antidepressant augmentation with lamotrigine, inositol, or risperidone. *Am J Psychiatry* 163; 210–216.

Oquendo MA, Currier D and Mann JJ. (2006) Prospective studies of suicidal behavior in major depressive and bipolar disorders: what is the evidence for predictive risk factors? *Acta Psychiatr Scand* 114; 151–158.

O'Rourke H and Fudge JL. (2006) Distribution of serotonin transporter labeled fibers in amygdaloid subregions: implications for mood disorders. *Biol Psychiatry* 60; 479–490.

Pace TWW, Mletzko TC, Alagbe O, Musselman DL, Nemeroff CB, Miler AH and Heim CM. (2006) Increased stress-induced inflammatory responses in male patients with major depression and increased early life stress. *Am J Psychiatry* 163; 9, 1630–1633.

Papakostas GI and Fava M. (2007) A meta-analysis of clinical trials comparing milnacipran, a serotonin-norepinephrine reuptake inhibitor, with a selective serotonin reuptake inhibitor for the treatment of major depressive disorder. *Eur Neuropsychopharmacology* 17; 32–36.

Papakostas GI, Shelton RC, Smith J and Fava M. (2007) Augmentation of antidepressants with atypical antipsychotic medications for treatment-resistant major depressive disorder: a meta-analysis. *J Clin Psychiatry* 68; 6, 826–831.

Parsey RV, Kent JM, Oquendo MA, Richards MC, Pratap M, Cooper TB, Arawngo V and Mann JJ. (2006) Acute occupancy of brain serotonin transporter by sertraline as measured by [^{11}C] DASB and positron emission tomography. *Biol Psychiatry* 59; 821–828.

Patkar AA, Masand PS, Pae CU, Peindl K, Hooper-Wood C, Mannelli P and Ciccone P. (2006) A randomized, double-blind, placebo-controlled trial of augmentation with an extended release formulation of methylphenidate in outpatients with treatment resistant depression. *J Clin Psychopharmacol* 26; 653–656.

Perlis RH, Ostacher MJ, Pael JK, Marangell LB, Zhang H, Wisniewski SR, Keter TA, Miklowitz DJ and Otto MW, Gyulai L, Reilly-Harrington NA, Sachs GS and Thase ME. (2006) Predictors of recurrence in bipolar disorder: primary outcomes from the systematic treatment enhancement program for bipolar disorder (STEP-BD). *Am J Psychiatry* 163; 217–224.

Pitchot W, Hansenne M, Pinto E, Reggers J, Fuchs S and Ansseau M. (2005) 5-hydroxytryptamine 1A receptors, major depression and suicidal behavior. *Biol Psychiatry* 58; 854–858.

Rapaport MH, Gharabawi GM, Canuso CM, Mahmoud RA, Keller MB, Bossie CA, Turkos I, Lasser RA, Loescher A, Bouhours P, Dunbar F and Nemeroff CB. (2006) Effects of risperidone augmentation in patients with treatment resistant depression: results of open label treatment followed by double blind continuation. *Neuropsychopharmacology* 31; 2505–2513.

Roberson-Nay R, McClure EB, Monk CS, Nelson EE, Guyer AE, Fromm SJ, Charney DS, Leibenluft E, Blair J, Ernst M and Pine DS. (2006) Increased amygdala activity during successful memory encoding in adolescent major depressive disorder: a fMRI study. *Biol Psychiatry* 60; 966–973.

Robertson B, Wang L, Diaz MT, Aiello M, Gersing K, Beyer J, Mukundan Jr S, McCarthy G and Doraiswamy PM. (2007) Effect of bupropion extended release on negative emotion processing in major depressive disorder: a pilot functional magnetic resonance imaging study. *J Clin Psychiatry* 68; 261–267.

Rush AJ, Trivedi MH, Wisniewski SR, Stewart JW, Nierenberg AA, Thase ME, Ritz L, Biggs MM, Warden D, Luther JF, Shores-Wilson K, Niederehe G and Fava M. (2006) Bupropion-SR, sertraline, or venlafaxine XR after failure of SSRIs for depression. *N Engl J Med* 354; 12, 1231–1242.

Sanacora G, Kendell SF, Levin Y, Simen AA, Fenton LR, Coric V and Krystal JH. (2007) Preliminary evidence of riluzole efficacy in antidepressant-treated patients with residual depressive symptoms. *Biol Psychiatry* 61; 822–825.

Santana N, Bortolozzi A, Serrats J, Mengod G and Artigas F. (2004) Expression of serotonin 1A and serotonin 2A receptors in pyramidal and GABAergic neurons of the rat prefrontal cortex. *Cereb Cortex* 14; 1100–1109.

Schaefer HS, Putnam KM, Benca RM and Davidson RJ. (2006) Event-related functional magnetic resonance imaging measures of neural activity to positive social stimuli in pre- and post-treatment depression. *Biol Psychiatry* 60; 974–986.

Schechter LE, Ring RH, Beyer CE, Hughes ZA, Khawaja X, Malberg JE and Rosenzweig-Lipson S. (2005) Innovative approaches for the development of antidepressant drugs: current and future strategies. *NeuroRx* 2; 4, 590–611.

Schramm E, van Calker D, Dykierek P, Lieb K, Kech S, Zobel I, Leonhart R and Berger M. (2007) An intensive treatment program of interpersonal psychotherapy plus pharmacotherapy for depressed inpatients: acute and long-term results. *Am J Psychiatry* 164; 768–777.

Schreiber R, Vivian J, Hedley L, Szczepanski K, Secchi RL, Zuzow M, van Laarhoven V, Moreau JL, Martin JR, Sik A and Blokland A. (2007) Effects of the novel 5-HT6 receptor antagonist RO4368554 in rat models or cognition and sensorimotor gating. *Eur Neuropsychopharmacol* 17; 277–288.

Shang Y, Gibbs MA, Marek GJ, Stiger T, Burstein AH, Marek K, Seibyl JP and Rogers JF. (2007) Displacement of serotonin and dopamine transporters by venlafaxine extended release capsule at steady state. *J Clin Psychopharmacol* 27; 1, 71–75.

Shelton RC, Haman KL, Rapaport MH, Kiev A, Smith WT, Hirschfeld RMA, Lydiard RB, Zajecka JM and Dunner DL. (2006) A randomized, double-blind, active control study of sertraline versus venlafaxine XR in major depressive disorder. *J Clin Psychiatry* 67; 11, 1674–1681.

Siegle GJ, Thompson W, Carter CS, Steinhauer SR and Thase ME. (2007) Increased amygdala and decreased dorsolateral prefrontal BOL responses in unipolar depression: related and independent features. *Biol Psychiatry* 61; 198–209.

Skidmore FM, Rodriguez RL, Fernandez HH, Goodman WK, Foote KD and Okun MS. (2006) Lessons learned in deep brain stimulation for movement and neuropsychiatric disorders. *CNS Spectr* 11; 7, 521–537.

Takano A, Suzuki K, Kosaka J, Ota M, Nozaki S, Ikoma Y, Tanada S and Suhara T. (2005) A dose finding study of duloxetine based on serotonin transporter occupancy. *Psychopharmacology* 185; 395–399.

Talbot PS and Laruelle M. (2002) The role of in vivo molecular imaging with PET and SPECT in the elucidation of psychiatric drug action and new drug development. *Eur Neuropsychopharmacol* 12; 503–511.

Tarazi FI, Baldessarini RJ, Kula NS and Zhang K. (2003) Long-term effects of olanzapine, risperidone, and quetiapine on ionotropic glutamate receptor types: implications for antipsychotic drug treatment. *J Pharmacol Exp Ther* 306; 1145–1151.

Thase ME. (2006) The failure of evidence based medicine to guide treatment of antidepressant nonresponders. *J Clin Psychiatry* 67; 12, 1833–1855.

Thase ME, Clayton AH, Haight BR, Thompson AH, Modell JG and Johnston JA. (2006) A double-blind comparison between bupropion XL and venlafaxine XR. *J Clin Psychopharmacol* 25; 5, 482–488.

Thase ME, Corya SA, Osuntokun O, Case M, Henley DB, Sanger TM, Watson SB and Dube S. (2007) A randomized, double-blind comparison of olanzapine/fluoxetine combination, olanzapine, and fluoxetine in treatment resistant major depressive disorder. *J Clin Psychiatry* 68; 2, 224–236.

Thase ME, Friedman ES, Biggs MM, Wisniewski SR, Trivedi MH, Luther JF, Fava M, Nierenberg AA, McGrath PJ, Warden D, Niederehe G, Hollon SD and Rush AJ. (2007) Cognitive therapy versus medication in augmentation and switch strategies as second step treatments: a STAR*D report. *Am J Psychiatry* 164; 739–752.

Thase ME, Macfadden W, Weisler RH, Chang W, Paulsson B, Khan A and Calabrese JR. (2006) Efficacy of quetiapine monotherapy in bipolar I and II depression. *J Clin Psychopharmacol* 26; 600–609.

Trivedi MH, Fava M, Wisniewski SR, Thase ME, Quitkin F, Warden D, Ritz L, Nierenberg AA, Lebowitz BD, Biggs MM, Luther JF, Shores-Wilson K and Rush AJ. (2006) Medication augmentation after the failure of SSRIs for depression. *N Engl J Med* 354; 1243–1252.

Trivedi MH, Rush AJ, Wisniewski SR, Nierenberg AA, Wawrden D, Ritz L, Norquist G, Howland RH, Lebowitz B, McGrath PJ, Shores-Wilson K, Biggs MM, Balasubramani GK and Fava M. (2006) Evaluation of outcomes with citalopram for depression using measurement based care in STAR*D: implications for clinical practice. *Am J Psychiatry* 163; 28–40.

Valenstein M, McCarthy JF, Austin KL, Greden JF, Young EA and Blow FC. (2006) What happened to lithium? Antidepressant augmentation in clinical settings. *Am J Psychiatry* 163;1219–1225.

Vanover KE, Weiner DM, Makhay M, Veinbergs I, GardellLR, Lameh J, Del Tredici AL, Piu F, Schiffer HH, Ott TR, Burstein ES, Uldam AK, Thygesen MB, Schlienger N, Andersson CM, Son TY, Harvey SC, Powell SB, Geyer MA, Tolf BR, Brann MR and Davis RE. (2006) Pharmacological and behavioral profile of ACP-103, a novel 5-HT2A receptor inverse agonist. *J Pharmacol Exp Ther* 317; 910–918.

Wagner KD, Kowtch RA, Emslie GJ, Findling RL, Wilens TE, McCague K, D'Souza J, Wamil A, Lehman RB, Berv D and Linden D. (2006) A double-blind, randomized, placebo-controlled trial of oxcarbazepine in the treatment of bipolar disorder in children and adolescents. *Am J Psychiatry* 163; 1179–1186.

Weisler RH, Cutler AJ, Ballenger JC, Post RM and Ketter TA. (2006) The use of antiepileptic drugs in bipolar disorders: a review based on evidence from controlled trials. *CNS Spectr* 11; 10, 788–799.

Weissman MM. (2007) Cognitive therapy and interpersonal psychotherapy: 30 years later. *Am J Psychiatry* 164; 5, 693–696.

West AR, Floresco SB, Charara A, Rosenkranz JA and Grace AA. (2003) Electrophysiological interactions between striatal glutamatergic and dopaminergic systems. *Ann N Y Acad Sci* 1003; 53–74.

Wisniewski SR, Fava M, Trivedi MH, Thase ME, Warden D, Niederehe G, Friedman ES, Biggs MM, Sackeim HA, Shores-Wilson K, McGrath PJ, Laori PW, Miyahara S and Rush AJ. (2007) Acceptability of second-step treatments to depressed outpatients: a STAR* D report. *Am J Psychiatry* 164; 753–760.

Wozniak J, Biederan J, Mick E, Waxmonsky J, Hantsoo L, Best C, Cluette-Brown JE and Laposata M. (2007) Omega-3 fatty acid monotherapy for pediatric bipolar disorder: A prospective open-label trial. *Eur Neuropsychopharmacol* 17; 440–447.

Yatham LN, Goldstein JM, Vieta E, Bowden CL, Grunze H, Post RM, Suppes T and Calabrese JR. (2005) Atypical antipsychotics in bipolar depression: potential mechanisms of action. *J Clin Psychiatry* 66; Suppl 5, 40–48.

Zarate CA, Singh JB, Carlson PJ, Brutsche NE, Ameli R, Luckenbaugh DA, Charney DS and Manji HK. (2006) A randomized trial of an N-methyl-D-aspartate antagonist in treatment resistant major depression. *Arch Gen Psychiatry* 63; 856–864.

Zarate CA, Singh JB, Quiroz JA, DeJesus G, Denicoff KK, Luckenbaugh DA, Manji HK and Charney DS. (2006) A double-blind, placebo-controlled study of memantine in the treatment of major depression. *Am J Psychiatry* 163; 153–155.

Zimmerman M, McGlinchey JB, Posternak MA, Friedman M, Attiullah N and Boerescu D. (2006) How should remission from depression be defined? The depressed patient's perspective. *Am J Psychiatry* 163; 148–150.

Index

Page numbers followed by '*f*' indicate figures; page numbers followed by '*t*' indicate tables.

5HIAA (5-hydroxy-indole acetic acid), 31
in cerebrospinal fluid, 36
"able stabilizers", 265, 265*f*
acamprosate
in combos for bipolar disorder, 263
acetylcholine receptors, TCA and, 150*f*
activity-dependent spine formation, by estradiol, 162*f*
adatanserin, 122
adolescence
antidepressants for, 67*f*
mania in, 260
affective disorders, 2. *See also* mood disorders
affective spectrum disorders, 104
norepinephrine and, 94
"affective storms", in children, 260
aggressiveness, 252*f*
Agilect/Azilect (rasaligine), 127*t*
for Parkinson's disease, 130
agitation, 95
agomelatine (Valdoxan), 122, 206
icon, 209*f*
agoraphobia, in children, 261
akathisia
from paroxetine withdrawal, 85
from SSRIs, 78
alertness, 198
loss
bupropion for, 104
as SSRI side effect, 78
alpha 1 adrenergic receptors
TCA and, 147, 151*f*

alpha 2 antagonists
icon, 107*f*
and norepinephrine, 108*f*
and serotonin, 108*f*, 109*f*
as serotonin norepinephrine disinhibitors, 106, 110*f*
alpha 2 delta ligands, 236
alpha 2 receptors
on axon terminal, 26*f*
blockade of, 107*f*
somatodendritic, 23, 27*f*
alpha-L-glutamyl transferase, 175
alprazolam (Xanax)
and CYP 450 3A4, 156
and sedation, 157
ALS (amyotrophic lateral sclerosis)
riluzole for, 233*f*
amantadine
for bipolar disorder, 243
icon, 244*f*
mechanism of action
on GABA, glutamate, sigma, and dopamine, 224*t*
VSSCs, synaptic vesicles, and carbonic anhydrase, 223*t*
possible actions in bipolar disorder, 246*f*
putative clinical actions, 221*t*, 222*t*
amibegron, 210
amitriptyline (Elavil, Endep, Tryptizol, Loroxyl), 120, 145*t*
amoxapine (Asendin), 120, 145*t*
amphetamines, 124, 127*t*
action
MAO inhibitors with, 127*t*
with MAOIs, and hypertension, 141*t*

breast-feeding
  depression and treatment during,
    167
  lithium and, 260
Buckeye bipolar bullets, 263, 264*f*
bulimia, fluoxetine (Prozac) for, 81
bupropion
  metabolites, 101, 102*f*
  potency for CYP450 2D6 inhibition,
    153
  with sertraline, 84
buspirone, 199, 205
  and CYP 450 3A4, 156
  mechanism of action augmentation, 201*f*,
    202*f*, 203*f*

caffeine
  interactions with fluvoxamine, 152
calcium channel blockers
  L-type, 245, 246*f*
  mechanism of action
    on GABA, glutamate, sigma, and
      dopamine, 224*t*
    VSSCs, synaptic vesicles, and carbonic
      anhydrase, 223*t*
  putative clinical actions, 221*t*, 222*t*
California careful cocktail, 263, 264*f*
California rocket fuel, 204*f*
California sunshine, 265*f*, 266
carbamazepine (Equetro), 157, 226
  actions as mood stabilizer, 231*f*
  binding site of, 230*f*
  and CYP 450 3A4, 156
  icon, 228*f*
  interaction with MAOIs, 143*t*
  for manic phase of bipolar disorder,
    220
  mechanism of action
    on GABA, glutamate, sigma, and
      dopamine, 224*t*
    VSSCs, synaptic vesicles, and carbonic
      anhydrase, 223*t*
  putative clinical actions, 221*t*, 222*t*
  and sedation, 157
  vs. valproate, 227
  and VSSCs, 255*f*
carbonic anhydrase, topiramate and, 235
cardiac arrhythmias
  from combining 3A4 substrates with
    inhibitors, 157
  as tricyclic antidepressant side effect,
    152*f*
cerebrospinal fluid, 5HIAA in, 36
"cheese reaction", tyramine and, 133
cheese, tyramine content of, 135*f*

childbearing years, depression during,
  164
children. *See also* autism
  "affective storms" in, 260
  antidepressants for, 67*f*
  bipolar disorder and mood stabilizers, 260
circuits
  apathy, 41*f*
  appetite, 46*f*
  depressed mood, 40*f*
  in depression, 37–44
  elevated/irritable mood, 49*f*
  fatigue, 43*f*
  goal-directed activity, 53*f*
  guilt, 47*f*
  malfunctioning
    and depression symptoms, 191
  for mania, 44–55
  mania symptom, 50*f*
  mapping mania symptoms onto, 53
  matching mania symptoms to, 48*f*
  psychomotor symptoms, 45*f*
  sleep, 42*f*, 51*f*
  suicide, 46*f*
  weight, 46*f*
  worthlessness, 47*f*
citalopram, 86
  icon, 86*f*
  potency for CYP450 2D6 inhibition, 153
clinical practice
  antidepressants in, 187
clomipramine (Anafranil), 145*t*, 153*f*
  inhibition of serotonin reuptake pump,
    146
clonidine, 169
clozapine, 107*f*
  in combos for bipolar disorder, 261
Coaxil (tianeptine, Stablon), 145*t*
codeine
  and CYP450 2D6 inhibitors, 156
cognitive behavioral therapy (CBT), 187
cognitive functioning
  in depression, 100
"combos" (combination of medications)
  for bipolar disorder treatment, 261
COMT (catechol-O-methyl transferase),
  24*f*
  and dopamine degradation, 92
  and norepinephrine, 22
concentration, 194
  and malfunctioning circuits, 193*f*
conduct disorder
  mania vs., 260, 261
constipation
  from NET inhibition, 95

cortex. *See also* dorsolateral prefontal cortex (DLPFC); orbitofrontal cortex; prefrontal cortex; ventromedial prefrontal cortex
   limbic, noradrenergic receptor stimulation in, 95
corticotrophin release factor 1 (CRF1) antagonists, 211
cost-based selection of antidepressants, 190, 190*f*
cyclobenzapine
   interaction with MAOIs, 143*t*
cyclothymic temperament, 4, 7*f*
   with major depressive episodes, 11, 12*f*
cytochrome P450 (CYP450) enzyme systems
   CYP450 1A2 substrates, 151, 153*f*
      inhibition, 153*f*
      inhibition consequences, 154*f*
   CYP450 2D6, 152
      inhibition, 87, 155*f*
      inhibition consequences, 155*f*
      paroxetine as substrate and inhibitor, 85
      substrates, 154*f*
      and venlafaxine conversion, 96, 96*f*
   CYP450 3A4, 156
      combining inhibitors with substrates, 157
      substrates and inhibitors, 156*f*
   inducers, 157
   pharmacokinetic actions, 151

DBH (dopamine beta hydroxylase), 22
decongestants
   and blood pressure, 141
   interaction with MAOIs, 142*f*
   interactions with drugs boosting sympathomimetic amines, 139
deep brain stimulation, 186, 186*f*
delusions
   link to nucleus accumbens, 252*f*
dementia. *See also* Alzheimer's disease
   bipolarity in, 15, 15*f*
demethylation, 153*f*
dendrites
   spine formation, estrogen and trophic actions on, 160
Deplin (L-methylfolate), 177
   for bipolar disorder, 247
depressed mood
   circuits, 40*f*
   thyroid hormones and, 181*f*
depression
   in bipolar disorder
      history, 19*f*
      response to antidepressants, 20*f*
      sleep disturbances in, 51*f*
      symptoms, 19*f*
      vs. unipolar depression, 16, 17*t*, 18, 18*f*

bipolar vs. unipolar, treatment, 249
chronic pain with
   duloxetine for, 99
comorbid psychiatric illness with, 195
disease progression in, 67
estrogen interaction with monoamines, 169*f*
in females
   during childbearing years and pregnancy, 164
   during menopause, 168*f*, 171
   over life cycle, estrogen and, 162
   during perimenopause, 167, 168*f*
   during postpartum period, 167
   SNRIs for, 171*f*
   SSRIs for, 170*f*
hypotheses for etiology, 36–37
incidence across female life cycle, 163*f*
incidence across male life cycle, 164*f*
major, 3*f*, 4
   antidepressant combinations as standard, 199
   common comorbidities, 198*f*
   progressive nature of, 20*f*
   relapse rates, 66*f*
   remission rates, 65*f*
   symptom-based algorithm, 193*f*, 194*f*
with mixed hypomania, 13
mixed states of mania and, 15*t*
monoamine hypothesis, 68
   normal monoamine neurotransmitter activity, 35*f*
   reduced monoamine neurotransmitter activity, 35*f*
monoamine receptor hypothesis, 36*f*
on mood chart, 2, 2*f*
mood stabilizers for treating, 217*f*
neuroimaging of brain activation in, 55*f*
neuronal response to sadness vs. happiness, 56*f*
neurotransmitter receptor hypothesis, 36
overlap with mania, 55
risk across female life cycle, 163*f*
symptoms, 37, 38*f*, 44
   matching to circuits, 39*f*
   residual, 65*f*
treatment
   combination of medications, 200*f*
   MTHF vs. folic acid, 175
   residual symptoms after, 191
unipolar, distinguishing from bipolar depression, 16, 17*t*, 18, 18*f*
depression pharmacy, 187, 188*f*
depressive temperament, 8*f*
Deprimyl (lofepramine, Gamanil), 145*t*